Cardiothoracic Surgical Critical Care

Editor

BRYAN BOLING

CRITICAL CARE NURSING CLINICS OF NORTH AMERICA

www.ccnursing.theclinics.com

Consulting Editor
JAN FOSTER

September 2019 • Volume 31 • Number 3

1600 John F. Kennedy Boulevard • Suite 1800 • Philadelphia, Pennsylvania, 19103-2899

http://www.theclinics.com

CRITICAL CARE NURSING CLINICS OF NORTH AMERICA Volume 31, Number 3
September 2019 ISSN 0899-5885, ISBN-13: 978-0-323-70868-5

Editor: Kerry Holland
Developmental Editor: Laura Fisher

© **2019 Elsevier Inc. All rights reserved.**

This periodical and the individual contributions contained in it are protected under copyright by Elsevier, and the following terms and conditions apply to their use:

Photocopying
Single photocopies of single articles may be made for personal use as allowed by national copyright laws. Permission of the Publisher and payment of a fee is required for all other photocopying, including multiple or systematic copying, copying for advertising or promotional purposes, resale, and all forms of document delivery. Special rates are available for educational institutions that wish to make photocopies for non-profit educational classroom use. For information on how to seek permission visit www.elsevier.com/permissions or call: (+44) 1865 843830 (UK)/(+1) 215 239 3804 (USA).

Derivative Works
Subscribers may reproduce tables of contents or prepare lists of articles including abstracts for internal circulation within their institutions. Permission of the Publisher is required for resale or distribution outside the institution. Permission of the Publisher is required for all other derivative works, including compilations and translations (please consult www.elsevier.com/permissions).

Electronic Storage or Usage
Permission of the Publisher is required to store or use electronically any material contained in this periodical, including any article or part of an article (please consult www.elsevier.com/permissions). Except as outlined above, no part of this publication may be reproduced, stored in a retrieval system or transmitted in any form or by any means, electronic, mechanical, photocopying, recording or otherwise, without prior written permission of the Publisher.

Notice
No responsibility is assumed by the Publisher for any injury and/or damage to persons or property as a matter of products liability, negligence or otherwise, or from any use or operation of any methods, products, instructions or ideas contained in the material herein. Because of rapid advances in the medical sciences, in particular, independent verification of diagnoses and drug dosages should be made.

Although all advertising material is expected to conform to ethical (medical) standards, inclusion in this publication does not constitute a guarantee or endorsement of the quality or value of such product or of the claims made of it by its manufacturer.

Critical Care Nursing Clinics of North America (ISSN 0899-5885) is published quarterly by Elsevier Inc., 360 Park Avenue South, New York, NY 10010-1710. Months of issue are March, June, September, and December. Business and Editorial Offices: 1600 John F. Kennedy Blvd., Suite 1800, Philadelphia, PA 19103-2899. Periodicals postage paid at New York, NY and additional mailing offices. Subscription prices are $160.00 per year for US individuals, $406.00 per year for US institutions, $100.00 per year for US students and residents, $206.00 per year for Canadian individuals, $510.00 per year for Canadian institutions, $230.00 per year for international individuals, $510.00 per year for international institutions and $115.00 per year for Canadian and international students/residents. To receive student/resident rate, orders must be accompanied by name of affiliated institution, data of term, and the *signature* of program/residency coordinator on institution letterhead. Orders will be billed at individual rate until proof of status is received. Foreign air speed delivery is included in all *Clinics* subscription prices. All prices are subject to change without notice. **POSTMASTER:** Send address changes to *Critical Care Nursing Clinics of North America*, Elsevier Health Sciences Division, Subscription Customer Service, 3251 Riverport Lane, Maryland Heights, MO 63043. **Customer Service: 1-800-654-2452 (US and Canada); 314-447-8871 (outside US and Canada). Fax: 314-447-8029. E-mail:** JournalsCustomerService-usa@elsevier.com **(for print support) and** JournalsOnlineSupport-usa@elsevier.com **(for online support).**

Reprints. For copies of 100 or more of articles in this publication, please contact the Commercial Reprints Department, Elsevier Inc., 360 Park Avenue South, New York, New York, 10010-1710; Tel.: 212-633-3874, Fax: 212-633-3820, and E-mail: reprints@elsevier.com.

Critical Care Nursing Clinics of North America is covered in *MEDLINE/PubMed (Index Medicus), International Nursing Index, Nursing Citation Index, Cumulative Index to Nursing and Allied Health Literature, and RNdex Top 100.*

Contributors

CONSULTING EDITOR

JAN FOSTER, PhD, APRN, CNS
Formerly, Associate Professor, College of Nursing, Texas Woman's University, Houston, Texas; Currently, President, Nursing Inquiry and Intervention, Inc, The Woodlands, Texas

EDITOR

BRYAN BOLING, DNP, AGACNP-BC
Advanced Practice Provider, Division of Critical Care, Department of Anesthesiology, University of Kentucky, Lexington, Kentucky

AUTHORS

DANIEL L. ARELLANO, MSN, RN, ACNP-BC, CCRN, CEN
Department of Undergraduate Studies, Cizik School of Nursing, University of Texas Health Science Center at Houston, Division of Anesthesiology, Critical Care, and Pain Medicine, Department of Critical Care, University of Texas MD Anderson Cancer Center, Houston, Texas

MONICA BECK, MSN, RN, OCN
Clinical Assistant Professor, University of Alabama in Huntsville, Huntsville, Alabama

RACHEL BEECH, RN, MSN, CPNP-AC
Pediatric Nurse Practitioner, Heinrich A. Werner Division of Pediatric Critical Care, University of Kentucky, Kentucky Children's Hospital, Lexington, Kentucky

BARBARA BIRRIEL, PhD, ACNP-BC, FCCM
Assistant Research Professor, The Pennsylvania State University College of Nursing, Hershey, Pennsylvania

TANYA BRONZELL-WYNDER, DNP, CRNP
Nurse Practitioner, Lung Center Service Line, Temple University Hospital, Philadelphia, Pennsylvania

MELISSA CALLANS, MSN, CRNP, CCDS, FHRS
Nurse Practitioner, Department of Cardiac Electrophysiology, Pennsylvania Hospital, University of Pennsylvania Health System, Clinical Instructor, AGACNP Program, University of Pennsylvania School of Nursing, Philadelphia, Pennsylvania

KEVIN C. CARNEY, MSN, CRNP
Nurse Practitioner, Manager, Lung Center Service Line, Temple University Hospital, Philadelphia, Pennsylvania

KIRSTAN CLAY-WEINFELD, MSN, CRNP, AGACNP-BC, CCRN-CSC-CMC
Nurse Practitioner, Department of Cardiac Electrophysiology, Pennsylvania Hospital, University of Pennsylvania Health System, Philadelphia, Pennsylvania

KATRINA D'ANGELO, MSN, AGACNP-BC
Nurse Practitioner, Heart and Vascular Intensivist Service, Penn State Health Milton S. Hershey Medical Center, Hershey, Pennsylvania

AMY DONNELLAN, RN, DNP, CPNP-AC
Pediatric Nurse Practitioner, Cardiac Intensive Care Unit, The Heart Institute, Cincinnati Children's Hospital Medical Center, Cincinnati, Ohio

CANDICE FALLS, PhDc, MSN, ACNP-BC
Acute Care Nurse Practitioner, Internal Medicine-Cardiology, University of Kentucky, Lexington, Kentucky

JOHNNA FORMAN, RN, MSN, PPCNP-BC
Pediatric Nurse Practitioner, Heinrich A. Werner Division of Pediatric Critical Care, University of Kentucky, Kentucky Children's Hospital, Lexington, Kentucky

KAREN GRONEK, MSN, CRNP
Nurse Practitioner, Department of Cardiovascular Surgery, Temple University Hospital, Philadelphia, Pennsylvania

HONG GU, RN, MSN, CCRN
Clinical Operations Leader, Northwestern Medicine–Central DuPage Hospital, Winfield, Illinois

TONJA M. HARTJES, DNP, ACNP-BC, FNP-BC, CNS, CCRN-CSC, CNEcl, FAANP
University of Florida, College of Nursing, Gainesville, Florida

HALEY HOY, PhD, ACNP
Associate Professor, University of Alabama in Huntsville, Huntsville, Alabama; Acute Care Nurse Practitioner, Vanderbilt Medical Center, Nashville, Tennessee

JEFFREY HUML, MD, FCCP, SCCM
Medical Director for Critical Care, Northwestern Medicine–Central DuPage Hospital, Winfield, Illinois

ALEXANDER JOHNSON, MSN, RN, ACNP-BC, CCNS, CCRN
Critical Care Clinical Nurse Specialist, Northwestern Medicine–Central DuPage Hospital, Winfield, Illinois

ANDREW R. KOLODZIEJ, MD, FACC
Assistant Professor of Medicine, Gill Heart Institute, University of Kentucky, Lexington, Kentucky

KATHLEEN KOPP, BSN, MAOL, RN, CCRN
University of Minnesota Medical Center, Minneapolis, Minnesota

DONNA LESTER, DNP, ACNP-BC, MS, CC-CNS
University of Florida, College of Nursing, Gainesville, Florida

S. JILL LEY, MS, RN, CNS, FAAN
Clinical Nurse Specialist, Surgical & Interventional, California Pacific Medical Center, Clinical Professor, University of California, San Francisco, California

THUY LYNCH, PhD, RN
Assistant Professor, University of Alabama in Huntsville, Huntsville, Alabama

P. LYNN McGUGAN, DNP, ACNP-BC, CCRN-CSC
CTICU, Duke University Hospital, ACNP, Durham, North Carolina

MICHAEL PETTY, PhD, RN, APRN, CNS, CCNS, FHFSA
Adjunct Clinical Assistant Professor, School of Nursing, University of Minnesota Medical Center, Minneapolis, Minnesota

LUCY SLUGANTZ, RN, BSN
Registered Nurse, Pediatric Intensive Care Unit, University of Kentucky, Kentucky Children's Hospital, Lexington, Kentucky

JILLIAN STEVENSON, RN, BSN, CCRN
Staff Registered Nurse, Northwestern Medicine–Central DuPage Hospital, Winfield, Illinois

KELLY A. THOMPSON-BRAZILL, DNP, ACNP-BC, CCRN-CSC, FCCM
Assistant Professor, Director, Adult-Gerontology Acute Care Nurse Practitioner Program, Georgetown University School of Nursing and Health Studies, Washington, DC; Nurse Practitioner, WakeMed Heart and Vascular Cardiothoracic Surgery, Raleigh, North Carolina

Contents

> The incidence and prevalence of structural heart disease has risen due to the longevity of the population, placing an economic burden on society. Over the past 20 years, treatment options for structural heart disease has significantly evolved. Advances in technology and interventional techniques have now shifted therapeutic options to include minimally invasive approaches to correct valvular heart disease. Patients with congenital heart defects are candidates for minimally invasive approaches to correct valvular heart disease. An interdisciplinary team approach using a fusion of multimodal imaging is the best approach for the treatment of this complex patient population.

> Heart failure is a progressive condition that continues to increase in both incidence and prevalence despite pharmacologic treatment. The high rate of morbidity and mortality associated with advanced heart failure has led to exploration of additional treatments, which include surgical interventions to improve outcomes. Heart transplant remains the gold standard but, because of the persistent donor shortage and increasing number of patients with advanced heart failure, mechanical circulatory support is gaining acceptance and can be used as a bridge to heart transplant for those eligible or as destination therapy.

> Lung transplantation is an established treatment of select patients with end-stage pulmonary disease. Lung transplantation should be considered for patients with end-stage pulmonary disease who have an expected 2-year survival of less than 50% without lung transplant and an expected 5-year survival of greater than 80% after transplant. This article reviews routine postsurgical intensive care unit management, along with management of complications such as acute kidney injury, atrial arrhythmias, deep vein thrombosis, primary graft dysfunction, hyperammonemia syndrome, and thrombocytopenia. Finally, management of long-term issues, including diabetes mellitus, hypertension, and bronchial stenosis, is discussed.

> Lung cancer is the leading cause of cancer-related death and the second most diagnosed cancer in the United States. Surgical intervention is most applicable to early-stage lung cancer diagnoses and considered the best curative option. Multiple surgical techniques are now available, including wedge resection, segmentectomy, lobectomy, and pneumonectomy. Robotics and video-assistance are commonly used in wedge resection and sometimes used for segmentectomy. Regardless of the technique, focused clinical management of the patient following lung cancer surgery by nurses and nurse practitioners remains a priority. Future innovations affecting the surgical treatment of lung cancer include immunotherapy and oncogenomics.

> This article discusses the anatomy and physiology of tetralogy of Fallot (TOF) and TOF variants. Indications for surgical repair, morbidity/mortalities, and surgical repair techniques are also reviewed. The article concludes with review of common postoperative complications and management strategies for arrhythmias, right ventricular dysfunction, low cardiac output, and residual defects.

> The hemodynamic monitoring landscape is rapidly evolving from pressure-based and static parameters to more blood flow–based and dynamic parameters. Consensus guidelines for cardiac surgery state that the pulmonary artery catheter is neither required nor helpful in most patients. In the meantime, critical care has been searching for the alternatives to the pulmonary artery catheter and protocols for use. Best available evidence for any protocol developed suggests the inclusion of stroke volume optimization to determine fluid responsiveness. Additional strategies to using stroke volume to optimize hemodynamics, including case studies, are discussed.

> This article reviews the use of vasoactive medications prescribed in the postoperative management of patients who have undergone cardiac surgery. With a focus on the influence these medications have on the physiologic contributors to cardiac output and blood pressure, insight into decision making related to use, titration, and discontinuation of these medications is provided. Case studies offer vignettes to demonstrate the application of knowledge gleaned from the article.

Cardiac arrhythmias are common after cardiac surgery and have profound sequelae. Bradycardias are typically transient and have reversible causes; however, persistent atrioventricular block is an indicator for permanent pacemaker implantation after valvular surgery. Transcatheter aortic valve surgery is associated with even higher rates of permanent pacemaker implantation. Atrial fibrillation, the most common postoperative arrhythmia, is associated with ischemic stroke, myocardial infarction, congestive heart failure, and short-term mortality. Ventricular arrhythmias have extremely high in-hospital mortality, as well as long-term mortality for those who survive the initial event. Implantable cardioverter-defibrillators have been shown to reduce long-term mortality for these patients.

Opioid analgesics are the historical mainstay for postoperative cardiothoracic surgery pain relief. Although opioids are efficacious, they are linked with adverse effects, including sedation and respiratory depression. Emerging research is helping clinicians move toward evidence-based, opioid-sparing management strategies, including peripheral nerve blocks and multimodal analgesia. Good communication is essential to understanding patients' perceptions of pain and attitudes toward different pain-relief methods. Preoperatively educating patients and families on expected nociception and treatment options decreases postprocedural pain. Discussing use of nonopioid analgesics for mild pain and instructions on tapering opioid medications at discharge may prevent future misuse.

This article reviews acute kidney injury following cardiothoracic surgery, addressing the full spectrum of the perioperative environment including preoperative, intraoperative, and postoperative factors for acute kidney injury. Topics discussed include pathophysiology, risk prediction scoring, diagnosis, prevention, treatment, and new directions for research.

Venoarterial (VA) extracorporeal membrane oxygenation (ECMO) may provide adequate blood flow and perfusion in postcardiotomy cardiogenic shock patients. This article discusses patient assessment and management with anticoagulation, sedation, ventilation, and nutrition. Complications may occur, including bleeding, hemolysis, infection, acute kidney injury, stroke, left ventricular distention, limb ischemia, and upper body hypoxia. Patients may recover enough myocardial function to be weaned from ECMO or may be transitioned to a ventricular assist device or transplant. Quality of life may be affected by VA ECMO but may be no different than patients with other chronic health issues.

Cardiac surgical patients risk arrest from tamponade, profound bleeding, and hypovolemia, typically occurring within hours of intensive care admission and associated with diminished response to cardiopulmonary resuscitation (CPR). The Society of Thoracic Surgeons' evidence-based Expert Consensus Statement establishes a new standard for postsurgery arrest management, prioritizing defibrillation or pacing before CPR, restricting epinephrine use, and calling for prompt resternotomy if initial efforts fail. The protocol is summarized in a simple algorithm replacing advanced cardiac life support. This US cardiac surgical resuscitation standard is aligned with worldwide guidelines. Important information for protocol adoption and training is provided.

Patients undergoing cardiothoracic surgery face a small but significant mortality risk. Despite this, end-of-life care specific to this population has received little attention. This article examines current literature on end-of-life care in cardiothoracic surgery and in critical care. Recommendations for management at the end of life are made based on the available evidence.

CRITICAL CARE NURSING CLINICS OF NORTH AMERICA

SERIES OF RELATED INTEREST

Nursing Clinics of North America
http://www.nursing.theclinics.com

THE CLINICS ARE AVAILABLE ONLINE!
Access your subscription at:
www.theclinics.com

Preface

Cardiothoracic Surgical Critical Care

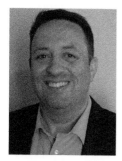

Bryan Boling, DNP, AGACNP-BC
Editor

Heart and lung diseases are two of the leading causes of death in the United States and worldwide. Despite advances in medical care, for many patients, surgery still represents their best hope for improved quality of life and even survival. Owing to the very nature of cardiothoracic surgery, the majority of these patients will spend time in the intensive care unit (ICU), either before or after their operations. Critical care nurses and a growing number of advanced practice nurses are directly involved in the care of these patients.

Advances in cardiothoracic surgery continue to expand treatment options for people with heart and lung disease. Newer techniques have made surgery available to patients who were previously not viable candidates. In many cases, these therapies are able to extend the life of patients who would previously not have survived. However, as the patient population increases, it also grows increasingly sicker at baseline. In addition, the cardiothoracic ICU has become more and more complex, with the addition of new technology for patient monitoring and care. This means that the patients we care for in the cardiothoracic ICU are of higher and higher acuity, and the amount of knowledge that critical care nurses must possess grows every day.

This issue covers the breadth of cardiothoracic surgical critical care, including newer techniques and therapies for heart disease, surgical options for the management of lung disease, and surgical options for the correction of congenital cardiac defects. Common postoperative complications and new technologies for the management of the postoperative patient are also discussed. We also explore the cutting edge of cardiac emergency management and the future of cardiac resuscitation. Finally, we can't discuss the topic of cardiothoracic surgical critical care without acknowledging that sometimes curative therapies are simply not available. Despite our best efforts,

Crit Care Nurs Clin N Am 31 (2019) xiii–xiv
https://doi.org/10.1016/j.cnc.2019.06.001
0899-5885/19/© 2019 Published by Elsevier Inc.

ccnursing.theclinics.com

sometimes patients do not survive, and helping patients have a dignified, pain-free death can be as important a part of critical care nursing as any curative therapy that we can offer.

Bryan Boling, DNP, AGACNP-BC
Division of Critical Care
Department of Anesthesiology
University of Kentucky
UK Medical Center
800 Rose Street, Suite N204
Lexington, KY 40536, USA

E-mail address:
bryan.boling@uky.edu

Minimally Invasive Surgical Options with Valvular Heart Disease

Tonja M. Hartjes, DNP, ACNP-BC, FNP-BC, CNS, CCRN-CSC, CNE$_{cl}$*,
Donna Lester, DNP, ACNP-BC, MS, CC-CNS

KEYWORDS

- Minimally invasive • Cardiac surgery • TAVR • MitraClip • TAPR • PPVI

KEY POINTS

- The incidence and prevalence of structural heart disease has risen due to the longevity of the population, placing an economic burden on society.
- Over the past 20 years, treatment options for structural heart disease has significantly evolved.
- Advances in technology and interventional techniques have now shifted therapeutic options to include minimally invasive approaches to correct valvular heart disease.
- Patients with congenital heart defects are candidates for minimally invasive approaches to correct valvular heart disease.
- An interdisciplinary team approach using a fusion of multimodal imaging is the best approach for the treatment of this complex patient population.

BACKGROUND

The incidence and prevalence of structural heart disease has risen due to the longevity of the population, placing an economic burden on society. Over the past 20 years, treatment options for structural heart disease and especially valvular disorders have significantly evolved. Advances in technology and interventional techniques have now shifted therapeutic options to include minimally invasive approaches to correct valvular heart disease. Valvular heart disease differs from person to person according to: (1) the type of valve (inflow vs outflow valve, native vs prosthetic), (2) condition of valve/type of valvular disease (congenital vs acquired, presence and degree of regurgitation or stenosis, paravalvular leak), (3) anatomic location of valve within the chest, and (4) potential risk factors including certain comorbid conditions and diseases. Typically, this complex population requires an interdisciplinary team approach

Disclosure: The authors have nothing to disclose.
University of Florida, College of Nursing, PO Box 100187, Gainesville, FL 32610-0187, USA
* Corresponding author.
E-mail address: tonjahartjes@gmail.com

(eg, cardiologist, surgeon, advanced practice provider, structural valve coordinator, radiologist, insurance coder) and a significant preoperative workup using a fusion of multimodal imaging and strict follow-up care.[1]

Minimally Invasive Valvular Surgery Options

Minimally invasive surgical repair has several advantages in comparison with traditional open procedures and patients should be informed of these options. Advantages include: (1) smaller incisions and trauma, which decreases pain postoperatively, (2) decreased intensive care and total hospital length of stay, (3) reduction in complications, and (4) reduced cost.[2–6] Older adults who were once deemed high risk/inoperable or too frail for cardiac surgery now have an option. In addition, younger candidates may also benefit from minimally invasive surgery, which will cause less discomfort, shorter lengths of stay, and have them returning to work sooner.[5] Minimally invasive operative approaches include: (1) ministernotomy, (2) hemisternotomy, (3) thoracotomy, (4) robotic or endoscopic, and (5) transcatheter procedures. This article will focus on the transcatheter approaches of minimally invasive cardiac surgery of the aortic and mitral valves (MVs). The preoperative workup, indications and contraindications, potential complications, postoperative care, and outcomes are discussed. A brief overview of the newer pulmonary and tricuspid transcatheter procedures is also discussed.

Incidence

The most common form of acquired valvular disease in developing countries is aortic stenosis (AS), which occurs because of degeneration. Approximately one-third of people with AS require surgical intervention.[7] As age increases so does the incidence of AS; it is 2% to 4% in people older than 65 years and 12.4% in those older than 75 years.[7,8] Symptomatic AS—defined as accompanied by syncope, chest pain, or heart failure—carries a poor prognosis when treated medically.[9] The continued life expectancy for persons with symptomatic AS is 2 years if accompanied by heart failure, 3 years with syncope, and 5 years with angina.[8]

The incidence of mitral regurgitation (MR) is 6% in people greater than 65 year old and rises steeply with age.[10] The origin is related to the degenerative apparatus (eg, primary), cardiomyopathy, or coronary artery disease (eg, secondary).[11] Existing guidelines support surgical intervention, with expected high surgical success when the person is symptomatic, or if the person is asymptomatic with reduced left ventricular function.[12]

AORTIC VALVE DISEASE

Persons with aortic valve disease present with a variety of symptoms, including shortness of breath, syncope, palpitations, fatigue, dizziness, orthopnea, and/or chest pain. On physical assessment they may be hypertensive, tachycardic, and have a crescendo-decrescendo systolic ejection murmur. The diagnosis is supported by a transthoracic echocardiography, which determines the severity of AS, presence of valve calcification, and distribution.[8] Surgical repair is indicated in patients with AS who have peak aortic velocity greater than 4 m/s, a mean gradient greater than 40 mm Hg, and valve area less than 1 cm^2.[13] Surgical approach options are traditional sternotomy, mini-aortic valve replacement with ministernotomy, minithorocotomy, and transcatheter aortic valve replacement (TAVR) delivered through femoral, transapical, subclavian, and transaortic vessels.[14]

Determining the best approach for surgery depends on several factors. Surgical aortic valve replacement (SAVR) risk stratification score is determined by the Society of Thoracic Surgeons Predicted Risk of Mortality (STS-PROM). If the score is greater than 50% probability of death, then the person is considered too high risk for SAVR.[15] Factors not reviewed in the STS-PROM scoring system, which are considered absolute contraindications, include a calcified aorta that will not allow cross-clamping without vessel damage, and previous chest damage, such as that caused by radiation.[15] Relative factors to also consider are possible previous bypass graft injury, pulmonary hypertension, right ventricle dysfunction, and liver failure.[15] Minimal surgical incisions, such as ministernotomy or thoracotomy, are other viable options if preoperative scans, anatomy, and the patient's risk factors are amenable.

In the past, persons with an STS-PROM score of greater than 50% were declined SAVR and their only options were medical therapy or hospice. With the advent of new technology, the TAVR for AS has given hope to high-risk/inoperable patients. Currently, the indications are being adjusted for intermediate-risk persons with STS score at 3% to 8%,[16] and being studied in those with aortic regurgitation.[17]

The cost of the actual valve is about $32,000 for the transcatheter valves (eg, SAPIEN by Edwards Lifescience and CoreValve by Medtronic) versus $7000 for valves used in SAVR.[2] Even though the cost of the transcatheter valves are high, costs overall were equivalent to SAVR, given the shorter intensive care unit and overall hospital length of stay.[5] Quality of life, physical capability, and New York Heart Association functional class improved significantly following TAVR.[3]

Multiple devices have been approved by the US Food and Drug Administration and new devices continue to evolve that will change indications or improve the safety profile. These include delivery methods such as balloon-expandable, self-expanding, and mechanically expanding. The valve material is continually changing and can be made of nitinol, porcine, or bovine tissue, pericardium, or a combination of materials that will individualize the device to the person depending on several factors, such as annulus size, heart anatomy, vascular system, and personal risk factors.[15] The technology will continue to progress as surgeons evaluate patients, their outcomes, and delivery options.

Preprocedural workup is significant and includes several studies to assist with determining the optimal approach, valve sizing, complication risk, or contraindications

Table 1	
Transcatheter aortic valve preprocedure imaging modalities	
Test	**Reason**
Cardiac catheterization or computed tomography coronary angiography (CTCA)	Evaluate presence of coronary artery disease Evaluate presence of pulmonary hypertension
Transesophageal echocardiography	Evaluate severity of AS Evaluate aortic valve (AV) anatomy (including annulus size), gradients, hemodynamics such as stroke volume index and concomitant valvular disease
CT angiography chest/abdomen/pelvis	Determine calcium score Evaluate diameter of aorta from groin to the AV position Measurement of AV annulus size, sinus of Valsalva size, sinotubular junction diameter, coronary ostia height
Carotid ultrasound	Assess stroke risk

(Table 1). Contraindications to TAVR can include[18]: (1) myocardial infarction with intervention less than 30 days, (2) stroke or transient ischemic attack within 6 months, (3) severe MR, (4) endocarditis, mass, or thrombus, and (5) active gastrointestinal bleed.

The procedure is performed in a hybrid operating room, most commonly using a transfemoral approach provided that vascular access of adequate size for the sheath and delivery device can be obtained. The femoral catheter accesses the valve area retrograde through the aortic arch. A transvenous pacing wire is used to ventricularly pace the heart at a rate of 180 to 220 beats per minute to minimize heart motion and lower aortic pressure to optimally deploy the aortic valve. Postimplantation, a transesophageal echocardiogram (TEE) evaluates the placement and functionality of the new valve.

A transfemoral approach is not always feasible among patients with severe peripheral vascular disease. According to Dunne and colleagues,[19], about one-third of patients with TAVR do not have adequate femoral diameter access for the procedure. The iliofemoral artery access should be at least 5 mm in diameter and assessed on the preoperative workup with the computed tomographic scan. Even as we discuss these parameters, smaller devices and percutaneous access are being developed, but until then the other options are transapical, subclavian, and direct aortic approach. The transapical approach requires a 3-inch chest incision at the fifth or sixth intercostal space with rib retraction. Access is directly through the left ventricular apex and requires closure with purse string sutures reinforced with pledgets and a left pleural chest tube.

Postoperative management of the patient with TAVR is based on the possible complications seen within 30 days and documented in the Surgical Replacement and Transcatheter Aortic Valve Implantation and Placement of Aortic Transcatheter Valve trials.[20] These complications include (1) hypotension, (2) bradycardia or asystole, (3) atrial fibrillation, and (4) paravalvular leak.

Hypotension is commonly due to volume depletion and can produce conduction disturbances such as heart block or tachyarrhythmias. Administration of intravenous fluids should be used cautiously in those patients with compromised heart function. Vasopressors may be necessary once volume status has been corrected. The provider should also evaluate for possible vascular complications such as dissection of vessel at access site or pericardial tamponade.

Arrhythmias such as bradycardia or heart block should be addressed with transvenous pacing and can occur at any time in the first 48 hours postprocedure. This complication is the most common and may require implantation of a permanent pacemaker.[15] Close monitoring with telemetry is necessary, and preoperative medications that block the sinoatrial or atrioventricular node may need to be withheld and reassessed after discharge in the clinic setting.

Atrial fibrillation occurs in about 11% of the persons within 30 days.[21,22] Electrolyte monitoring and replacement of potassium and magnesium are important in the postoperative phase. Institution of beta blockers is common preoperatively in patients with AS, so early initiation postoperatively is crucial.

Other complications seen are paravalvular leak or thrombosis, acute kidney injury, myocardial infarction, and stroke.[22–24] The overall risk of major stroke is 2.4%. This risk is greatest in the first 30 days postoperatively (4.1%).[6] Incidence of complications is declining with improvement of the delivery systems, devices, surgical techniques, and physician experience, and with the use of conscious sedation versus general anesthesia.[6]

Discharge planning should begin before admission and include the family, to assure for a timely discharge to home or a rehabilitation facility. Medications should include aspirin indefinitely and Plavix for 6 months.[15] If the person was on preoperative oral anticoagulation, this may also be resumed. Several trials are ongoing to study the duration of antiplatelet therapy post-TAVR and the use of anticoagulation to include direct oral anticoagulants and left atrial appendage closure devices, especially in those patients with atrial arrhythmias. Follow-up echocardiogram should be performed within 30 days of implantation.

MITRAL VALVE DISEASE

Patients with MV disease exhibit symptoms such as shortness of breath, fatigue, palpitations, orthopnea, and peripheral edema. On physical examination they may be tachycardic, with atrial arrhythmias, pulmonary edema, or pleural effusions and a diastolic murmur. Five functional components of the MV are evaluated: (1) leaflets, (2) annulus, (3) chordae tendinae, (4) papillary muscles, and (5) left ventricular function.[14] Indications for surgical intervention are prolapse, regurgitation, or annulus calcification/stenosis. Less invasive surgical options include: (1) lower hemisternotomy, (2) right lateral mini-thorocotomy, (3) endoscopic or port access, (4) transcatheter MV implantation (only investigational at this time), and (5) MitraClip, based on the Alfieri stitch concept, which is approved for prohibitive-risk MV regurgative surgery.[6]

The causes of MV disease has shifted over the years, from ischemic and rheumatic, with the advent of antibiotics and early revascularization, to predominately degenerative processes.[23] Indications for MV repair include (1) symptomatic severe MR and (2) asymptomatic disease with reduced left ventricular (LV) function or normal LV function with high probability of success.[12] Choosing the treatment approach depends on the 5 functional components, STS mortality evaluation, risk factor evaluation of morbidity and mortality and experienced hybrid operating room staff. Preprocedural workup needs to include several studies to assist with determining the optimal approach, valve sizing, complication risk, or contraindication (**Table 2**).

The MitraClip is only indicated for significant 3+ MR of a degenerative nature with a prohibitive risk of MV surgery of greater than 8% on STS mortality. Contraindications are (1) intolerance to procedural anticoagulation and postoperative antiplatelet therapy, (2) active endocarditis or rheumatic MV disease, and (3) evidence of thrombus in the heart, inferior vena cava, or femoral vein.

The MitraClip operative procedure is performed in a hybrid operating room under modified sedation.[14] A catheter is placed through septum into the left atrium. The

Table 2	
Transcatheter mitral valve preprocedure imaging modalities	
Test	**Reason**
Cardiac catheterization or computed tomography coronary angiography (CTCA)	Evaluate presence of coronary artery disease
Transesophageal echocardiography	Evaluate severity of MV disease MV anatomy and morphology, hemodynamics, LV function, and concomitant valvular disease
CT angiography chest/abdomen/pelvis	Measure diameter of aorta from groin to the aortic valve position Measurement of MV annulus size
Pulmonary function tests	Assess pulmonary risk of ventilation liberation
Carotid ultrasound	Assess stroke risk

clip is advanced through the left atrium into the left ventricle just below the leaflets. The clip is retracted and closed to hold the leaflets together to reduce MR and will allow flow on both sides of the clip. Once optimized, the clip is deployed.

Postoperative management of the patient who has undergone MV repair includes minimizing sedation to promote early extubation within 6 hours, chest tube removal when output is <100 mL in 8 hours, pacing wire removal within 1 day, and continued diuresis for 3 to 5 days.[14] The practitioner needs to evaluate for the onset of possible complications such as bleeding, infection, arrhythmias, mechanical leaflet malfunction or structural degeneration, paravalvular leak, congestive heart failure, and leg ischemia in those whom femoral vessel cannulation was used. Discharge planning should include medication instructions regarding antiplatelet or anticoagulation management, daily weights, diet restrictions such as sodium, and exercise restrictions for the first 2 weeks. Follow-up includes an office visit at 2 weeks and TEE in 30 days.[14]

OPTIONS FOR PULMONIC AND TRICUSPID VALVULAR DISEASE

Over the past 2 decades, most research and advancement in minimally invasive surgical options for valvular heart disease has occurred within aortic and MV transcatheter approaches. Options for pulmonary and tricuspid transcatheter heart valves (THVs) are in their early stages.

Pulmonary valve anomalies are typically associated with congenital heart disease (CHD). CHD occurs in 5 to 8 per 1000 live births; 20% may experience pulmonary valve disease or right ventricular outflow track (RVOT) conditions such as tetralogy of Fallot, truncus arteriosus, or pulmonary atresia. Surgical intervention is typically required within the first months of life and repeat surgical interventions are expected over the child's lifetime.[25] Pulmonary valve anomalies or right ventricular outflow tract dysfunction are typically seen in persons with CHD.[25] Persons present with symptoms of right ventricular volume overload resulting from pulmonary regurgitation (PR) and RVOT dysfunction. This continues and will eventually cause right ventricular dilation, tricuspid regurgitation (TR), and annular dilation. This results in exercise intolerance, heart failure, arrhythmias, right/left ventricle dysfunction, and risk of sudden cardiac death.[1] Diagnosis is confirmed with transthoracic echocardiography, which determines the presence of a CHD and severity of the PR.

Persons with CHD often require early and recurrent surgical intervention throughout their lifetime related to progressive RVOT dysfunction, pulmonary stenosis (PS), PR, and anastomotic stenosis of a conduit.[25] Surgical repair and the subsequent reoperations are associated with an increased morbidity and mortality.[25] When stenosis occurs after surgery, a balloon or open valvuloplasty may be performed. A nonsurgical transcatheter intervention was created in 2000; the percutaneous pulmonary valve implantation (PPVI) for right ventricular to pulmonary artery stenosis or PR. In addition, a transcatheter pulmonary valve replacement (TPVR), with a right internal jugular or transfemoral approach, is available for RVOT dysfunction when PS and PR are present, thus expanding the lifespan of the conduit.[1] Both techniques can use either the Melody THV by Medtronic or the Edwards Lifesciences SAPIEN pulmonic THV. Preplanning includes various imaging modalities (**Table 3**).

Overall, both techniques have demonstrated improved right ventricular volumes and pressures, with reversed right-sided pressures and LV remodeling, improved functional capacity, resolved PR and normalized RVOT gradients.[1,25] The PPVI technique has demonstrated good short-term and long-term outcomes. These data were published by the US Investigational Device Exemption (IDE) trial, reporting a 5-year freedom from reimplantation of 76% and explant of 92%.[25] TPVR short-term

Table 3
Transcatheter pulmonic valve preprocedure imaging modalities

Test	Reason
Transesophageal echocardiography or CT angiography	Further characterize or evaluate the valve[1,25]
Cardiac magnetic resonance (CMR)	Evaluates bioprosthetic or transcatheter heart valves if already in place. In addition, CMR may be used to determine right ventricular volume and RVOT morphology, which is paramount when determining the timing of intervention in chronic PR[1,25]
Coronary angiography	Evaluate coronary anatomy (varies in the CHD population)
CTA-fluoroscopy and TEE-fluoroscopy	Preplanning the precise location and anatomy, as well as real-time during the procedure[1,25]

outcomes demonstrate clinical improvement of symptoms and durability of the device. Between 2011 and 2014, the US IDE study revealed a >90% 1-year freedom from reintervention or valvular dysfunction.[1]

Complications for both techniques include: (1) stent fracture (up to 30% occurrence), (2) endocarditis (2.4% risk of occurrence per year), (3) valvular dysfunction, (4) coronary compression, and (5) RVOT tear or rupture with predeployment and postdeployment balloon dilations. Reoccurrence of valvular dysfunction should be evaluated for stent fracture or endocarditis. Paravalvular leaks are uncommon compared with TAVR.[1,25]

TR is an often underrecognized or undertreated condition in the United States. Less than 1% of persons with TR undergo surgery annually, despite a 1-year mortality of 36.1%.[26] In addition, reoccurrence of significant TR can occur in as many as 60% of persons by 5 years.[26] Persons with tTR are typically treated with a valve annuloplasty. Off-label use of TAVR technology has been used for transcatheter tricuspid valve intervention for persons with degenerated bioprostheses, but has yielded mixed results.[26] This is due in part to the mechanical and clinical challenges in quantifying the degree of tTR and any subsequent improvement after intervention, identifying tricuspid landing zones and truly determining the impact of TR in the face of pulmonary hypertension, atrial fibrillation, and left heart disease.[26]

SUMMARY

Significant strides have occurred in minimally invasive surgery techniques over the past 20 years, which have reduced pain, complications, length of stay, and costs for persons undergoing cardiac surgery. Driven by demand and cost, these minimally invasive techniques are now adjunct to the medical therapy for valvular heart disease. Considered safe and cost-effective, future transcatheter technologies include the development of new devices, the advancement of pulmonary and tricuspid THV options, the pursuit of transcatheter perfection with regard to improvements in complication rates, and the durability of THVs and reduction in reintervention rates, as well as expansion of the population eligible for the procedures. Research regarding THV long-term outcomes is limited because the technologies are new. Further study evaluating the durability of the valves and valve-in-valve replacement is required.

REFERENCES

1. Ruiz CE, Klinger C, Perk G, et al. Transcatheter therapies for the treatment of valvular and paravalvular regurgitation in acquired and congenital valvular heart disease. J Am Coll Cardiol 2015;66(2):169–83.
2. Johnson SR. Nonsurgical heart valve procedure spurs cost concerns. Modern Healthcare; 2014. Available at: https://www.modernhealthcare.com/article/20140329/MAGAZINE/303299961. Accessed January 2, 2019.
3. Mohammadi M, Hill C, Chaney S. Is transcatheter aortic valve replacement a safe treatment for elderly persons with severe aortic stenosis. J Am Assoc Nurse Pract 2016;28(7):387–92.
4. Irace FG, Rose D, Ascoli R, et al. Video assistance in mitral valve surgery: reaching the "Thru" port access. J Vis Surg 2015;1:13.
5. Atluri P, Stetson RL, Hung G, et al. Minimally invasive mitral valve surgery is associated with equivalent cost and shorter hospital stay when compared with traditional sternotomy. J Thorac Cardiovasc Surg 2016;151(2):385–8.
6. Shemin R. The future of cardiovascular surgery. Circulation 2016;133:2712–5.
7. Popma JJ, Adams DH, Reardon MJ, et al. Transcatheter aortic valve replacement using a self-expanding bioprosthesis in persons with severe aortic stenosis at extreme risk for surgery. J Am Coll Cardiol 2014;63(19):1972–81.
8. Badiani S, Bhattacharyya S, Lloyd G. Role of echocardiography before transcatheter aortic valve implantation. Curr Cardiol Rep 2016;18:38.
9. Vranckx P, Windecker S, Welsh RC, et al. Thrombo-embolic prevention after transcatheter aortic valve implantation. Eur Heart J 2017;3(45):3341–50.
10. Sorajja P, Leon MB, Adams DH, et al. Transcatheter therapy for mitral regurgitation: clinical challenges and potential solutions. Circulation 2017;136:404–17.
11. Prendergast BD, DeBonis M. Valve repair: a durable surgical option in degenerative mitral regurgitation. Circulation 2017;135:423–5.
12. Herrmann HC, Maisano F. Transcatheter therapy of mitral regurgitation. Circulation 2014;130:1712–22.
13. Nishimura RA, Otto CM, Bonow RO, et al. 2014 AHA/ACC guideline on the management of persons with valvular heart disease. J Am Coll Cardiol 2014;63(22):e57–185.
14. Wolfe JA, Malaisrie SC, Farivar RS, et al. Minimally invasive mitral valve surgery II: surgical technique and postoperative management. Innovations 2016;11:251–9.
15. Karycki M. Transcatheter aortic valve replacement. Nurs Crit Care 2019;14(1):22–30.
16. Berger D. Evolution of a TAVR program. Crit Care Nurs Q 2018;41(4):360–8.
17. Pellikka PA, Dangas G. TAVR for severe aortic regurgitation. J Am Coll Cardiol 2017;70(22):2764–5.
18. O'Leary GM. Transcatheter aortic valve replacement. Nurs Crit Care 2019;11(5):36–42.
19. Dunne B, Tan D, Chu D, et al. Transapical versus transaortic transcatheter aortic valve implantation: a systematic review. Ann Thorac Surg 2015;100:354–61.
20. Reynolds MR, Magnusen EA, Wang K, et al. Cost-effectiveness of transcatheter aortic valve replacement compared with standard care among inoperable persons with severe aortic stenosis, PARTNER Cohort B. Circulation 2012;125(9):1102–9.
21. Leon MB, Smith CR, Mack M, et al. Transcatheter aortic-valve implantation for aortic stenosis in persons who cannot undergo surgery. N Engl J Med 2010;363:1597–607.

22. Reardon MJ, Van Mieghem NM, Popma JJ, et al. Surgical or transcatheter aortic-valve replacement in the intermediate-risk persons. N Engl J Med 2017;376: 1321–31.

23. Vakamudi S, Jellis C, Mick S, et al. Sex differences in the etiology of surgical mitral valve disease. Circulation 2018;138:1749–51.

24. Coli A, Manzan E, Besola L, et al. One year outcomes after transapical echocardiography-guided mitral valve repair. Circulation 2018;138:843–5.

25. Anasari MM, Cardoso R, Garcia D, et al. Percutaneous pulmonary valve implantation: present status and evolving future. J Am Coll Cardiol 2015;66(20): 2246–55.

26. O'Neill W, O'Neill B. Transcatheter tricuspid valve intervention: the next frontier. J Am Coll Cardiol 2015;65(12):1196–8.

Surgical Approaches in Heart Failure

Candice Falls, PhDc, MSN, ACNP-BC[a],*, Andrew R. Kolodziej, MD[b]

KEYWORDS

- Heart failure • Mechanical circulatory support • Heart transplant
- Total artificial heart

KEY POINTS

- Heart failure is a common condition that continues to increase in incidence and prevalence.
- Heart transplant remains the gold standard for treatment of advanced heart failure.
- Durable mechanical circulatory support options are available for patients who are not transplant candidates or cannot wait for transplant.

INTRODUCTION

Heart failure is a progressive condition that continues to increase in both incidence and prevalence, accounting for more than 2% to 3% of the national health care budget.[1–6] Despite improvements in treatment of end-stage heart failure, the costs per quality-adjusted year is still greater than $400,000.[7] The high rate of morbidity and mortality associated with advanced heart failure has led to exploration of additional treatments, which include surgical interventions to improve outcomes.[8–11] This article focuses on the most common surgical interventions that have shown improvement in morbidity and mortality for patients with heart failure.

EPIDEMIOLOGY OF HEART FAILURE

The epidemiology of heart failure has been extensively studied for the past several decades with a large contribution of literature stemming from the Framingham Heart Study. Major findings in the 1980s noted that the rate of heart failure increases with age and is higher in men than in women. In addition, hypertension, coronary artery disease, and diabetes mellitus are associated with increased risk of heart failure. In the

Disclosure: The authors have nothing to disclose.
[a] Internal Medicine-Cardiology, University of Kentucky, 1000 South Limestone Pavilion A 08. 176, Lexington, KY, USA; [b] Gill Heart Institute, University of Kentucky, 900 South Limestone, CTW 320, Lexington, KY 40536, USA
* Corresponding author.
E-mail address: Cdharv0@uky.edu

1980s the prevalence of heart failure was 24 per 1000 in men and 25 per 1000 in women, with a median survival time of 1.7 years in men and 3.2 years in women.[12]

Longitudinal analysis of the Framingham Study noted in the 1990s that heart failure continued to increase in incidence and prevalence, affecting about 1% of persons in their 50s, with progressive increases to about 10% of persons in their 80s.[13] The incidence also increased with age, from 0.2% in persons 45 to 54 years old to 4% in those aged 85 to 94 years. Mortality was noted to be around 37% within 2 years of diagnosis.[13–16]

Continued analysis of epidemiologic data from the Framingham Study in the 2000s further supported the burden of heart failure affecting more than 5 million Americans, with more than 550,000 new cases a year.[17,18] Median survival for men and women was noted to be similar to the 1990s, with a 5-year survival rate of 25% of men and 38% of women. Hypertension was noted to be the most common cause of heart failure, followed by myocardial infarction, valvular heart disease, and diabetes.[17–19]

At present, heart failure affects more than 5.7 million Americans, with more than 670,000 new cases a year.[20] Readmissions related to heart failure continue to remain a burden, with rates of 20% at 1 month and 50% at 6 months, with more than 43% of patients being hospitalized more than 5 times or more within 5 years of being diagnosed.[21] Heart failure–related admissions account for 56.7% of all heart failure episodes, with heart failure being the most common reason for hospitalization in adults aged 85 years and older and the second most common for adults aged 65 to 84 years.[18–22] Approximately 15% to 35% of patients with end-stage heart failure have a 1-year mortality. Hypertension and diabetes remain the top comorbidities linked to the high prevalence of heart failure.[21,22]

PATHOPHYSIOLOGY OF SYSTOLIC HEART FAILURE

Heart failure is defined as "a complex clinical syndrome that results from any structural or functional impairment of ventricular filling or ejection of blood."[22] This condition can ultimately lead to decreased exercise tolerance as well as symptoms of dyspnea at rest and/or exertion as well as fatigue and edema with variable severity. However, the premise of heart failure physiology is increased intracardiac filling pressures, which is further explained later in the article.

Although there are 2 basic varieties of heart failure, systolic as well as diastolic, this article focuses on systolic heart failure. Systolic heart failure, whether treated according to guideline-directed approach or not, ultimately leads to advancement of myocardial dysfunction with end organs being affected, which brings up the concept of advanced heart failure. This entity is associated with refractory heart failure symptoms despite medical therapy as well as persistently increased intracardiac filling pressures, inability to exercise, as well as recurrent hospitalizations, which in turn is associated with increased mortality.[23] At this stage there are further options in treatment of heart failure, such as inotropic support, but inevitably surgical treatment, such as heart transplant or mechanical circulatory support, may be required.

Strength of myocardial contraction has been shown to be related to the preload and thus the stretch of the fibers, which was first described by Otto Frank in the nineteenth century. This finding was elegantly confirmed a century later by Ernest Starling and colleagues when they showed that increasing venous return and subsequent filling of heart chambers increased stroke volume. Thus a principle described by "the ability of the heart to change its force of contraction and therefore stroke volume in response to changes in venous return and subsequent chamber filling pressure"[24] came to be known as the Frank-Starling principle and is shown in **Fig. 1.**

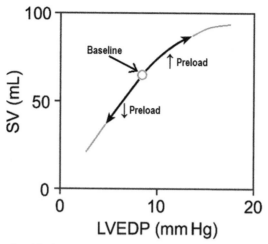

Fig. 1. Effects of preload (volume status) on left ventricular filling pressures and ventricular function: Frank-Starling principle. LVEDP, left ventricular end-diastolic pressure; SV, stroke volume.

Note that the myocardium does not operate on the single Frank-Starling curve but its function is defined by multiple curves, as noted in **Fig. 2**. These curves represent myocardial physiology based on its afterload as well as inotropic state.

In order to improve the understanding of heart failure pathophysiology, it is important to understand the Frank-Starling curve, its principle of preload, and how this correlates with intracardiac filling pressures and thus the concept of pressure-volume loops.

Looking at the Frank-Starling curve, it is possible to visualize the effects of increased preload in the form of left ventricular end-diastolic pressure (LVEDP) on the stroke volume. In a normal functioning heart, the higher the LVEDP, the higher the stroke volume, with the curve theoretically not reaching its plateau, as shown by **Fig. 1**. In

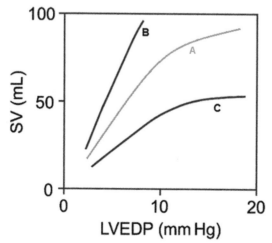

Fig. 2. Frank-Starling graph showing effects of inotrope on stroke volume relative to left ventricular filling pressures. A) normal contractility B) increased contractility C) decrease contractility.

contrast, increased inotropy increases the slope of this line, making the myocardium more responsive and sensitive to preload with higher rate of stroke volume increase compared with the amount of preload increase, as denoted by line B in **Fig. 2**. Decreased inotropy, as in heart failure, seems to reach a plateau point of the curve at lower LVEDP, as represented by line C in **Fig. 2**.

To further visualize this principle, looking at pressure-volume loops it becomes evident that when venous return is increased, there is increased filling of the ventricle leading to an increase in end-diastolic volume (**Fig. 3**). If the ventricle now contracts at this increased preload, the ventricle empties to the same end-systolic volume, thereby increasing its stroke volume, which is defined as end-diastolic minus end-systolic volume, provided that the afterload and inotropy are held constant. The increased stroke volume is seen as an increase in the width of the pressure-volume loop. The normal ventricle is therefore capable of increasing its stroke volume to match physiologic increases in venous return; however, this is not the case for ventricles that are in failure.

In a failing heart and thus systolic dysfunction, there is evidence of downward and rightward shift of the Frank-Starling curve, indicating loss of inotropy with resultant increase in left ventricle (LV) filling pressures. Initially there are multiple compensatory mechanisms in place to maintain stroke volume, such as increased preload associated with neurohormonal upregulation and retention of sodium leading to increased

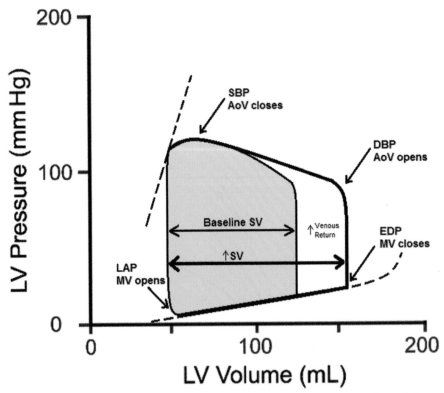

Fig. 3. Pressure-volume loop as it relates to increased preload (venous return) and left ventricular function (stroke volume). AoV, aortic valve; DBP, diastolic blood pressure; EDP, end-diastolic pressure; LAP, left atrial pressure; LV, left ventricle; MV, mitral valve; SBP, systolic blood pressure.

blood volume and thus increased filling pressures. Subsequently, these compensatory mechanisms result in chamber remodeling manifested by dilatation, which initially is in essence another compensatory phenomenon.[25] This remodeling ultimately leads to decreased stroke volume and persistently increased filling pressures and volume overload. These physiologic phenomena are shown in **Fig. 4**.

PRINCIPLE OF TREATING ADVANCED HEART FAILURE

The premise of treating heart failure is through control of congestion and thus preload because it has been shown that most symptoms and recurrent hospitalizations in patients with heart failure are related to congestive exacerbation.[26] In addition, an important concept in treating heart failure is controlling afterload. This control in turn can be achieved through neurohormonal blockade, which ultimately leads to decrease in intracardiac filling pressures.[25–27] The strategy of achieving neurohormonal blockade through medical therapy by using the combination of angiotensin-converting enzyme inhibitors or angiotensin receptor blockers with β-blockers as well as more recently angiotensin receptor–neprilysin inhibitor, have reached a class I recommendation by the American College of Cardiology Foundation/American Heart Association/Heart Failure Society of America Task Force.[28]

Luckily for those patients who are refractory or intolerant to guideline-directed medical therapy, clinicians are now able to either replace the organ or support it with implantable pumps. Replacing the organ improves the physiology drastically but, holding true to the hemodynamic principle of heart failure, the premise of treatment is to offload the heart, decreasing intracardiac filling pressures through decreasing volume overload and improving the Frank-Starling forces such that it restores the pressure-volume loop position to the right, with concomitant improvement in stroke volume.

SURGICAL OPTIONS
Heart Transplant

Despite advances in pharmacologic as well as device therapy for chronic systolic heart failure, long-term morbidity and mortality remain unacceptably high. Five-year

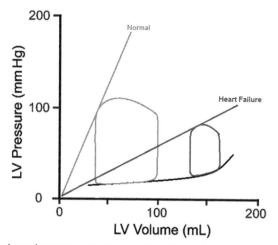

Fig. 4. Pressure-volume loop representing results of heart failure.

mortality for patients with advanced heart failure is about 80%[29] and thus further surgical approaches are necessary. One of those options, and a gold standard treatment of advanced end-stage systolic heart failure, is heart transplant. The fundamental indication for heart transplant is poor quality of life as well as rapidly progressive physiology such as cardiogenic shock.

Since the first orthotropic, interhuman heart transplant performed on December 3, 1967, at the Groote Schuur Hospital in Cape Town, South Africa, by Dr Christiaan Neethling Barnard, great progress has been made. By end of 1968, 102 transplants had been performed in 17 countries and 52 centers. Only a third of these patients lived longer than 3 months. It was not until 1980, with the use of cyclosporine, borrowed from renal transplantation, that ultimate successful progress resulted in improved survival.[30] To date, worldwide, about 3500 heart transplants are performed annually. Most of these are performed in the United States (2000–2300 annually) with an average 1-year survival rate of 90% with conditional half-life of 13.2 years.[31–33] Heart transplant remains the gold standard of advanced heart failure treatment of carefully selected patients. **Box 1** summarizes indications and contraindications for heart transplant.

SURGICAL CONSIDERATIONS

Orthotopic placement (organ placed in the anatomically original position) is the most commonly used placement of the donor heart during surgery. There are 2 main techniques of anastomosing the recipient vasculature/structures to the donor heart: bicaval and biatrial techniques. The biatrial technique is the most widely used approach to orthotropic heart transplant, although this depends on the transplant surgeon (**Fig. 5**).

MEDICAL CONSIDERATIONS

As noted in **Fig. 6**, early graft failure in the first year is the most common cause of posttransplant complications, including death. Graft failure downtrends with the first year, primarily caused by acute rejection, whereas infectious complications associated with aggressive immunosuppression begin to develop during that time period. Ultimately, resurgence of graft failure as well as concomitant cardiac allograft vasculopathy in addition to malignancy predominate long-term outcomes.[33]

MECHANICAL CIRCULATORY SUPPORT

Even though over the last 5 decades heart transplant has been the gold standard of care for carefully selected patients with end-stage heart disease, challenges continue to exist in this patient population. These challenges include complications associated with posttransplant care but, more importantly, the increasing number of potential recipients compared with the number of donor organs.[33] Approximately 117,000 people need a lifesaving organ. Every 10 minutes someone is listed for transplant and every 22 minutes someone dies while waiting for an organ.[34] Because of this limiting factor, there has been an increase in technological advances to be able to keep patients with end-stage, advanced heart failure alive in order to ultimately offer them the gold standard of care. This technology is mechanical circulatory support, both short as well as long term.

Interest in mechanical circulatory support dates back to the 1950s, during the time of development of cardiopulmonary bypass and open-heart surgery.[35] The first successful implantation of a left ventricular assist device (LVAD) was completed in 1966

Box 1
Indications and contraindications for heart transplant

Indications
  Significant, life-limiting heart failure:
  • Persistent New York Heart Association class III or IV symptoms despite maximal guideline-
    directed medical therapy
  Decreased exercise tolerance (peak oxygen uptake [Vo_2] ≤14 mL/kg/min for patients not on
  β-blockers and peak Vo_2 ≤12 mL/kg/min for patients on β-blockers)
  Recurrent life-threatening LV arrhythmias despite optimized medical antiarrhythmic therapy
  Refractory cardiogenic shock requiring mechanical circulatory support (LVAD, TAH)
  Cardiogenic shock requiring continuous parenteral inotropic therapy
  Patient with end-stage congenital DLCO heart disease with heart failure
  Refractory angina despite maximal medical therapy and not amenable to percutaneous or
  surgical revascularization
  Severe hypertrophic or restrictive cardiomyopathy with end-stage heart failure symptoms
  Severe cardiac allograft vasculopathy in transplanted patients with evidence of graft failure

Contraindications
  Age greater than 70 years
  BMI greater than 35 kg/m²
  TPG greater than 15 mm Hg, PVR greater than 5 Wood units or pulmonary artery pressure
  greater than 60 mm Hg with 1 of the above or the inability to achieve PVR less than 2.5 Wood
  units with vasodilator or inotropic therapy
  Primary lung disease with impaired pulmonary function tests (FEV_1<40% or predicted,
  FVC<50%, or normal DLCO<40%)
  Uncontrolled diabetes (HbA1c>7.5%)
  eGFR<30
  Hepatic cirrhosis
  Severe peripheral vascular disease not amenable to revascularization
  Active infections except LVAD-related infections (HIV, hepatitis B and hepatitis C, although
  now a relative contraindication)
  Active drug use: must be abstinent 6 months
  Noncompliance or lack of caregiver or social support
  Dementia or mental retardation

Abbreviations: BMI, body mass index; eGFR, estimated glomerular filtration rate; FEV_1, forced
expiratory volume in 1 second; FVC, forced vital capacity; HbA1c, glycosylated hemoglobin;
HIV, human immunodeficiency virus; LVAD, left ventricular assist device; PVR, pulmonary
vascular resistance; TAH, total artificial heart; TPG, transpulmonary gradient.

Data from Mehra MR, Canter CE, Hannan MM, et al. The 2016 International Society for Heart
Lung Transplantation listing criteria for heart transplantation: a 10-year update. J Heart Lung
Transplant 2016;35(1):1–23.

---

by Dr DeBakey. A paracorporeal (external) circuit was able to provide mechanical support for 10 days after the surgery.[35] The lack of heart donors and contraindications to
heart transplant further stimulated the necessity for development of this technology.
The first successful long-term implantation of an artificial LVAD was conducted in
1988 by Dr William F. Bernhard of Boston Children's Hospital Medical Center.[36]

Initially pulsatile pumps were the standard of care given that pulsatility is a necessary physiologic phenomenon. Both the Randomized Evaluation of Mechanical Assistance for the Treatment of Congestive Heart Failure (REMATCH) and Investigation of
Non-Transplant Eligible Patients Who Are Inotrope Dependent (INTrEPID) trials evaluated the role of pulsatile pumps in patients with advanced heart failure who were inel-
igible for heart transplant and noted 48% reduction in mortality compared with optimal
medical therapy.[37,38] The caveat, and ultimately the demise of pulsatile pumps, was
their durability. A device with a durability of about 24 months could only serve as a

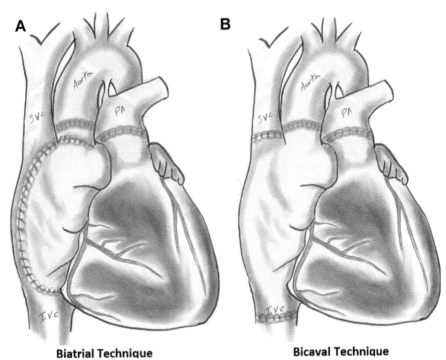

Fig. 5. (*A, B*) Two different approaches for anastomosis during orthotropic heart transplant. IVC, inferior vena cava; PA, pulmonary artery; SVC, superior vena cava.

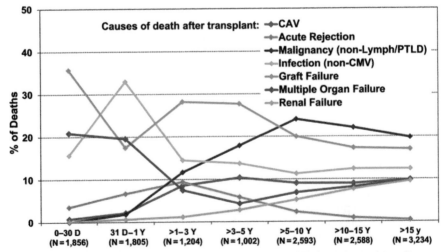

Fig. 6. Relative incidence of leading causes of death for adult heart transplants (January 2009–June 2016). CAV, cardiac allograft vasculopathy; CMV, cytomegalovirus; PTLD, post-transplant lymphoproliferative disorder. (*From* Kirklin JK, Pagani FD, Kormos RL, et al. Eighth annual INTERMACS report: special focus on framing the impact of adverse events. J Heart Lung Transplant 2017;36(10):1080–6; with permission.)

prolonged bridge to transplant for patients who were too sick and thus required implementation of mechanical circulatory support in order to improve end-organ function and eventually be placed on a heart transplant list. What about the patients who were not transplant candidates to begin with? Further endeavors with other devices gave rise to continuous-flow pumps. Progress was made in 1987 when a variation of a continuous-flow device was implanted in a pediatric patient as bridge to transplant. Dr Frazier in his case report states that this procedure "prompted us to speculate about broader application of nonpulsatile flow, to the development of fully implantable devices for long-term cardiovascular support of the terminal heart disease patient ... *The potential for long-term benefit lies in meeting the requirements of the circulatory system with a nonpulsatile pump.*"[39] Interest in more durable devices has led to the HeartMate II pump (a continuous-flow LVAD), replacing pulsatile technology after a study showed that continuous-flow LVADs improve survival from disabling stroke and device failure compared its predecessor (Heartmate XVE).[40]

At present, all devices on the market are continuous-flow pumps based on an axial or centrifugal mechanism (**Fig. 7**). The axial-flow rotary pump consists of a rotating, screwlike propeller within a tube housing. The energy from the rotating element increases blood pressure and flow. The centrifugal pump with spinning blades captures and throws fluid forward, which results in essentially pulseless physiology, depending on the residual left ventricular function.[41]

Because temporary devices such as extracorporeal membrane oxygenation are discussed elsewhere in this issue, this the focus here is primarily on durable devices, namely LVADs, as well as on a brief discussion of total artificial heart technology. LVADs unload the LV and thus, because blood is withdrawn directly from the left atrium (LA)/LV (considering there is no mitral stenosis), pulmonary capillary wedge pressure and LVEDP decrease. This decrease is shown by the Pressure-Volume loop being shifted leftward, as noted in **Figs. 8**A-D and **8**E. Although it appears that stroke volume decreases even though there is significant left ventricular unloading, as noted by the pressure-volume loop, at the same time, arterial pressure increases, as noted in **Figs. 8**B and C. Although peak LV pressure and arterial pressure become increasingly dissociated compared with systemic, arterial blood pressure significantly increases and thus, ultimately, improving end-organ perfusion often results in reversal of end-organ dysfunction (see **Figs. 7**B-8D and E; **Table 1**).[42]

Four major indications for LVAD implantation exist (**Box 2**):

1. Bridge to transplant
2. Destination therapy

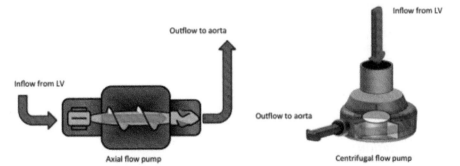

Fig. 7. The mechanism of axial (eg, HeartMate II) versus centrifugal (HeartWare, HeartMate III) pump hemodynamics. (*From* Lim HS, Howell N, & Ranasinghe A. The physiology of continuous-flow left ventricular assist devices. J Card Fail. 2017;23(2):170; with permission.)

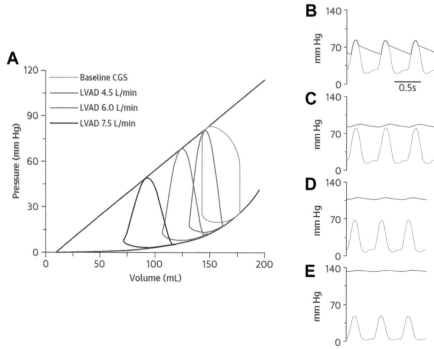

Fig. 8. (*A*) Flow-dependent changes of the pressure-volume loop with LV-to-aortic pumping. The loop becomes triangular and shifts progressively leftward (indicating increasing degrees of LV unloading). Corresponding LV and aortic pressure waveforms at baseline (*B*), 4.5 L/min (*C*), 6.0 L/min (*D*), and 7.5 L/min (*E*). With increased flow, there are greater degrees of LV unloading and uncoupling between aortic and peak LV pressure generation. CGS, cardiogenic shock. (*From* Burkhoff D, Sayer G, Doshi D, et al. Hemodynamics of mechanical circulatory support. J Am Coll Cardiol 2015;66:2671; with permission.)

3. Bridge to recovery
4. Bridge to decision

Bridge to transplant remains the most common indication for implantation of LVADs. As mentioned earlier, because of the growing population of patients with advanced HF and stagnant numbers of donor organs, improved durability of the newer devices offers select patients increased survival and improvement of quality of life. This improvement ultimately may let those patients remain candidates for transplant in the future. Alternatively, destination therapy is offered to particularly selected patients with advanced HF who are not candidates for heart transplant **Fig. 9**.

TEMPORARY OPTIONS

Temporary options are listed in **Table 2**.

DURABLE OPTIONS

There are basically 2 types of devices used: paracorporeal (percutaneous ventricular assist devices) and totally implantable devices (LVADs or biventricular assist devices) (**Table 3**).

Level	Symptoms	Signs and Hemodynamics	Need for LVAD
Table 1 INTERMACS profiles			
1	"Crash and burn"	Critical cardiogenic shock	Within hours
2	"Sliding on inotropes"	Progressive decline on inotropic support	Within days
3	Dependent stability	Stable but inotropic dependent	Elective over weeks to months
4	"Frequent flyer"	Resting symptoms, although remains home on oral therapy with frequent hospitalizations	Variable urgency, dependent on nutrition and organ function
5	Housebound	Exertion intolerant	Variable urgency, dependent on nutrition and organ function
6	"Walking wounded"	Exertion limited to symptoms, although still responding to oral guideline-directed medical therapy	Variable urgency, dependent on nutrition and organ function
7	Advanced NYHA III symptoms	NYHA class II or III, responding to oral guideline-directed medical therapy	Not currently indicated

Abbreviation: NYHA, New York Heart Association.

TOTAL ARTIFICIAL HEART

The first successful implantation of total artificial heart (TAH), which led to subsequent heart transplants, was performed in 1969. Subsequent successful implantations did not occur until the beginning of 1980.[43] Since that time there have been many models that have been implanted but only 1 has withstood the test of time:

Box 2
Indications and contraindications for mechanical support

Indications

Severe symptomatic heart failure despite optimal medical therapy

Left ventricular ejection fraction that is less than or equal to 25%

Exercise oxygen uptake [Vo_2] that is less than or equal to 12 mL/kg/min

Continuous intravenous inotropes or intra-aortic balloon pump therapy to prevent symptomatic hypotension, decreasing renal function, or worsening pulmonary congestion

Contraindications

Blood clotting disorders

Liver cirrhosis

Severe lung disease

Other comorbid conditions that result in less than 1-year survival

Data from Miller LW, Guglin M. Patient selection for ventricular assist devices: a moving target. J Am Coll Cardiol. 2013;61(12):1209-21.

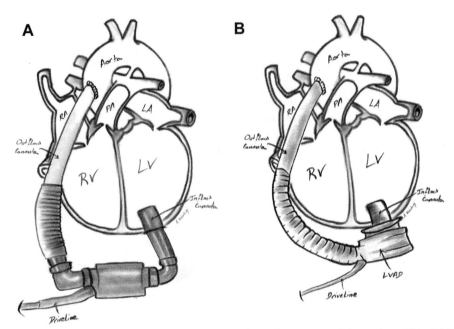

Fig. 9. (*A*) Axial-flow device. (*B*) Centrifugal flow device. RA, right atrium; RV, right ventricle.

SynCardia TAH (SynCardia Systems, Inc., Tucson, AZ; **Fig. 10**). This device is an intracorporeal, pneumatically driven biventricular system, which completely replaces the failing heart. The use of TAH as a bridge to transplant has shown a 79% survival to transplant, versus 46% in patients not receiving a TAH in a small observational prospective study.[44] **Box 3** summarizes indications and contraindications for TAH implantation.

SURGICAL CONSIDERATIONS

Because the human body generates a significant amount of scar tissue around the device, reentry for future heart transplant becomes significantly more difficult. For this reason, the device as well as proximal vasculature are covered by a Gore-Tex material

Table 2 Temporary devices		
Device	**Mechanism**	**Duration**
IABP	Counterpulsation	Days
Impella	Axial flow	Days
ECMO	Continuous flow	Days to weeks
Centrimag	Centrifugal	Weeks
Tandem Heart	Centrifugal	Days

Abbreviations: ECMO, extracorporeal membrane oxygenation; IABP, intra-aortic balloon pump.

Table 3 Durable devices		
Device	Mechanism	Indications
HeartMate II	Axial flow	BTT, DT
HeartMate III	Centrifugal flow	BTT
HeartWare	Centrifugal flow	BTT, DT
TAH	Pulsatile	BTT

Abbreviations: BTT, bridge to transplant, DT, destination therapy; TAH, total artificial heart.

in order to facilitate future reentry and minimize the necessity for dissecting the structures.[45]

MEDICAL CONSIDERATIONS

The most recent analysis of the INTERMACS registry reveals that about 80% of people are alive after 1 year. Another analysis shows that survival to transplant was 68.3%, with strokes occurring in 7.9% of the population.[34]

Postimplant management is based on proper anticoagulation as well as management of end-organ dysfunction. The most common organs involved are the liver and kidneys, with renal dysfunction being related to lack of natriuretic peptides (A and B types). Level of postoperative end-organ dysfunction depends on severity of decompensated state before implantation.

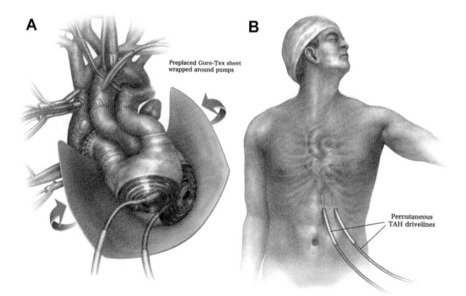

Fig. 10. (*A*) Gore-Tex (Gore Medical, Flagstaff, AZ) sheets are sewn into the pericardial well with a few 4-0 Prolene sutures. After coming off bypass, and achieving hemostasis, the sheets can be wrapped around the ventricles to prevent harm on reentry. (*B*) Percutaneous lines exit 6 to 8 cm from left subcostal margin. (*From* Morris RJ. The Syncardia total artificial heart: implantation technique. Oper Tech Thorac Cardiovasc Surg 2012;17(2):164; with permission.)

Box 3
Indications and contraindications for total artificial heart implantation

Indications

Patients who are heart transplant candidates with severe biventricular failure and imminent risk of death (INTERMACS profiles 1 and 2) in setting where suitable donor is not available

Bridge to transplant in patients in need of retransplant experiencing graft failure not responding to conventional therapy: severe and diffuse coronary artery vasculopathy

Patients with infiltrative or hypertrophic cardiomyopathy and associated low-output failure versus cardiogenic shock; These are patients not amenable to left ventricular systolic device.

Patients who experienced ventricular tachycardia storm or malignant arrhythmias despite multiple ablations and medical therapy

Contraindications

Patients ultimately not deemed to be transplant candidates

Data from Arabia F. Total artificial heart. In: Kobashigawa JA, editor. Clinical guide to heart transplantation. Cham, Switzerland: Springer; 2017. p. 227–236.

SUMMARY

Heart failure continues to increase in incidence and prevalence despite pharmacologic therapy and additional therapies such as cardiac resynchronization therapy and remains the most common cause of hospitalization. Heart failure is associated with poor quality of life and has an overall 1-year mortality of 20%. Because of the morbidity, mortality, and costs associated with heart failure, surgical advances are becoming more widely accepted.

Although heart transplant remains the gold standard, organ availability remains a major limitation. Because of the persistent donor shortage and increasing number of patients with advanced heart failure, mechanical circulatory support is gaining acceptance and can be used as a bridge to heart transplant for those eligible or as destination therapy. The current strategy for the management of patients with advanced heart failure with reduced ejection fraction is to initially screen for heart transplant, with destination therapy ventricular assist device considered as secondary treatment of those who do not qualify for heart transplant. Regardless of which option is decided on, the benefits of heart transplant or ventricular assist devices outweigh those of pharmacologic treatment of heart failure alone. Heart transplant and ventricular devices improve symptoms and survival in advanced heart failure with a 1-year survival of 90% and should be considered in patients who qualify.

REFERENCES

1. Bensimhon D, Adams G, Whellan D, et al. Effect of exercise training on ventricular function, dyssynchrony, resting myocardial perfusion, and clinical outcomes in patients with heart failure: a nuclear ancillary study of Heart Failure and A Controlled Trial Investigating Outcomes of Exercise TraiNing (HF-Action); design and rationale. Am Heart J 2007;154:46–53.
2. Boummel R, Rijnsoever E, Borleffs J, et al. Effect of cardiac resynchronization therapy in patients with New York Heart Association function class IV heart failure. Am J Cardiol 2010;106:1146–51.
3. Ellenbogen K, Kay G, Wilkoff B. Device therapy for congestive heart failure. Philadelphia: Elsevier Inc; 2004. p. 1–45.

4. Kenny T. The nuts and bolts of cardiac resynchronization therapy. Malden (MA): Blackwell Futura; 2007. p. 1–62.

5. Kron J, Conti J. Cardiac resynchronization therapy for treatment of heart failure in the elderly. Clin Geriatr Med 2007;23:193–203.

6. Whellan D, O'Connor C, Lee K, et al. Heart failure and a controlled trial investigating outcomes of exercise training: design and rationale. Am Heart J 2007; 153:201–11.

7. Iyengar A, Kwon OJ, Tamrat M, et al. The in-hospital cost of ventricular assist device therapy: implications for patient selection. ASAIO J 2017;63(6): 725–30.

8. Long E, Swain G, Mangi A. Comparative survival and cost effectiveness of advanced therapies for end-stage heart failure. Circ Heart Fail 2014;7:470–8.

9. Mishra V, Fiane A, Geiran O, et al. Hospital costs fell as numbers of LVADs were increasing: experiences from Oslo University Hospital. J Cardiothorac Surg 2012; 7:76.

10. Wozniak C, Stehlik J, Bradley C, et al. Ventricular assist devices or inotropic agents in status 1A patients? Survival analysis of the united network of organ sharing database. Ann Thorac Surg 2014;97:1364–72.

11. Pulikottil-Jacob R, Suri G, Connock M, et al. Comparative cost-effectiveness of the HeartWare versus HeartMate II left ventricular assist devices used in the United Kingdom National Health Service bridge-to-transplant program for patients with heart failure. J Heart Lung Transplant 2014;33(4):350–8.

12. Ho KK, Pinsky JL, Kannel WB, et al. The epidemiology of heart failure: the Framingham Study. J Am Coll Cardiol 1993;22(4 Supplement 1):A6–13.

13. Mosterd A, Hoes AW. Clinical epidemiology of heart failure. Heart 2007;93(9): 1137–46.

14. Kannel WB, Belanger AJ. Epidemiology of heart failure. Am Heart J 1991;121(3): 951–7.

15. Kannel WB. Incidence and epidemiology of heart failure. Heart Fail Rev 2000; 5(2):167–73.

16. McMurray JJ, Stewart S. Epidemiology, aetiology, and prognosis of heart failure. Heart 2000;83(5):596–602.

17. Masip J, Formiga F, Fernández-Castañer M, et al. First hospital admission due to heart failure: in-hospital mortality and patient profile. Rev Clin Esp 2019;219(3): 130–40.

18. Bui AL, Horwich TB, Fonarow GC. Epidemiology and risk profile of heart failure. Nat Rev Cardiol 2011;8(1):30.

19. Pfuntner A, Wier LM, Stocks C. Most frequent conditions in US hospitals, 2011: statistical brief# 162 2006.

20. Roger V, Go A, Lloyd-Jones D, et al. Heart disease and stroke statistics 2012 update: a reports from the American heart association. Circulation 2011;112–5.

21. Miller LW, Guglin M. Patient selection for ventricular assist devices: a moving target. J Am Coll Cardiol 2013;61(12):1209–21.

22. Uchmanowicz I, Kuśnierz M, Wleklik M, et al. Frailty syndrome and rehospitalizations in elderly heart failure patients. Aging Clin Exp Res 2018;30(6): 617–23.

23. Okumura N, Jhund PS, Gong J, et al, PARADIGM-HF Investigators and Committees. Importance of clinical worsening of heart failure treated in the outpatient setting: evidence from the prospective comparison of ARNI with ACEI to determine impact on global mortality and morbidity in heart failure trial (PARADIGM-HF). Circulation 2016;133:2254–62.

24. Klabunde RE. Cardiovascular physiology concepts. 2nd edition 2012.

25. Dzau VJ, Colucci WS, Hollenberg NK, et al. Relation of the renin-angiotensin-aldosterone system to clinical state in congestive heart failure. Circulation 1981;63:645–51.

26. Zile MR, Bennett TD, St John Sutton M, et al. Transition from chronic compensated to acute decompensated heart failure: pathophysiological insights obtained from continuous monitoring of intracardiac pressures. Circulation 2008; 118:1433–41.

27. Packer M. The neurohormonal hypothesis: a theory to explain the mechanism of disease progression in heart failure. J Am Coll Cardiol 1992;20:248–54.

28. Yancy CW, Jessup M, Bozkurt B, et al. 2016 ACCF/AHA/HFSA focused update on new pharmacological therapy for heart failure: an update of the 2013 ACCF/AHA guideline for the management of heart failure. J Am Coll Cardiol 2016;68: 1476–88.

29. Yancy CW, Jessup M, Bozkurt B, et al. 2013 ACCF/AHA guideline for the management of heart failure. J Am Coll Cardiol 2013;62(16):e147–239.

30. Stolf NAG. History of heart transplantation: a hard and glorious journey. Braz J Cardiovasc Surg 2017;32(5):423–7.

31. Lund LH, Edwards LB, Dipchand AI, et al. The registry of the International Society for Heart and Lung Transplantation: thirty-third adult heart transplantation report-2016; focus theme: primary diagnostic indications for transplant. J Heart Lung Transplant 2016;35:1158–69.

32. Cook JA, Shah KB, Quader MA, et al. The total artificial heart. J Thorac Dis 2015; 7(12):2172.

33. Lund LH, Khush KK, Wia MAS, et al. The registry of the International Society for heart and lung transplantation: thirty-fourth adult heart transplantation report—2017. J Heart Lung Transplant 2017;36(10):1037–46.

34. Kirklin JK, Pagani FD, Kormos RL, et al. Eighth annual INTERMACS report: special focus on framing the impact of adverse events. J Heart Lung Transplanta 2017;36(10):1080–6.

35. DeBakey ME. Left ventricular bypass pump for cardiac assistance. Clinical experience. Am J Cardiol 1971;27:3–11.

36. Kirklin JK, Naftel DC. Mechanical circulatory support: registering a therapy in evolution. Circ Heart Fail 2008;1(3):200–5.

37. Rose EA, Moskowitz AJ, Packer M, et al. The REMATCH trial: rationale, design, and end points. Ann Thorac Surg 1999;67(3):723–30.

38. Rogers JG, Butler J, Lansman SL, et al, INTrEPID Investigators. Chronic mechanical circulatory support for inotrope-dependent heart failure patients who are not transplant candidates: results of the INTrEPID Trial. J Am Coll Cardiol 2007;50(8): 741–7.

39. Frazier OH, Bricker JT, Macris MP, et al. Use of a left ventricular assist device as a bridge to transplantation in a pediatric patient. Tex Heart Inst J 1989;16: 46–50.

40. Slaughter MS, Rogers JG, Milano CA, et al. Advanced heart failure treated with continuous-flow left ventricular assist device. N Engl J Med 2009;361(23): 2241–51.

41. Lim HS, Howell N, Ranasinghe A. The physiology of continuous-flow left ventricular assist devices. J Card Fail 2017;23(2):169–80.

42. Burkhoff D, Sayer G, Doshi D, et al. Hemodynamics of Mechanical Circulatory Support. J am Col Cardiol 66:2664–74.

43. Frazier OH, Akutsu T, Cooley DA. Total artificial heart (TAH) utilization in man. Trans Am Soc Artif Intern Organs 1982;28:534–8.
44. Copeland JG, Smith RG, Arabia FA, et al. Cardiac replacement with a total artificial heart as a bridge to transplantation. N Engl J Med 2004;351:859–67.
45. Morris RJ. The Syncardia total artificial heart: implantation technique. Oper Tech Thorac Cardiovasc Surg 2012;17(2).

Lung Transplant for the Critical Care Nurse

Kevin C. Carney, MSN, CRNP[a],*, Tanya Bronzell-Wynder, DNP, CRNP[a],
Karen Gronek, MSN, CRNP[b]

KEYWORDS

- Lung transplant • Respiratory failure • Immunosuppression • ECMO
- Cardiothoracic surgery

KEY POINTS

- Lung transplant is an established therapy for select patients with end-stage pulmonary disease, with improvement in both survival and quality of life.
- This article reviews the indications and contraindications of lung transplant, along with physiologic parameters that warrant a referral for transplant.
- Immediate postoperative management, along with use of antibiotics and immunosuppressive medications is covered.
- Short- and long-term complications after transplant are discussed, along with tailored management strategies.

INTRODUCTION

In 1963, Dr James Hardy performed the first human lung transplant. Although the patient's oxygenation and symptoms of dyspnea improved, the recipient survived 18 days before succumbing to renal failure.[1] Over the next 18 years, approximately 40 lung transplants took place, with most recipients dying within 30 days posttransplant because of infectious issues or anastomotic complications.

After the development of the immunosuppressive medication, cyclosporine, in 1976, Dr Bruce Reitz performed the first successful heart-lung transplant in 1981[2] and Dr Joel Cooper the first successful single lung transplant in 1983.[3] Today, lung transplantation has become an established treatment of select patients with end-stage pulmonary disease, with approximately 4000 procedures taking place each year worldwide.

Disclosure Statement: The authors have nothing to disclose.
The authors have no financial conflicts of interest and have not received funding for this article.
[a] Lung Center Service Line, Temple University Hospital, 6th floor Rock Pavilion, 3401 North Broad Street, Philadelphia, PA 19140, USA; [b] Department of Cardiovascular Surgery, Temple University Hospital, 2nd floor Rock Pavilion, 3401 North Broad Street, Philadelphia, PA 19140, USA
* Corresponding author.
E-mail address: kevin.carney@tuhs.temple.edu

SURVIVAL AND QUALITY OF LIFE

As of 2016, median survival for adult recipients exceeded 6 years, and for those who survived at least the first year posttransplant, conditional median survival exceeded 8 years. When looking at transplant eras, median survival improved from 4.3 years in the period between 1990 and 1998 to 6.5 years from 2009 to 2016 (**Fig. 1**).[4] Expectedly, bilateral lung transplant recipients had better survival than single lung recipients (**Fig. 2**) with survival of 59% versus 48% at 5 years.[4]

In addition to increased survival, patients who undergo lung transplant demonstrate dramatic improvements in quality of life (QOL), particularly in measures of physical health and functioning.[5]

DIAGNOSES AND TIMING OF REFERRAL

Lung transplantation should be considered for patients with end-stage pulmonary disease who have an expected 2-year survival of less than 50% without lung transplant and an expected 5-year survival of greater than 80% after transplant, assuming the allograft is functioning normally.[6] The most common diagnoses for lung transplantation worldwide are chronic obstructive pulmonary disease (COPD) (approximately 35%), interstitial lung disease (approximately 30%), and cystic fibrosis (approximately 17%).[4]

At time of referral, most patients report intermittent dyspnea with activities of daily living and are unable to climb one flight of steps without shortness of breath. See **Box 1** for disease specific criteria to help clinicians identify appropriate patients for referral to a Lung Transplant Program.

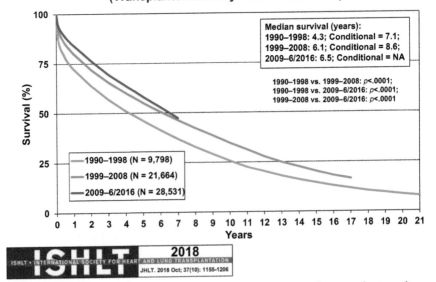

Fig. 1. Kaplan-Meier survival for adult lung transplant recipients by transplant era (transplants: January 1990–June 2016). (*From* International Society for Heart and Lung Transplantation. Adult lung transplantation statistics. Available at: https://ishltregistries.org/downloadables/slides/2018/lung_adult.pptx; with permission.)

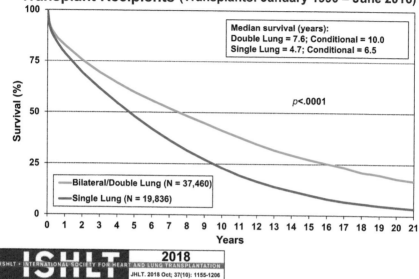

Fig. 2. Kaplan-Meier survival by procedure type for primary transplant recipients (transplants: January 1990–June 2016). (*From* International Society for Heart and Lung Transplantation. Adult lung transplantation statistics. Available at: https://ishltregistries.org/downloadables/slides/2018/lung_adult.pptx; with permission.)

Box 1
Physiologic parameters at time of referral

- COPD—FEV1 less than 25% predicted, +/− evidence of hypercapnia, +/− elevated pulmonary artery pressures, or history of mechanical ventilation.

- Cystic fibrosis—same criteria as COPD; in addition, increased antibiotic resistance and/or incomplete recovery from exacerbations, recurrent hemoptysis, pneumothoraces, and loss of body weight.

- Pulmonary fibrosis—FVC less than 60% predicted, DLCO less than 40%, elevated pulmonary artery pressure, and ANY oxygen requirement.

- Pulmonary hypertension—NYHA class III or IV despite multiple medical therapies, right arterial pressure greater than 15 mm Hg, pulmonary arterial pressure greater than 50 mm Hg, cardiac index less than 2 L/min/m², uncontrolled syncope, hemoptysis, pericardial effusions or progressive right heart failure.

Abbreviations: DLCO, diffusing capacity of the lungs for carbon monoxide; FEV1, food expiratory volume in the first second of expiration; FVC, forced vital capacity; NYHA, New York Heart Association.

Data from Weill D, Benden C, Corris PA, et al. A consensus document for the selection of lung transplant candidates: 2014—An update from the Pulmonary Transplantation Council of the International Society for Heart and Lung Transplantation. J Heart Lung Transplant. 2015;34(1):1-15.

After a patient is referred to Lung Transplant Program, medical information is reviewed by a Transplant Nurse Coordinator or Medical Director for evidence of end-stage pulmonary disease without any absolute contraindications listed later (**Box 2**). If the referred patient meets both criteria, a new patient visit is scheduled, medical information is confirmed, and the risks/benefits of lung transplant are discussed with the patient before the evaluation for transplant is initiated.

OLDER PATIENTS

Although there is no established upper limit for candidate age, transplant programs often consider the "physiologic age" before evaluating for lung transplant. In 2016, approximately 20% of lung transplant recipients were aged 66 years or older (**Fig. 3**).[4] In the United States, most transplant programs will evaluate potential candidates as old as 70 years of age, with some centers evaluating patients up to age 75 years and a select few centers evaluating patients older than 75 years.

LUNG TRANSPLANT EVALUATION

The evaluation consists of objective measures of organ function along with a psychosocial assessment, including cognition, history of psychiatric disorders or substance abuse, compliance issues, and level of social support. This evaluation is performed on an outpatient basis unless the patient is acutely ill.

When the evaluation is complete, the results are presented at a multidisciplinary team meeting attended by Surgeons, Pulmonologists, Transplant Nurse Coordinators, Speech Therapists, Physical Therapists, Social Workers, Dieticians, Psychologists, and other consulting Physicians. After this discussion, the patient usually falls into one of the following categories:

Box 2
Absolute contraindications to listing for lung transplant

- Recent history of malignancy (2–5 years cancer free, depending on type/stage/treatment).
- Untreatable significant dysfunction of another major organ system (eg, heart, liver, and kidney) unless combined organ transplantation can be performed.
- Acute medical instability.
- Chronic infection with highly virulent and/or resistant microbes.
- Class II or III obesity (body mass index $\geq$35.0 kg/m^2).
- Current nonadherence or a history of repeated nonadherence to medical therapy and/or psychological conditions associated with the inability to adhere with complex medical therapy.
- Absence of an adequate or reliable social support system.
- Severely limited functional status with poor rehabilitation potential.
- Illicit substance abuse or dependence.

Data from Weill D, Benden C, Corris PA, et al. A consensus document for the selection of lung transplant candidates: 2014—An update from the Pulmonary Transplantation Council of the International Society for Heart and Lung Transplantation. J Heart Lung Transplant. 2015;34(1):1-15.

Adult and Pediatric Lung Transplants
Recipient Age by Year (Transplants: January 1987 – June 2017)

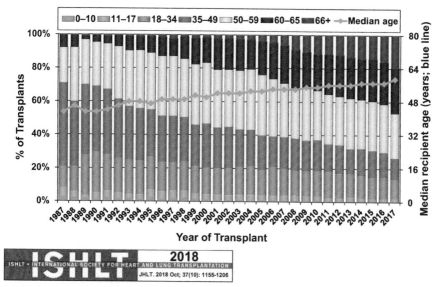

Fig. 3. Adult and pediatric lung transplants: Recipient age by year (transplants: January 1987–June 2017). (*From* International Society for Heart and Lung Transplantation. Overall lung transplantation statistics. Available at: https://ishltregistries.org/downloadables/slides/2018/lung_overall.pptx; with permission.)

- Ready to list for transplant.
- Deny for listing because of an absolute contraindication identified during the evaluation.
- Defer a decision, pending resolution of outstanding medical, social, or functional issues identified during the evaluation.

LISTING FOR LUNG TRANSPLANT AND WAITLIST MANAGEMENT

In the United States, once the decision is made to list a patient as a candidate for lung transplant, demographic and clinical information are entered by the transplant program into a national database maintained by the Organ Procurement and Transplantation Network. For potential recipients aged 12 years and older, these clinical variables create the patient's Lung Allocation Score (LAS).[7] Patients and clinicians can access the LAS calculator at https://optn.transplant.hrsa.gov/resources/allocation-calculators/las-calculator/.[8]

To maintain/update the patient's LAS, certain variables including the need for assisted ventilation, oxygen requirements, and current Pco_2 (optional) need to be updated as frequently as every 2 weeks for patients with an LAS greater than 50 and every 6 months for LAS less than 50.[7] Other variables, including spirometry, 6-minute walk, and serum creatinine need to be updated at least every 6 months.[7]

Candidates are seen by their Transplant Clinician every 2 to 3 months to evaluate their suitability for transplant and to collect objective data to accurately calculate the LAS. Candidates and their families are reminded that the transplant team must be notified immediately of any hospitalizations or deterioration in pulmonary or general health status.

DONOR/RECIPIENT MATCHING

In the United States, Donor blood type and Recipient LAS determine the order of donor/recipient matching. Once a family consents to organ donation, offers are sent electronically to the transplant centers of the first 20 candidates with the highest LAS who reside within 250 nautical miles of the donor hospital. This change was made in November 2017, to increase availability of lungs to patients at increased risk of dying without a lung transplant.[9]

Transplant centers have 60 minutes to reply electronically by entering a "provisional yes" or "no" based on the clinical information provided. The patient with the highest LAS and "provisional yes" is offered the lung. If the transplant center declines the lung because of size disparity or clinical concerns, the patient with the next highest LAS and "provisional yes" is offered the lung. This sequence continues until a transplant center verbally accepts the lungs.

SUPPORTIVE THERAPIES

Venovenous (VV) extracorporeal membrane oxygenator (ECMO) may be used as a "bridge" to lung transplant in the setting of hypercarbic and/or hypoxemic respiratory failure despite optimal ventilator support. Intraoperative cardiopulmonary bypass (CPB) and venoarterial (VA) ECMO are indicated in the setting of hemodynamic instability due to moderate to severe right ventricular dysfunction.[10]

The decision of CPB versus VA-ECMO is often a surgeon's preference; however, the use of VA-ECMO decreases the risk of bleeding and subsequent blood transfusion[11–13] when compared with CPB. In addition, use of ECMO decreases the risk of hemolysis[10] and improves long-term survival in comparison to CPB, which activates the inflammatory response,[10,14] delays extubation, prolongs intensive care unit (ICU) time, and increases the risk of primary graft dysfunction (PGD).[12,13]

Although beneficial, VA- and VV-ECMO are associated with reversible thrombocytopenia, bleeding, critical illness neuropathy, acute kidney injury (AKI), infection, and potential limb ischemia due to decreased perfusion.[15] Limb ischemia prevention in a noncentrally cannulated patient includes an hourly neurovascular assessment, use of distal perfusion cannulas, regional oximetry monitoring, and anticoagulation.[16,17] Consult to Vascular Surgery should be initiated immediately with any clinical concern for compartment syndrome, acute limb ischemia, or thrombosis.

SURGICAL APPROACH

The most common approach for a single or bilateral sequential lung transplant is the anterolateral thoracotomy. Other surgical approaches include a transverse thoracotomy for a single lung transplant and a median sternotomy for a combined heart and lung transplant, lung transplant with concomitant coronary artery bypass surgery, or if CPB is indicated.

INDUCTION THERAPY

Approximately 80% of patients undergo induction therapy at the time of transplant (**Fig. 4**), with improvement in long-term survival compared with no induction therapy (**Fig. 5**). The 2 most common induction agents are basiliximab (Simulect) and alemtuzumab (Campath). Basiliximab binds to the interleukin 2 receptor of an activated T cell,

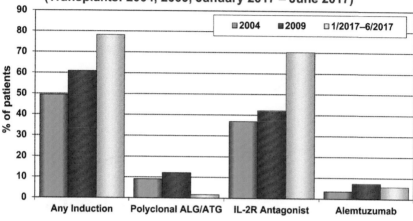

Fig. 4. Induction immunosuppression (transplants: 2004, 2009, January 2017–June 2017). (*From* International Society for Heart and Lung Transplantation. Adult lung transplantation statistics. Available at: https://ishltregistries.org/downloadables/slides/2018/lung_adult.pptx; with permission.)

decreasing T-cell replication, thereby decreasing the incidence of acute cellular rejection.[18,19] This medication is given in 2 separate doses, once during the operative procedure before the release of cross-clamp and again on postoperative day 4.

Alemtuzumab's mechanism of action is through antibody and cell-mediated lysis of T and B lymphocytes.[18,19] Because of its profound and long-standing immunosuppressive effects, patients with a prior history of cancer, an active infection at time of transplant or cytomegalovirus (CMV) mismatch (donor CMV+ and recipient CMV−), should use an alternative induction agent.[18,19] Alemtuzumab is given as one dose during the operative procedure before release of cross-clamp.

IMMUNOSUPPRESSION MANAGEMENT (MAINTENANCE THERAPY)

Immunosuppressive medications are prescribed to all solid organ recipients to allow "tolerance" of the transplanted organ. Tolerance is when the transplanted organ is seen as "self" by the recipient's immune system; this is accomplished by prescribing medications that remove or suppress T lymphocytes before release of cross-clamp (Induction Therapy, discussed earlier) and by blocking communication between T-helper cells and antigen-presenting cells.[18,19]

The 3 main drug categories used for maintenance therapy include calcineurin inhibitors (CNIs), antiproliferatives, and corticosteroids. CNIs consist of cyclosporine (Neoral) or tacrolimus (Prograf). CNIs work by preventing the synthesis of interleukin 2, which suppress T-lymphocyte function and replication.[18,19] Although this drug class is the backbone of solid-organ immunosuppressive therapy, significant side effects

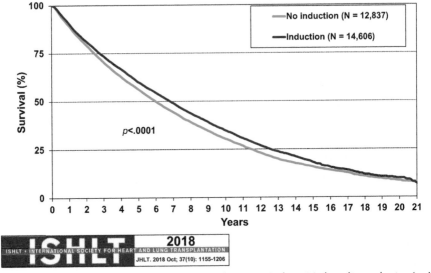

Fig. 5. Survival by induction usage conditional on survival to 14 days (transplants: April 1994–June 2016). (*From* International Society for Heart and Lung Transplantation. Adult lung transplantation statistics. Available at: https://ishltregistries.org/downloadables/slides/2018/lung_adult.pptx; with permission.)

including nephrotoxicity, neurotoxicity, diabetes, infection, and electrolyte imbalances are common. This drug class also interacts with common medications that may increase or lower the level of CNIs, leading to allograft loss or increased toxicity.

Antiproliferatives, or antimetabolites, include mycophenolate mofetil (CellCept) and azathioprine (Imuran).[18,19] These medications work by producing cytostatic effects on B and T lymphocytes and can cause the following side effects: nausea, vomiting, diarrhea, and leukopenia.[18,19]

Corticosteroids (prednisone and methylprednisolone) work by inhibiting production of T lymphocytes. Side effects include hyperglycemia, muscle myopathy, peptic ulcers, and osteoporosis.[18,19] **Fig. 6** lists the different immunosuppressive combinations used after transplant.

PROPHYLAXIS AGAINST OPPORTUNISTIC INFECTION

Because transplant recipients take 2 or 3 immunosuppressive medications to allow for tolerance of the allograft, they are at increased risk for bacterial, fungal, and viral infections. Pneumocystis jiroveci pneumonia (PJP), aspergillosis, and CMV are the most virulent opportunistic infections, and lung transplant patients receive the following therapies either life-long or for a center-specific period of time.

For PJP prophylaxis, patients receive sulfamethoxazole/trimethoprim (STX, Bactrim DS) 3 times a week, which decreases the incidence of PJP by 85% in transplanted patients.[20] If the patient has an allergy to sulfa, atovaquone (Mepron), 750 mg, twice a day or dapsone, 100 mg, daily are oral alternatives. Before initiating therapy, patients should be screened for glucose-6-phosphate dehydrogenase deficiency, which can

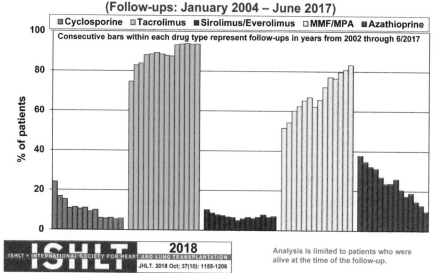

Fig. 6. Maintenance immunosuppression at time of 1-year follow-up (follow-ups: January 2004–June 2017). (*From* International Society for Heart and Lung Transplantation. Adult lung transplantation statistics. Available at: https://ishltregistries.org/downloadables/slides/2018/lung_adult.pptx; with permission.)

lead to hemolytic anemia and jaundice when subjected to certain foods and medications, including STX and dapsone.[21] Side effects of STX include hyperkalemia, hyponatremia, and renal tubular acidosis, whereas atovaquone can cause nausea, vomiting, diarrhea, and insomnia. Dapsone side effects include nausea, loss of appetite, and skin rash.

For fungal prophylaxis, voriconazole (VFEND), 200 mg, twice daily or weekly inhaled amphotericin B (Abelcet) are used to help prevent invasive or disseminated aspergillosis. Side effects of these medications include leg fatigue, hallucinations, visual changes, and transaminitis,[22] and use of voriconazole will also significantly increase levels of CNIs.

For patients with a moderate risk (recipient CMV+) or high risk (donor CMV+ and recipient CMV−) of CMV infection after transplant, intravenous ganciclovir (Cytovene) or oral valganciclovir (Valcyte) are used.[19] These medications are dosed by weight and creatinine clearance. If the patient and recipient are both CMV negative, and therefore a low-risk for CMV infection, the patient should be treated with acyclovir (Zovirax) for herpesvirus prophylaxis.

IMMEDIATE POSTTRANSPLANT MANAGEMENT
Ventilator Management and Extubation

Inhaled nitric oxide (INO) is used intraoperatively in the setting of significant pulmonary artery hypertension (HTN) to decrease the risk of right ventricular dysfunction.[22] In the ICU, INO is generally weaned to 5 parts per million (PPM), then slowly to 1 PPM, before discontinuing therapy once pulmonary arterial pressures and oxygenation are satisfactory. Inhaled prostacyclin is used as an alternative to INO and also to improve hypoxemia in the setting of PGD.

The goals of mechanical ventilation postoperatively are to improve alveolar recruitment and oxygenation while decreasing the risk of acute lung injury; this is done by reducing the fraction of inspired oxygen ratio (Fio_2) to maintain an oxygen saturation greater than 92%, optimizing positive end-expiratory pressure (PEEP), and using a "low-stretch" tidal volume of 6 cc/kg/min.

Once hemodynamics and oxygen status is stable, sedation is minimized, and a neurologic assessment is performed hourly. When the patient is awake and following commands, weaning parameters are obtained and a rapid shallow breathing index (RSBI) is calculated by dividing the respiratory rate by the tidal volume. An RSBI less than 105 breaths/min/L is associated with a decreased rate of reintubation.[23] Before extubation, bedside bronchoscopy is performed for airway inspection and to clear secretions and donor airway slough.

HEMODYNAMIC ASSESSMENT AND MANAGEMENT

In addition to the respiratory assessment mentioned earlier, monitoring preload, afterload, and end organ function is done hourly. Preload may be increased by administering volume, in the form or albumin, or decreased with diuretics. In the setting of anemia with hemodynamic instability, packed red blood cells are administered; however, blood products are uncommon in a standard lung transplant recipient. Afterload support may include the use of vasodilators, vasopressors, sedation, and PEEP. Finally, serial measures of lactate and hourly measure of urine and chest tube output are monitored.

PRIMARY GRAFT DYSFUNCTION

PGD is described as a diffuse radiographic infiltrate, in the absence of other causes, that develops in the first 72 hours after lung transplant and is categorized by measuring the partial pressure of oxygen and Fio_2 (P/F ratio)[24]; Grade 0 demonstrates a normal chest radiograph and any P/F ratio; diffuse radiographic allograft infiltrates and a P/F ratio greater than 300 is classified as grade 1, a ratio 200 to 300 as grade 2, and a ratio less than 200 as grade 3.[25] Associated time is measured postoperatively at 0, 24, 48, and 72 hours.

Donor characteristics that increase the risk of PGD include prior smoking, aspiration, chest trauma, heavy alcohol consumption, thromboembolism, and fat emboli.[26] In the recipient, risk factors include a body mass index (BMI) greater than 25 kg/m², previous cardiothoracic surgery, extensive intraoperative blood transfusion, prolonged ischemic time, and a pretransplant diagnosis of pulmonary arterial HTN, idiopathic pulmonary fibrosis, or sarcoidosis.[26] Recipients of African American descent and female gender have been noted in one study[27] but was not definitive in others.[25,26] Finally, the use of an undersized donor lung compared with the recipient's thoracic space increases the risk of PGD.

Postoperatively, pneumonia, aspiration, ventilator-associated injury, and hypotension can also contribute to injury to the donor lung.[25] Technically challenging and difficult recipient lung explantation, for example in sarcoidosis or previous pleurodesis, can prolong ischemic time contributing to PGD.

Suspected PGD is treated as discussed earlier with supportive management including protective lung ventilation strategy, diuretics, avoidance of hypoxemia with use of INO, and ECMO in severe PGD if necessary.

PERIOPERATIVE ANTIBIOTICS

Perioperative antibiotic include gram-positive coverage against methicillin-resistant *Staphylococcus aureus* with vancomycin (Vancocin) and gram-negative coverage against *Pseudomonas aeruginosa* with a fourth-generation cephalosporin or broad-spectrum penicillin such as piperacillin-tazobactam (Zosyn). Empirical antibiotic selection is center specific and should consider recipient preoperative infection history along with local resistance patterns. Special care for candidates with cystic fibrosis/bronchiectasis is warranted because of likely colonization with MDR-resistant organisms.[28]

Perioperative antibiotics are dosed by recipient weight and creatinine clearance and ordered for at least 72 hours to allow for final cultures from the donor and the recipient's explanted lung. After 72 hours, antibiotics are stopped or adjusted, occasionally with the guidance of transplant infectious disease. In the event of an open chest, antibiotics are extended until the chest is closed, and an intravenous antifungal agent is also added.

The most common secondary infection, clostridium difficile, is prevalent in greater than 10% of lung transplants.[29] Because of the risk of morbidity and mortality, treatment is initiated on suspicion with oral vancomycin.

POSTOPERATIVE COMPLICATIONS
Acute Kidney Injury

AKI after lung transplantation is prevalent. In one study, greater than 74% of those in the ICU posttransplantation developed AKI, with approximately 2% requiring hemodialysis 1 year post-transplant.[30] Prevention of nephrotoxicity includes careful monitoring of CNI and vancomycin levels, as supratherapeutic levels of CNI can lead to onset of AKI.[31] Avoiding hypotension and adequate volume resuscitation perioperatively is the goal of this and any postsurgical patient.

Electrolyte Imbalances

Patients posttransplant are at an increased risk of electrolyte imbalances, caused by the fluid shifts and insensible losses that occur during surgery and side effects of immunosuppressive medications. Monitoring and replacing potassium, magnesium, sodium, and phosphorus can limit complications including cardiac dysfunction, rhabdomyolysis, and blood cell dysfunction.

Atrial Arrhythmias/Atrial Fibrillation

Risk factors for atrial arrhythmias (AA) include hyperlipidemia, age greater than 55 years, restrictive lung disease, HTN, male gender, prior smoking, left atrial enlargement, and coronary artery disease.[32] After lung transplant, the incidence of atrial fibrillation (AF) is as high as 35% and is associated with increased hospital length of stay and mortality.[33] Selective beta blockers, such as metoprolol (Lopressor), are often used to prevent/treat AF, whereas calcium channel blockers, such as diltiazem (Cartia) are used cautiously because they will increase levels of CNI.

Rate control is the first-line strategy, and antiarrhythmic therapy with flecainide (Tambocor) and amiodarone (Cordarone) is reserved for patients who do not respond to standard treatment.[34] A consult to electrophysiology should be considered for nonresponders and for recipients with unstable AF and atrial flutter who may require cardioversion.

Use of anticoagulation is considered using CHA2DS2-VASc scoring, while weighing the risks of a significant bleed postsurgery.[35]

Hyperammonemia Syndrome

Hyperammonemia syndrome (HS) is a rare complication in the early posttransplant period, affecting less than 5% of lung transplant recipients, but is frequently fatal.[36,37] Cause is largely unknown; however, infections with Ureaplasma parvum and Mycoplasma hominis[38] have correlated. For this reason, ammonia levels and neurologic assessment are closely monitored.

HS should be considered in the setting of encephalopathy, seizure, or coma, and ammonia levels exceeding 200 mg/dL require immediate medical therapy, including bowel decontamination with lactulose, metronidazole (Flagyl), and rifaximin (Xifaxan), along with renal replacement therapy, nitrogen scavenger therapy (sodium benzoate), and removal of exogenous nitrogen from enteral or intravenous nutrition.[36,39]

Deep Vein Thrombosis

Lung transplant recipients are at high risk for pulmonary embolism and deep vein thrombosis (DVT), with incidence as high as 45% in patients with central line access.[40] Conversion to peripheral access along with use of subcutaneous enoxaparin (Lovenox) and early mobility is paramount.

Thrombocytopenia

In the setting of 50% decline in platelets, heparin-induced thrombocytopenia (HIT) should be considered.[41] Once suspected, heparin in any form should be discontinued and an HIT panel and serotonin release assay collected. Alternative anticoagulation with bivalirudin (Angiomax) is initiated, along with assessment of underlying liver or renal impairment. A hematology consult is strongly considered, and venous duplexes are performed to rule out DVT.

Postoperative lung transplant thrombocytopenia may be related to use of CPB or ECMO or drug induced by immunosuppressants, antivirals, or antibiotics.

NEUROLOGIC COMPLICATIONS

The most common postoperative neurologic complications after lung transplant include encephalopathy, cerebral vascular accident, and seizure.[42] Other complications include phrenic nerve injury (24%) and critical illness myopathy (30%).[43] Early identification and treatment of these complications will hopefully decrease morbidity and hospital length of stay and improve QOL.[44]

MALNUTRITION

Patients with end-stage respiratory disease are at high risk of pulmonary cachexia, and candidates should be assessed by a Registered Dietitian (RD) before listing to maximize their nutritional status. Postoperatively, an RD will calculate the recipient's nutritional needs and make recommendations for the provision of nutrients (oral, enteric, or intravenous). All recipients should be evaluated by the Speech and Language Pathologist following extubation to evaluate for dysphagia and laryngeal and vocal cord injuries before eating or drinking.

In the acute phase post–lung transplantation, which varies from 2 to 28 days, energy needs are calculated at 1.3 to 1.5 times the patient's basal energy expenditure or 25 to 35 kcal/kg of their estimated dry weight.[45] These patients also require between 1.3 and 2.5 g of protein per kilogram to allow for wound healing.[45]

GASTRO ESOPHAGEAL REFLUX DISEASE

Patients with chronic respiratory disease are at an increased risk of exacerbation secondary to gastro esophageal reflux disease (GERD), especially those with interstitial lung disease and cystic fibrosis.[46] After lung transplant, GERD and microaspiration have been identified as risk factors for the development of chronic lung allograft dysfunction (CLAD).[47] For patients with severe reflux despite maximal medical therapy, a total (Nissen) or partial (Belsey or Toupet) fundoplication is performed either before or after lung transplant to decrease these risks.

GASTROPARESIS

Gastroparesis affects approximately 23% of patients who undergo single lung transplant and as high as 91% of patients who undergo combined heart and lung transplant.[48] Posttransplant gastroparesis is often caused by damage to the vagus nerve during explantation, which negatively affects esophageal sphincter function and delays gastric emptying, contributing to microaspiration and the development of CLAD long-term.[49]

Gastroparesis is initially treated with medications such as metoclopramide (Reglan) or erythromycin (erythromycin ethylsuccinate) to increase motility, along with dietary modifications including 6 small, low-fat, and low-fiber meals. Other therapies include botox injections or pyloroplasty to dilate the lower esophageal sphincter.

POSTTRANSPLANT CONSTIPATION

Use of narcotics after lung transplant is required to manage surgical pain, allowing for early mobility and airway clearance techniques to decrease the risk of atelectasis and pneumonia. Opioids affect the gastrointestinal tract by binding to mu receptors, decreasing peristalsis, and delaying transit through the large intestine, which decreases water excretion, leading to hardened stool.[50] To avoid constipation and ileus, all patients should be placed on a bowel regimen with a stool softener such as docusate sodium (Colace) along with selective use of laxatives such as polyethylene glycol (Miralax).

WARD MANAGEMENT

After leaving the ICU, a vigorous postoperative rehabilitative course is continued with physical and occupational therapy. Consults to Physical Medicine and Rehabilitation are requested for patients who might require acute inpatient rehabilitation before discharge to home.

Oxygen is weaned to keep saturation greater than 92%, and while chest tubes remain in place, daily chest radiographs are performed and strict chest tube output is measured. Once chest tube output decreases to less than 150 cc/24 hours, they are removed.

When the patient is cleared by speech therapy to take food/liquid by mouth, immunosuppressive medications, antibiotics, and pain medications are converted to oral dosing when appropriate. For patients unable to take food/liquid by mouth, consults with the Registered Dietician and Surgery for feeding tube placement are initiated.

DISCHARGE PLANNING AND THE INTERDISCIPLINARY TEAM

To ensure patient and programmatic success, use of an interdisciplinary team consisting of transplant surgeons, pulmonologists, nurse practitioners and physician assistants, transplant coordinators, social workers, psychologists, physical and occupational therapists, speech therapists, registered dietician, case managers, bedside nurses, and pharmacists is paramount.[51] This team works closely to assure the transplant patient receives proper training, education, and support throughout their transplant journey.

The interdisciplinary team provides patient-centered care while considering the unique caregiver needs. Patient education is conducted in both group and individual settings, using different teaching methods to allow patients and their caregivers receive the necessary information in a format that is conducive to learning.[52]

COMORBIDITIES AFTER LUNG TRANSPLANT
Diabetes

The incidence of diabetes after lung transplant is between 25% and 30% at 1 year and increases to approximately 40% by post-op year five.[4] Two of the immunosuppressive medications, tacrolimus and prednisone, will increase blood sugars, whereas recipient age greater than 45 years and BMI greater than 30 increase the likelihood of diabetes posttransplant.[53]

Uncontrolled blood sugars after transplant can increase the risk of infections and delay wound healing, so tight glycemic control is imperative. In the ICU, continuous infusion of insulin should be given to keep blood sugars within 140 to 180 mg/dL, and after transfer to the floor service fasting blood sugars should be kept less than 140 mg/dL using a combination of short- and long-acting insulin.[54]

Although oral agents are typically avoided in the first 30 to 45 days after transplant, use of insulin sensitizers and secretagogues may be considered in select patients with normal renal function.[55] Lifestyle modifications, including a low-fat, low carbohydrate diet and 20 to 30 minutes of aerobic exercise most days of the week is encouraged, along with management of hyperlipidemia and HTN.

Hypertension

HTN affects 75 million people in America, or 1 in 3 adults, with only 54% of patients at their target blood pressure.[56] For patients aged younger than or equal to 60 years, target blood pressure is less than or equal to 140/90 mm Hg, and for patients aged 60 years, target blood pressure is less than or equal to 150/90 mm Hg.[56] Risk factors for developing hypertension include elevated BMI, African American descent, male sex, taking CNIs, and use of corticosteroids,[18] the last 2 of which affect all lung transplant recipients. The incidence of HTN 1 year after lung transplant is 52%, increasing to 83% at 5 years.[4]

Although the Eighth Joint National Committee recommends initial management of HTN with either a thiazide agent or an ACE/ARB, these drug categories should be avoided after transplant because of AKI and hyperkalemia[57] but could be considered once renal function has stabilized. Beta blockers, such as metoprolol (Lopressor), are mainly metabolized in the liver and are therefore a good first choice for HTN management and treatment of atrial arrhythmias as stated earlier. Calcium channel blockers, such as diltiazem (Calan), are metabolized via the CYP3A4 pathway leading to elevated drug levels of CNIs, and should be avoided if possible,[57] but nifedipine (Procardia) and amlodipine (Norvasc) can be used safely.

Bronchial Stenosis

Approximately 10% to 15% of patients develop bronchial stenosis after lung transplant, with approximately 35% of these patients developing recurrence.[58] Bronchial stenosis is mainly caused by ischemia of the donor bronchus but can also be caused by perioperative hypotension and infection. Symptoms of bronchial stenosis include dyspnea, stridor, cough, and wheeze, whereas pulmonary function testing demonstrates a reduced peak and forced expiratory flow, and chest computed tomography scan shows narrowing of the bronchus.[58] Because of these changes, patients are at higher risk of developing pneumonia. Treatment of bronchial stenosis includes bronchoscopy with dilation, +/− cautery, and airway stenting with temporary silicone stenting. Refractory cases may require retransplant.

SUMMARY

Lung transplantation is an established treatment of select patients with end-stage pulmonary disease. Survival posttransplant continues to increase, along with improvement in QOL. Lung transplantation should be considered for patients with end-stage pulmonary disease who have an expected 2-year survival of less than without lung transplant and an expected 5-year survival of greater than 80% after transplant. After lung transplant, patients are prescribed immunosuppressive medications to allow for tolerance of the transplanted organ, but these medications have numerous risks including chronic kidney injury and infection.

REFERENCES

1. Hardy JD, Webb WR, Dalton, et al. Lung homotransplantation in man: report of the initial case. JAMA 1963;12(21):1065–74.
2. Reitz BA, Wallwork JL, Hunt SA, et al. Heart-lung transplantation: successful therapy for patients with pulmonary vascular disease. N Engl J Med 1982;306: 557–64.
3. Toronto Lung Transplantation Group. Unilateral lung transplantation for pulmonary fibrosis. N Engl J Med 1986;314:1140–5.
4. Chambers D, Yusen R, Cherikh, et al. The registry of the international society for heart and lung transplantation: 34th adult lung and heart-lung transplant report. J Heart Lung Transplant 2017;36(10):1047–59.
5. Singer JP, Chen J, Blanc PD, et al. A thematic analysis of quality of life in lung transplant. Am J Transplant 2013;13(4):839–50.
6. Weill D, Benden C, Corris PA, et al. A consensus document for the selection of lung transplant candidates: 2014–an update from the Pulmonary Transplantation Council of the International Society for Heart and Lung Transplantation. J Heart Lung Transplant 2015;34(1):1–15.
7. Organ Procurement and Transplantation Network. Policy 10: Allocation of lungs. 134-162. Available at: https://optn.transplant.hrsa.gov/media/1200/optn_policies. pdf. Accessed October 5, 2018.
8. Organ Procurement and Transplantation Network. Lung Allocation system. Available at: https://optn.transplant.hrsa.gov/resources/allocation-calculators/las-calculator/. Accessed October 5, 2018.
9. Organ Procurement and Transplantation Network. Policy modification to lung distribution sequence. Available at: https://optn.transplant.hrsa.gov/news/policy-modification-to-lung-distribution-sequence. Accessed October 9, 2018.
10. Ko H, Weiss SJ. The need for extracorporeal support for lung transplantation: why and what does the future hold? J Cardiothorac Vasc Anesth 2017;31(2):409–10.
11. Mohite PN, Sabashnikov A, Patil NP, et al. The role of cardiopulmonary bypass in lung transplantation. Clin Transplant 2016;30(3):202–9.

12. Ius F, Kuehn C, Tudorache I, et al. Lung transplantation on cardiopulmonary support: venoarterial extracorporeal membrane oxygenation outperformed cardiopulmonary bypass. J Thorac Cardiovasc Surg 2012;144:1510–6.

13. Biscotti M, Yang J, Sonett J, et al. Comparison of extracorporeal membrane oxygenation versus cardiopulmonary bypass for lung transplantation. J Thorac Cardiovasc Surg 2014;148:2410–5.

14. Machuca TN, Collaud S, Mercier O, et al. Outcomes of intraoperative extracorporeal membrane oxygenation versus cardiopulmonary bypass for lung transplantation. J Thorac Cardiovasc Surg 2015;149:1152–7.

15. Magouliotis DE, Tasiopoulou VS, Svokos AA, et al. Extracorporeal membrane oxygenation versus cardiopulmonary bypass during lung transplantation: a meta-analysis. Gen Thorac Cardiovasc Surg 2018;66(1):38–47.

16. Cottini SR, Wenger U, Sailer S, et al. Extracorporeal membrane oxygenation: beneficial strategy for lung transplant recipients. J Extra Corpor Technol 2013; 45(1):16–20.

17. Stuart FP. Organ transplantation. Georgetown (TX): CRC Press; 2003.

18. Klein AA, Lewis CJ, Madsen JC, editors. Organ transplantation: a clinical guide. New York: Cambridge University Press; 2011.

19. Stern A, Green H, Paul M, et al. Prophylaxis for Pneumocystis pneumonia (PCP) in non-HIV immunocompromised patients. Cochrane Database Syst Rev 2014;(10):CD005590.

20. Lee SWH, Chaiyakunapruk N, Lai NM. What G6PD-deficient individuals should really avoid. Br J Clin Pharmacol 2017;83(1):211–2.

21. Neoh CF, Snell G, Levvey B, et al. Antifungal prophylaxis in lung transplantation. Int J Antimicrob Agents 2014;44(3):194–202.

22. Bhandary S, Stoicea N, Joseph N, et al. Pro: inhaled pulmonary vasodilators should be used routinely in the management of patients undergoing lung transplantation. J Cardiothorac Vasc Anesth 2017;31(3):1123–6.

23. Karthika M, Al Enezi FA, Pillai LV, et al. Rapid shallow breathing index. Ann Thorac Med 2016;11(3):167–76.

24. Christie JD, Carby M, Bag R, et al. Report of the ISHLT working group on primary lung graft dysfunction. J Heart Lung Transplant 2005;24:1454.

25. Snell GI, Yusen RD, Weill D, et al. Report of the ISHLT working group on primary lung graft dysfunction. J Heart Lung Transplant 2017;36:1097.

26. Diamond JM, Arcasoy S, Kennedy CC, et al. Report of the international society for heart and lung transplantation working group on primary lung graft dysfunction. J Heart Lung Transplant 2017;36:1104.

27. Liu Y, Liu Y, Su L, et al. Recipient-related clinical risk factors for primary graft dysfunction after lung transplantation: a systematic review and meta-analysis. PLoS One 2014;9:e92773.

28. Shoham S, Shah PD. Impact of multidrug-resistant organisms on patients considered for lung transplantation. Infect Dis Clin North Am 2013;27:343.

29. Paudel S, Zacharioudakis IM, Zervou FN, et al. Prevalence of Clostridium difficile infection among solid organ transplant recipients: a meta-analysis of published studies. PLoS One 2015;10:e0124483.

30. Monnier A, Krummel T, Collange O, et al. Prevalence of acute and chronic renal failure after lung transplantation. J Heart Lung Transplant 2015;34(4):S261.

31. Sikma MA, Hunault CC, van de Graaf EA, et al. High tacrolimus blood concentrations early after lung transplantation and the risk of kidney injury. Eur J Clin Pharmacol 2017;73(5):573–80.

32. Raghavan D, Gao A, Ahn C, et al. Contemporary analysis of incidence of post-operative atrial fibrillation. J Heart Lung Transplant 2015;34(4):563–70.

33. Orrego CM, Cordero-Reyes AM, Estep JD, et al. Atrial arrhythmias after lung transplant: underlying mechanisms, risk factors, and prognosis. J Heart Lung Transplant 2014;33(7):734–40.

34. Jesel L, Barrraud J, Lim HS. Early and late atrial arrythmias after lung transplantation-incidence, predictive factors and impact on mortality. Circ J 2017;81:660–7.

35. Chen JY, Zhang AD, Lu HY, et al. CHADS2 versus CHA2DS2-VASc score in assessing the stroke and thromboembolism risk stratification in patients with atrial-fibrillation: a systematic review and metanalysis. J Geriatr Cardiol 2013;10(3): 258–66.

36. Fernandez R, Ratliff A, Crabb D, et al. Ureaplasma transmitted from donor lungs is pathogenic after lung transplantation. Ann Thorac Surg 2017;103(2):670–1.

37. Bharat A, Cunningham SA, Scott Budinger GR, et al. Disseminated Ureaplasma infection as a cause of fatal hyperammonemia in humans. Sci Transl Med 2015; 7(284):284re3.

38. Chen C, Bain KB, Iuppa JA, et al. Hyperammonemia syndrome after lung transplantation: a single center Experience. Transplantation 2016;100(3):678–84.

39. Nguyen A, Tyson K. Idiopathic hyperammonemia after orthotopic lung transplantation. J Anest & Inten Care Med 2017;1(4):555566.

40. Evans CF, Iacono AT, Sanchez PG, et al. Venous thromboembolic complications of lung transplantation: a contemporary single-institution review. Ann Thorac Surg 2015;100(6):2033–9.

41. Assfalg V, Huser N. Heparin-induced thrombocytopenia in solid organ transplant recipients: the current scientific knowledge. World J Transplant 2016;6(1): 165–73.

42. Mateen FJ, Dierkhising RA, Rabinstein AA, et al. Neurological complications following adult lung transplantation. Am J Transplant 2010;10(4):908–14.

43. Gamez J, Salvado M, Martinez-deLa Ossa A, et al. Influence of early neurological complications on clinical outcome following lung transplant. PLoS One 2017; 12(3):e0174092.

44. Shigemura N, Sclabassi RJ, Bhama JK, et al. Early major neurologic complications after lung transplantation: incidence, risk factors, and outcome. Transplantation 2013;95(6):866–71.

45. Jomphe V, Lands L, Mailhot G. Nutritional requirements of lung transplant recipients: challenges and considerations. Nutrients 2018;10(6):790.

46. Patti MG, Vela MF, Odell D, et al. The intersection of GERD, aspiration, and lung transplantation. J Laparoendosc Adv Surg Tech A 2016;26(7):501–5.

47. Lo WK, Goldberg HJ, Wee, et al. Both pre-transplant and early post-transplant antireflux surgeries prevent development of early allograft injury after lung transplantation. J Gastrointest Surg 2016;20(1):111–8.

48. Cho A, Alhalabi L, Nunes F, et al. Incidence and impact of gastroparesis after lung transplantation. Chest 2017;152(4):A1101.

49. Mini-Series LT. Bronchiolitis obliterans syndrome (BOS) following lung transplant. Am J Respir Crit Care Med 2016;193:P19–20.

50. Müller-Lissner S, Bassotti G, Coffin B, et al. Opioid-induced constipation and bowel dysfunction: a clinical guideline. Pain Med 2017;18(10):1837–63.

51. Nancarrow SA, Booth A, Ariss, et al. Ten principles of good interdisciplinary team work. Hum Resour Health 2013;11(1):19.

52. Whittaker C, Dunsmore V, Murphy F, et al. Long-term care and nursing management of a patient who is the recipient of a renal transplant. J Ren Care 2012;38(4): 233–40.

53. Hackman KL, Snell GI, Bach LA. Prevalence and predictors of diabetes mellitus after lung transplantation: a prospective, longitudinal study. Diabetes Care 2014; 37(11):2919–25.

54. Shivaswamy V, Boerner B, Larsen J. Post-transplant diabetes mellitus: causes, treatment, and impact on outcomes. Endocr Rev 2015;37(1):37–61.

55. Goldberg PA. Comprehensive management of post-transplant diabetes mellitus: from intensive care to home care. Endocrinol Metab Clin North Am 2007;36(4): 907–22.

56. Merai R. CDC grand rounds: a public health approach to detect and control hypertension. MMWR Morb Mortal Wkly Rep 2016;65(45):1261–4.

57. Weir MR, Burgess ED, Cooper JE, et al. Assessment and management of hypertension in transplant patients. J Am Soc Nephrol 2015;26(6):1248–60.

58. Machuzak M, Santacruz JF, Gildea T. Airway complications after lung transplantation. Thorac Surg Clin 2015;25(1):55–75.

Surgical Treatment of Lung Cancer

Haley Hoy, PhD, ACNP[a],*, Thuy Lynch, PhD, RN[b], Monica Beck, MSN, RN, OCN[b]

KEYWORDS

- Small cell lung cancer • Non-small cell cancer • Lobectomy • Wedge resection
- Minimally invasive surgical technique • Low-dose computed tomography

KEY POINTS

- Lung cancer is the leading cause of cancer-related death in the United States.
- Multiple surgical techniques are now available but are generally limited to the early-stage lung cancer diagnoses.
- Surgical intervention is most applicable to early-stage (I–II) non-small cell lung cancer and is considered the best curative option.
- Effective clinical management of the patient following lung cancer surgery is critical.
- Future surgical intervention for lung cancer will likely be affected by promising developments in immunotherapy and oncogenomics.

INTRODUCTION
Incidence and Prevalence

Lung cancer is the leading cause of cancer-related death and the second most diagnosed cancer for both men and women in the United States[1,2] More than 25, 000 surgeries for lung cancer are performed every year in the United States.[3,4] Despite the decrease in lung cancer death in the past decades, more than 2 million new cases of lung cancer, or 11.6% of the world's total cancer incidence, were expected to be diagnosed in 2018. Lung cancer is estimated to cause 154,050 deaths in the United States in 2018, potentially accounting for 25% of all cancer deaths in the country.[5] The global geographic distribution of lung cancer demonstrates marked regional variation, with an age-standardized rate of 33.8 per 100,000, and it is the fourth most frequent cancer in women (13.5 per 100,000).[6] The National Institutes of Health estimate that cancer cost the United States $147.5 billion in 2015, $13.4 billion of which is attributed to lung cancer.[2]

Disclosure Statement: The authors have nothing to disclose.
[a] University of Alabama in Huntsville, Acute Care Nurse Practitioner, Vanderbilt Medical Center; [b] University of Alabama in Huntsville, 301 Sparkman Drive, Huntsville, Al 35899, USA
* Corresponding author. 55 Revere Way, Huntsville, AL 35801.
E-mail address: haley.hoy@uah.edu

Genetic Risk

Cigarette smoking and environmental pollution are major causes of lung cancer; however, numerous studies have shown that genetic factors also contribute to the development of lung cancer.[7] Environmental factors and somatic events are major factors contributing to the development of sporadic lung cancer.[7] Although cigarette smoking continues to be a primary risk factor, lung cancer incidence has been increasing in individuals who have never smoked.[8] Genetic factors are also a significant contributor, but only a few specific genes and other genetic factors that affect lung cancer have been identified.[9] Genetic abnormalities, such as epidermal growth factor receptor (EGFR), have been implicated in the development of lung cancer.[10] EGFR is a transmembrane receptor tyrosine kinase protein that is expressed in some normal epithelial, mesenchymal, and neurogenic tissue.[10] Overexpression of EGFR has been noted and linked to the pathogenesis of many human malignancies, including non-small cell lung cancer (NSCLC).[11]

Lung Cancer Surgery

The current treatment strategy for NSCLC depends on clinical staging. Surgical resection is generally considered the treatment of choice in patients with stage I or II disease whose condition allows for general anesthesia and a lung resection.[12] Surgery is also an accepted treatment modality in a reasonable proportion of patients with clinical stage IIIb and stage IV disease.[12] Although the standards of resections have changed over the past 20 years, there have been several advances in staging, and perioperative and anesthetic management, as well as some noticeable progress made in surgical techniques and approaches.[12]

Surgery and radiation can be curative in stage I NSCLC.[13] Untreated patients with stage I NSCLC have a 5-year survival of only 6% compared with an overall survival of 43% to 73% for all patients with stage I cancer.[14] Curative therapy should be offered to all patients for whom it is clinically appropriate. However, up to 20% of patients with early-stage NSCLC have been described as medically inoperable.[15] Although new technologies have extended into clinical practice over the past decade, it is uncertain whether these have led to increased access to treatment.

PROGNOSIS
Tumor, Nodal Involvement, Distant Metastasis Classification System

Lung cancer staging is critical to help determine which patients are candidates for surgical intervention. The treatment and prognosis of a lung cancer generally depend on the stage of advancement at the time of diagnosis. The staging of lung cancer has undergone significant development over the last century. Determining the stage is the most significant dividing line between patients who are candidates for surgical resection and those who are inoperable but may benefit from chemotherapy and/or radiation therapy.

The basis for staging NSCLC is the tumor, nodal involvement, distant metastasis (TNM) system.[16] The TNM classification has been amended on several occasions and amendments have been proposed based on a large international database developed by the International Association of for the Study of Lung Cancer.[17] The use of a consistent stage classification system is an essential aspect of management of patients with lung cancer.[16] The lung cancer stage classification was recently updated and published by the American Joint Commission on Cancer, and the T, N, and M components are specifically described in **Table 1**. Most lung cancers are initially detected by plain chest radiograph. Up until the 1970s, chest radiograph was the

Table 1
Definitions for tumor, nodal involvement, and distant metastasis (TNM) descriptors

T (primary tumor)	
T0	No primary tumor
Tis	Carcinoma in situ (squamous or adenocarcinoma)
T1	Tumor ≤3 cm
T1mi	Minimally invasive adenocarcinoma
T1a	Superficial spreading tumor in central airways[a]
T1a	Tumor ≤1 cm
T1b	Tumor >1 but ≤2 cm
T1c	Tumor >2 but ≤3 cm
T2	Tumor >3 but ≤5 cm or tumor involving: visceral pleura, main bronchus[b] (not carina), atelectasis to hilum[c]
T2a	Tumor >3 but ≤4 cm
T2b	Tumor >4 but ≤5 cm
T3	Tumor >5 but ≤7 cm or invading chest wall, pericardium, phrenic nerve; or separate tumor nodule(s) in the same lobe
T4	Tumor >7 or tumor invading: mediastinum, diaphragm, heart, great vessels, recurrent laryngeal nerve, carina, trachea, esophagus, spine; or tumor nodule(s) in a different ipsilateral lobe
N (regional) lymph nodes	
N0	No regional node metastasis
N1	Metastasis in ipsilateral pulmonary or hilar nodes
N2	Metastasis in ipsilateral mediastinal or subcarinal nodes
N3	Metastasis in contralateral mediastinal, hilar, or supraclavicular nodes
M (distant metastasis)	
M0	No distant metastasis
M1a	Malignant pleural or pericardial effusion or pleural or pericardial nodules or separate tumor nodule(s) in a contralateral lobe
M1b	Single extrathoracic metastasis
M1c	Multiple extrathoracic metastases (≥1 organ)

[a] Superficial spreading tumor of any size but confined to the tracheal or bronchial wall.
[b] Atelectasis or obstructive pneumonitis extending to hilum; such tumors are classified as T2a if greater than 3 but less than or equal to 4 cm, T2b if greater than 4 and less than or equal to cm.
[c] Pleural effusions are excluded that are cytologically negative, nonbloody, transudative, and clinically judged not be due to cancer.
From Detterbeck F. The eighth edition TNM stage classification for lung cancer: What does it mean on Main Street? J Thorac Cardiovasc Surg 2018;155(1):357; with permission.

only tool available for staging lung cancer. Unfortunately, plain radiograph is both insensitive and nonspecific in diagnosing the extent of disease within the chest. More advanced imaging is now available (see later discussion).

TYPES OF LUNG CANCER

Most lung cancers belong in 2 main pathologic categories: NSCLC (84% of all lung cancers) and small cell lung cancer (SCLC) (13% of all lung cancers),[18] as shown in **Table 2**. From here, there are many subtypes and variants; however, surgical intervention is most applicable to early-stage I and II NSCLC and is very rarely considered for

Table 2
Types of lung or bronchial cancers

Major Categories	Subcategories	Subtypes
NSCLC (84%)	Adenocarcinoma (40%) • Common in smokers and women • Often located in periphery of lung parenchyma • Often presents with fewer symptoms	Acinar Papillary Adenocarcinoma in situ (bronchoalveolar) Solid adenocarcinoma with mucin formation Mixed Variants (mucinous, signet ring, and clear cell)
	Squamous cell carcinoma (30%–35%) • Typically arises in more central location • Subtype most amenable to sputum cytology • Tumor cavitation and necrosis in 10% • Not amenable to treatment with vascular endothelial growth factor receptor inhibitors (VEGFs) Large cell (15%) • Undifferentiated tumor (no evidence of squamous or glandular maturation) • Diagnosis made by exclusion	
SCLC or Oat Cell (13%)	• 98% related to cigarette smoking • Arises in large central airways, metastasizes early, limiting the role of surgery • Neuroendocrine in origin • Aggressive • Most express c-KIT oncoprotein	

SCLC.[19] Surgical intervention, however, is considered the best curative option for early-stage I and II NSCLC.[20] Therefore, this article applies mostly to the treatment of NSCLC.

Clinical Manifestations

Although hemoptysis is frequently thought of as a primary presenting symptom for lung cancer, it actually only occurs in 7% to 10% of patients.[21] In a large, nationally representative cohort study that evaluated symptom prevalence for early-stage lung cancer, cough (n = 1055; 81.5%), dyspnea (n = 1052; 81.2%), pain (n = 756; 58.4%), fatigue (n = 964; 74.4%), depressive symptoms (n = 1030; 79.6%), and nausea or vomiting (n = 426; 32.9%) were found to be the primary symptoms.[22] Other symptoms may include hoarseness, weight loss, anorexia, pleural effusion, dysphagia, lymphadenopathy, and paraneoplastic syndromes.[23]

DIAGNOSTIC ASSESSMENT
Diagnostic Tissue Sampling

Several diagnostic techniques are available to identify the histopathology and the stage of disease, both of which drive the selection of treatment options. The principal criteria for selection of various diagnostic tissue sampling (tumor or lymph nodes) techniques is the least invasive technique with the highest probability of diagnostic yield. For example, sputum cytology is simple, low-risk, and least invasive, but typically selects for squamous cell carcinoma due to the characteristically central location of these tumors. Diagnostic tissue sampling techniques and imaging techniques are often combined to reduce risk and maximize yield. Improved lung cancer screening techniques, such as low-dose computed tomography (LDCT) are more frequently used to identify early-stage lung cancer, resulting in an increased incidence of solitary nodule detection (ie, <3 cm). However, this advancement has increased the challenges to obtaining adequate tissue sampling for diagnostic and staging purposes. Bronchoscopy is the most common technique, with or without additional imaging guidance. Nonbronchoscopic techniques include image-guided transthoracic needle biopsy and surgical resection.[24]

Radiographic Imaging

Radiographic imaging for lung cancer provides diagnostic, location, and staging information, and informs the selection of the diagnostic tissue sampling technique. Axial CT is the gold standard for staging because it provides 3-dimensional images of tumors and anatomic structures, and identifies lymphadenopathy. Chest radiograph is easy and cost-effective; however, as mentioned previously, the 2-dimensional images provide limited information. PET detects lymphadenopathy and the presence of metastasis by measuring and evaluating maximal standard uptake values (SUVs) of fluorodeoxyglucose; the higher the SUVs, the more likely it is that cancer is present. When PET imaging is fused with CT images, positive correlations between the images increase confidence in the interpretation. Bone scintigraphy and MRI have limited roles in diagnosis and staging, particularly if a PET scan reveals high SUVs. Moreover, imaging also provides information on the probability of surgical benefit, as well as the optimal specific surgical technique to be used.

SURGICAL TECHNIQUES

Surgical options for lung cancer include wedge resection, segmentectomy, lobectomy, and pneumonectomy. Brief definitions, benefits, and limitations of each type are described in **Table 3**. Both wedge resection and segmentectomy may be done using minimally assisted techniques, including video-assisted thoracoscopic surgery (VATS) or robotic-assisted thoracoscopic surgery (RATS) techniques. The fundamental difference between VATS and RATS is that the surgeon holds the instrument in VATS and the robot holds the instrument in RATS. Both are considered minimally invasive techniques and result in fewer surgical side effects for patients.[25]

As mentioned previously, surgery for early-stage lung cancer has the highest curative potential and remains the treatment of choice. Surgical options for lung cancer are generally reserved for patients with stage I to II (sometimes stage III) NSCLC and very rarely for SCLC. The role of surgical intervention in NSCLC N2 disease (metastasis in ipsilateral mediastinal or subcarinal nodes) remains controversial.[26]

CLINICAL MANAGEMENT

Postsurgical clinical management for lung cancer is similar to that for all thoracic surgeries. Although surgery is reserved for patients with early-stage lung cancer, when it is indicated, chest tube management, pain control, mobilization, and venous thromboembolic (VTE) prophylaxis remain clinical priorities.

The basics of chest tube management, although well-understood, can be overlooked in the complicated postsurgical setting. From a nursing standpoint, frequent observation of the patient with a chest tube is required. Moreover, emphasis on the importance of an occlusive dressing, the integrity of the drainage system, avoidance of aggressive manipulation or clamping of the tube, and assessment of air leaks are critical aspects of chest tube management.[27] Recent evidence suggests that early conversion to water seal may reduce the duration of air leaks; however, controversy remains regarding the management of chest tubes after pulmonary lobectomy.[28] Recent developments in digital chest tube management may shorten the duration of chest tube placement, but this too is controversial.[29]

Pain management, although closely related to chest tube care and mobilization, is unique following surgical treatment of lung cancer. Pain after thoracotomy has been described as the most severe postsurgical pain.[30] Furthermore, the failure to adequately address pain management can lead to additional complications after lung cancer surgery, including atelectasis and pneumonia. Pain control is generally achieved through epidural anesthesia, in addition to topical anesthetics, oral antiin-flammatories, and a general avoidance of opioids.[30]

Early mobilization after thoracic surgery has been well-studied and is now a gener-ally accepted standard of care.[31,32] Benefits of early mobilization include earlier extu-bation, improved pulmonary function, and decreased incidence of pulmonary embolism (PE) and deep venous thrombosis (DVT).[25]

VTE prophylaxis, although often protocolized, is a critical part of patient care following surgery for lung cancer. Although DVT and PE are potentially fatal compli-cations after any surgery, the incidence of these types of events are increased for patients undergoing thoracic surgery for malignant lung disease. Close observation and a low threshold for early evaluation should be maintained in these patients.[33] Pulmonary angiography remains the gold standard for detection of pulmonary embolus.[34]

COMPLICATIONS

As mentioned previously, complications following surgery for lung cancer are similar to those for all thoracic surgeries. For better understanding, they can be broadly classi-fied as thoracic and nonthoracic complications. Common thoracic complications include atelectasis, pulmonary edema, pneumonia, and respiratory failure. An impor-tant note is that nursing care, including mobility and vigilant airway clearance, can significantly affect all of these potential complications. Other thoracic complications that occur less commonly but that are important to be aware of following lung cancer surgery include phrenic nerve injury and postpneumonectomy syndrome. Phrenic nerve injury is an early complication after thoracotomy that can be the result of ice packs or direct mechanical trauma. This injury can make it more difficult to wean pa-tients from mechanical ventilation and can contribute to decreased cough and secre-tion clearance. Postpneumonectomy syndrome is a late postsurgical complication resulting from a mediastinal shift toward the side of the affected lung after surgical resection. Patients may present with dyspnea, stridor, and dysphagia; these may be mistaken for symptoms of other conditions. A high index of suspicion for postpneumo-nectomy syndrome should be maintained following surgical lung resection.[33]

Nonthoracic complications include DVT and PE, discussed previously, as well as vocal cord injury and cardiac herniation. Vocal cord injuries, although more common after esophagectomy and mediastinoscopy, may occur after thoracic surgery. When unilateral vocal cord dysfunction is present, symptoms may be mild and include voice changes and hoarseness. However, stridor or respiratory distress, more commonly seen with bilateral vocal cord dysfunction, should be treated as an emergency.[33] Prompt recognition of the complication in the postoperative period is critical. Cardiac herniation is a potentially fatal complication that can occur following an intrapericardial

Table 3
Surgical techniques

Surgical Options	Brief Definition	Benefits	Limitations
Wedge resection Typically done with video-assisted thoracoscopic surgery (VATS) or robotic-assisted thoracoscopic surgery (RATS)	Small nonanatomic wedge removed Smaller than segmentectomy	Preferred in patients with poor pulmonary reserve Fewer complications and shorter hospital stays	Generally not used in tumors >4 cm Location of tumor may preclude use of this option May be associated with higher rate of local recurrence
Segmentectomy (may be done via VATS and RATS)	Segment of lung removed but not an entire lobe	Larger parenchymal margins and yields increased number of lymph nodes	Larger than wedge resection but less than lobe If margins not clear, may need lobectomy
Lobectomy	Removal of an entire lobe of lung with regional lymph nodes	Gold standard for NSCLC Removal of entire lobe	Preserves pulmonary function[26] Low mortality rate
Pneumonectomy	Removal of entire lung and its lymph nodes	Option when cancer involves proximal vascular structures or bronchi	Higher mortality rate More complications

pneumonectomy without closure of the pericardium. Hemodynamic compromise is usually noticed during assessment of the patient during a change of position, cough, or chest tube manipulation.[35] This complication, when suspected, should be treated as a medical emergency.

RECENT INNOVATIONS

Innovations in the surgical treatment of lung cancer include relatively new minimally invasive surgical techniques, widespread use of spiral LDCT, and recent promising developments related to immunotherapy and oncogenomics.

Minimally invasive approaches (including robotics) (see **Table 3**) have been shown to be effective and achieve similar outcomes with fewer side effects.[25] Minimally invasive techniques, when appropriate, require fewer incisions and result in shorter lengths of stay and less pain for patients. However, patients with poor pulmonary function who cannot tolerate single-lung ventilation may not be candidates for minimally invasive techniques.[36]

The use of LDCT for lung cancer screening has been accepted as standard of care and is a recommendation by the US Preventative Services Task Force (USPSTF).[37] The USPSTF, after a comprehensive review, made recommendations in 2013 that all adults with a history of heavy smoking or current smokers between the age of 55 and 80 years should be screened annually with LDCT. This recommendation is supported by the Centers for Disease Control and is expected to reduce lung cancer mortality by 20%.[38] Long-term effects of this recommendation are pending the results of large scale trials currently underway.[39]

Immunotherapy, or use of the body's immune response, in the treatment of lung cancer is a recent important innovation related to surgical treatment of lung cancer. Immunotherapy has been used to make some tumors more amenable to resection, and antigen-specific cancer immunotherapy may be used as destination therapy in some metastatic lung cancers.[40] Additional research is underway to further define the best use of immunotherapy in lung cancer.

Oncogenomics is a subset of genomics that applies to cancer-associated genes. Oncogenomics and lung cancer can refer to both patient and tumor genomics, both of which affect risk stratification, survival, and the long-term prognoses of patients with lung cancer. Although not currently as well-understood in relation to lung cancer as other diseases, important research is ongoing in an effort to help patients and their providers make informed decisions in the future.[41]

SUMMARY

Lung cancer remains the leading cause of cancer-related death in the United States. Surgical intervention in the early stage is considered the best curative option, with more than 25, 000 surgeries performed annually. Multiple surgical techniques, including RATS and VATS techniques, in addition to concomitant immunotherapy, are now available. Nurses and nurse practitioners should familiarize themselves with treatment strategies and their sequelae because focused clinical management remains a priority.

ACKNOWLEDGMENTS

This article is dedicated to the memory of Thomas Lynch Jr. who tragically passed away at age 55 years after a diagnosis of non-small cell lung cancer.

REFERENCES

1. Centers for Disease Control and Prevention. Basic information about lung cancer. 2018. Available at: https://www.cdc.gov/cancer/lung/basic_info/. Accessed November 28, 2018.

2. American Lung Association. Lung cancer fact sheet. 2018. Available at: https://www.cancer.org/content/dam/cancer-org/cancer-control/en/booklets-flyers/lung-cancer-fact-sheet.pdf. Accessed November 28, 2018.

3. Park S, Park IK, Kim ER, et al. Current trends of lung cancer surgery and demographic and social factors related to changes in the trends of lung cancer surgery: an analysis of the national database from 2010 to 2014. Cancer Res Treat 2017;49(2):330–7.

4. International Agency for Research on Cancer. GLOBOCAN 2018: estimated cancer incidence, mortality and prevalence worldwide in 2018. 2018. Available at: http://gco.iarc.fr/today/data/factsheets/cancers/15-Lung-fact-sheet.pdf. Accessed December 20, 2018.

5. American Cancer Society. Key statistics for lung cancer. 2018. Available at: https://www.cancer.org/cancer/non-small-cell-lung-cancer/about/key-statistics.html. Accessed December 11, 2018.

6. Ferlay J, Shin HR, Bray F, et al. Estimates of worldwide burden of cancer in 2008: GLOBOCAN 2008. Int J Cancer 2010;127(12):2893–917.

7. Kanwal M, Ding X-J, Cao Y. Familial risk for lung cancer. Oncol Lett 2017; 13(2):535.

8. Cheng PC, Cheng YC. Correlation between familial cancer history and epidermal growth factor receptor mutations in Taiwanese never smokers with non-small cell lung cancer: a case-control study. J Thorac Dis 2015;7(3):281–7.

9. Lichtenstein P, Holm NV, Verkasalo PK, et al. Environmental and heritable factors in the causation of cancer–analyses of cohorts of twins from Sweden, Denmark, and Finland. N Engl J Med 2000;343(2):78–85.

10. Bethune G, Bethune D, Ridgway N, et al. Epidermal growth factor receptor (EGFR) in lung cancer: an overview and update. J Thorac Dis 2010;2(1):48–51.

11. Inamura K, Ninomiya H, Ishikawa Y, et al. Is the epidermal growth factor receptor status in lung cancers reflected in clinicopathologic features? Arch Pathol Lab Med 2010;134(1):66–72.

12. Howington JA, Blum MG, Chang AC, et al. Treatment of stage I and II non-small cell lung cancer: diagnosis and management of lung cancer, 3rd ed: American College of Chest Physicians evidence-based clinical practice guidelines. Chest 2013;143(5 Suppl):e278S–313S.

13. Vest MT, Herrin J, Soulos PR, et al. Use of new treatment modalities for non-small cell lung cancer care in the Medicare population. Chest 2013;143(2):429–35.

14. Scott WJ, Howington J, Feigenberg S, et al. Treatment of non-small cell lung cancer stage I and stage II: ACCP evidence-based clinical practice guidelines (2nd edition). Chest 2007;132(3 Suppl):234s–42s.

15. Mehta HJ, Ross C, Silvestri GA, et al. Evaluation and treatment of high-risk patients with early-stage lung cancer. Clin Chest Med 2011;32(4):783–97.

16. Detterbeck FC. The eighth edition TNM stage classification for lung cancer: what does it mean on Main Street? J Thorac Cardiovasc Surg 2018;155(1):356–9.

17. Rami-Porta R, Bolejack V, Giroux DJ, et al. The IASLC lung cancer staging project: the new database to inform the eighth edition of the TNM classification of lung cancer. J Thorac Oncol 2014;9(11):1618–24.

18. American Cancer Society. Cancer facts & figures 2014. 2014. Available at: http://www.cancer.org/research/cancerfactsstatistics/cancerfactsfigures2014/index. Accessed September 20, 2014.

19. Barnes H, See K, Barnett S, et al. Surgery for limited-stage small-cell lung cancer. Cochrane Database Syst Rev 2017;(4):CD011917.

20. Network NCC. Small cell lung cancer. NCCN clinical practice Guidelines in Oncology. New York: 2018(Version 1.2019-October 10, 2018).

21. von Gunten C, Buckholz G. Palliative care: overview of cough, stridor, and hemoptysis. UpToDate; 2018.

22. Walling AM, Weeks JC, Kahn KL, et al. Symptom prevalence in lung and colorectal cancer patients. J Pain Symptom Manage 2015;49(2):192–202.

23. Yarbro CH, Wujcik D, Gobel BH. Cancer nursing: principles and practice. 7th edition. Sudbury (MA): Jones and Bartlett Publishers; 2011.

24. Arias S, Lee H, Semaan R, et al. Use of electromagnetic navigational transthoracic needle aspiration (E-TTNA) for sampling of lung nodules. J Vis Exp 2015;(99):e52723.

25. Ceppa DP, Kosinski AS, Berry MF, et al. Thoracoscopic lobectomy has increasing benefit in patients with poor pulmonary function: a Society of Thoracic Surgeons Database analysis. Ann Surg 2012;256(3):487–93.

26. Rotman JA, Plodkowski AJ, Hayes SA, et al. Postoperative complications after thoracic surgery for lung cancer. Clin Imaging 2015;39(5):735–49.

27. Kane CJ, York NL, Minton LA. Chest tubes in the critically ill patient. Dimens Crit Care Nurs 2013;32(3):111–7.

28. Bertholet JW, Joosten JJ, Keemers-Gels ME, et al. Chest tube management following pulmonary lobectomy: change of protocol results in fewer air leaks. Interact Cardiovasc Thorac Surg 2011;12(1):28–31.

29. Takamochi K, Nojiri S, Oh S, et al. Comparison of digital and traditional thoracic drainage systems for postoperative chest tube management after pulmonary resection: a prospective randomized trial. J Thorac Cardiovasc Surg 2018; 155(4):1834–40.

30. Sparks A, Stewart JR. Review of pain management in thoracic surgery patients. J Anesth Clin Res 2018;9(4):817–20.

31. Yeung J, Melody T, Kerr A, et al. Randomised controlled pilot study to investigate the effectiveness of thoracic epidural and paravertebral blockade in reducing chronic post-thoracotomy pain: TOPIC feasibility study protocol. BMJ Open 2016;6(12):e012735.

32. Castro E, Turcinovic M, Platz J, et al. Eafrly mobilization: changing the mindset. Crit Care Nurse 2015;35:1–5.

33. Sengupta S. Post-operative pulmonary complications after thoracotomy. Indian J Anaesth 2015;59(9):618–26.

34. Barkley TW, Myers CM. Practice considerations for adult-gerontology acute care nurse practitioners. Hollywood (CA): Barkley and Associates; 2015.

35. Alimi F, Marzouk M, Mgarrech I, et al. Cardiac herniation after left intrapericardial pneumonectomy. Asian Cardiovasc Thorac Ann 2016;24(6):590–2.

36. Hennon MW, Demmy TL. Video-assisted thoracoscopic surgery (VATS) for locally advanced lung cancer. Ann Cardiothorac Surg 2012;1(1):37–42.

37. U.S. Preventive Services Task Force. Lung cancer screening. Available at: https://www.uspreventiveservicestaskforce.org/Page/Document/UpdateSummaryFinal/lung-cancer-screening. Accessed January 15, 2019.

38. Humphrey LL, Deffebach M, Pappas M, et al. Screening for lung cancer with low-dose computed tomography: a systematic review to update the US Preventive services task force recommendation. Ann Intern Med 2013;159(6):411–20.

39. Pinsky PF. Lung cancer screening with low-dose CT: a world-wide view. Transl Lung Cancer Res 2018;7(3):234–42.

40. Murala S, Alli V, Kreisel D, et al. Current status of immunotherapy for the treatment of lung cancer. J Thorac Dis 2010;2(4):237–44.

41. Vogelstein B, Papadopoulos N, Velculescu VE, et al. Cancer genome landscapes. Science 2013;339(6127):1546–58.

A Review of Tetralogy of Fallot and Postoperative Management

Johnna Forman, RN, MSN, PPCNP-BC[a],*,
Rachel Beech, RN, MSN, CPNP-AC[a], Lucy Slugantz, RN, BSN[b],
Amy Donnellan, RN, DNP, CPNP-AC[c]

KEYWORDS

- Tetralogy of Fallot • Pediatric cardiac intensive care unit • Surgical repair
- Postoperative management • Postoperative complications • Nursing care

KEY POINTS

- Tetralogy of Fallot (TOF) is the most common cyanotic congenital heart defect, affecting 7% to 10% of patients with congenital heart disease.
- TOF is caused by a morphologic abnormality in utero, resulting in a tetrad of defects that include ventricular septal defect, pulmonary stenosis, overriding aorta, and right ventricular hypertrophy.
- Multiple TOF variants exist with a wide spectrum of right ventricle outflow tract obstruction.
- Approximately 75% of infants require an elective surgical repair between 3 and 6 months, with the additional 25% requiring neonatal intervention.
- The most common postoperative complications include arrhythmias, right ventricle dysfunction, low cardiac output syndrome, and residual defects.

INTRODUCTION

Congenital heart disease (CHD) affects approximately 1% of live births, which are typically classified as either acyanotic or cyanotic.[1,2] Tetralogy of Fallot (TOF) is the most common cyanotic congenital heart defect.[1–3] Niels Stenson was the first to describe TOF in 1671.[2,3] However, the first complete description of TOF is credited to Etienne

Disclosure: The authors have nothing to disclose.
[a] Heinrich A. Werner Division of Pediatric Critical Care, University of Kentucky, Kentucky Children's Hospital, 800 Rose Street, MN 460, Lexington, KY 40536, USA; [b] Pediatric Intensive Care Unit, University of Kentucky, Kentucky Children's Hospital, 800 Rose Street, MN 460, Lexington, KY 40536, USA; [c] Cardiac Intensive Care Unit, The Heart Institute, Cincinnati Children's Hospital Medical Center, 3333 Burnet Avenue, MLC 1002, Cincinnati, OH 45229, USA
* Corresponding author.
E-mail address: johnna.otis3@uky.edu

Fallot, who published his findings in 1888.[2-4] Maude Abbott first introduced the term TOF in 1924.[2,3] TOF was the first cyanotic congenital heart defect surgically repaired, in 1945 by Alfred Blalock at Johns Hopkins University.[3-5] This article discusses TOF in more detail, including incidence, anatomy, variants, common syndromes, degree of right ventricle outflow tract obstruction (RVOTO), review of surgical repair, common postoperative complications, and management strategies.

REVIEW OF TETRALOGY OF FALLOT ANATOMY AND PHYSIOLOGY
Incidence

TOF represents approximately 7% to 10% of all congenital heart defects.[6,7] As stated earlier, TOF is the most common cause of cyanotic CHD, with an estimated occurrence of 1 in 3500 people or 0.23 to 0.63 cases per 1000 births.[2,5,7] The Centers for Disease Control and Prevention estimates that 1660 infants are born with TOF in the United States each year.[8,9] Boys and girls are equally affected and the precise cause of TOF remains unknown.[2,3]

Anatomy

TOF consists of a tetrad, or a group of 4 defects, which are ventricular septal defect (VSD), pulmonary stenosis (PS), overriding aorta, and right ventricular hypertrophy (RVH) (**Fig. 1**). This tetrad of defects results from a morphologic abnormality in utero causing an anterior and leftward displacement of the infundibular septum.[10] There is a wide spectrum of anatomic variability that exists within the tetrad of defects, as well as the degree of RVOTO.[4]

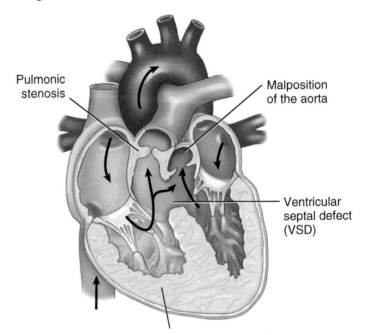

Pulmonic stenosis

Malposition of the aorta

Ventricular septal defect (VSD)

Right ventricular hypertrophy

Fig. 1. Tetralogy of Fallot. (*From* Shiland BJ. Cardiovascular system. In: Mastering healthcare terminology, 6th edition. St. Louis: Elsevier; 2019; with permission.)

A VSD is a hole or opening in the ventricular septum between the left ventricle (LV) and right ventricle (RV) of the heart. The VSD in TOF results from the malalignment and the anterior leftward displacement of the infundibular septum, creating a large and nonrestrictive VSD. In approximately 5% of patients with TOF, additional VSDs may occur. Typically, these additional VSDs occur in the muscular septum.[4]

PS occurs when blood flow from the RV to the pulmonary artery (PA) is inhibited. In TOF, PS is attributed to subpulmonary obstruction and involvement of the pulmonary valve (PV). Subpulmonary obstruction results from the narrowing of the right ventricular outflow tract (RVOT) caused by the anterior and leftward deviation of the infundibular septum and the relationship of the muscle bands that extend from the septum to the right ventricular free wall.[4,6] The PV annulus is smaller than normal in most cases of TOF. The leaflets of the PV are often thickened with restricted movement, and the PV is bicuspid 58% of the time.[4] In addition, it is common for the PA and/or the PA branches to be diminutive, causing suprapulmonary obstruction. Symptoms and degree of RVOTO experienced by patients with TOF depend on the severity of subvalvar, valvar, and supravalvar obstruction of the PV.[4,6]

An overriding aorta occurs when the aorta overrides the ventricular septum and is connected to both the LV and RV, also resulting from the maligned anterior and leftward displacement of the infundibular septum. In the setting of significant RVOTO, shunting of blood occurs across the VSD from the RV to LV, and the overriding aorta promotes the ejection of deoxygenated blood into systemic circulation.[6]

RVH occurs when the musculature of the RV becomes thickened. RVH is not present at birth but develops as a sequela to the morphologic abnormality that occurred in utero. After birth, RVH develops progressively because of the combination of systemic pressures in the RV, RVOTO, and presence of a large, nonrestrictive VSD.[11]

Tetralogy of Fallot Variants

Variations of TOF exist, including TOF with pulmonary atresia (TOF/PA) and TOF with absent PV.[10] In TOF/PA, the anatomy is similar to TOF; however, the RVOTO is extreme and pulmonary blood flow (PBF) is supplied from the systemic arterial circulation via a patent ductus arteriosus (PDA) or major aortopulmonary collateral arteries (MAPCAs).[10,12] More than half of all neonates with TOF/PA present with cyanosis as the PDA closes.[10] Patency of the PDA is maintained with the initiation of prostaglandin E1 (PGE1) therapy until surgical palliation or repair. Absence of a systolic ejection murmur, a typical physical finding in TOF, should raise suspicion for pulmonary atresia. Neonates with TOF/PA with a large PDA or MAPCAs may have a continuous murmur on physical examination.[10] Surgical palliation or complete repair is completed during the neonatal period for TOF/PA because of PDA dependency.[10,12]

TOF with absent PV can be distinguished from TOF/PA by the severity of the RVOTO. In TOF with absent PV, the RVOTO is less severe.[12] Underdeveloped nonfunctional leaflets serve as the PV with significant pulmonary insufficiency (PI).[12] As a result of free PI, the main PA and secondary branches are dilated, sometimes to the extreme, causing proximal and distal airway compression. Ultimately, TOF with absent PV syndrome is primarily a lung disease. If airway compromise is severe, early surgical repair may be required with LeCompte maneuver to reduce central airway compression.[12]

Common Syndromes

Approximately 25% of patients with TOF have other associated chromosomal abnormalities. TOF is most often associated with 22q11.2 deletion syndrome and trisomy 21.[2,3,6,7] Microdeletions in the region of 22q11 occur in 20% of patients with TOF and 40% of patients with TOF/PA.[7,10] Microdeletions in the region of 22q11 also occur in 83% of patients with velocardiofacial syndrome and 94% of patients with DiGeorge syndrome.[10] TOF is also associated with trisomy 18 and 13 and other less common chromosomal abnormalities.[3,6,7] The estimated risk of reoccurrence in families is 3%.[6,7] Extracardiac defects associated with these syndromes also affect the long-term outcomes of patients with TOF.[3]

Physiology

As mentioned earlier, the presentation of TOF can vary greatly depending on the degree of RVOTO (**Table 1**). Infants with mild RVOTO maintain normal oxygen saturations and may develop signs and symptoms of pulmonary overcirculation.[10] As pulmonary vascular resistance (PVR) decreases during the first few weeks to months of life, infants with mild RVOTO may shunt blood from the LV to the RV across the VSD. Over time, the left-to-right shunt across the VSD may result in symptoms of congestive heart failure (CHF).[10] Because infants with mild RVOTO maintain normal oxygen saturations, they are often referred to as pink tets.[10]

Infants with moderate RVOTO maintain near-normal ratios of pulmonary to systemic blood flow and oxygen saturation percentages in the low 90s.[10] Because infants with moderate RVOTO maintain near-normal ratios of pulmonary to systemic blood flow, they often do not develop pulmonary overcirculation or CHF. Typically, infants with moderate RVOTO still remain pink in appearance and maintain normal growth and development.[10]

Infants with severe RVOTO have markedly decreased PBF and increased systemic blood flow. Severe RVOTO causes deoxygenated blood to shunt from the RV to the LV across the VSD. Infants with severe RVOTO often rely on a PDA or MAPCAs for PBF. These infants typically have oxygen saturation percentages in the 70s and appear cyanotic or blue.[10]

Infants with TOF are also at risk of experiencing hypercyanotic episodes, also known as tet spells. Hypercyanotic episodes are caused by an acute change in the ratio of pulmonary and systemic blood flow.[10] During a hypercyanotic episode, there is an increase in PVR and decrease in systemic vascular resistance (SVR), which leads to deoxygenated blood shunting from the RV to the LV across the VSD and results in profound desaturation.[10] These episodes are classically characterized by extreme irritability/crying, hyperpnea, profound cyanosis, pallor, lethargy, absence of murmur, and loss of consciousness.[3,10] Hypercyanotic episodes can result in a metabolic acidosis that causes further increase in PVR and worsens the degree of right-to-left shunt across the VSD.[10] If PBF cannot be reestablished via medical management, infants with severe hypercyanotic episodes may require urgent surgical intervention for either palliation or complete repair.[3,4,10]

REVIEW OF SURGICAL REPAIR AND TECHNIQUE
Indications for Surgery

Timing of surgical intervention depends on several factors, including ductal dependency, severity of obstruction within the subpulmonary outflow tract, frequency of hypercyanotic spells, and degree of cyanosis. Most neonates with TOF (>75%) can wait until 3 to 6 months of age for elective surgical repair.[3,12] Neonates with low birth weight, those who are PDA dependent requiring PGE1 infusion, or those who are having frequent hypercyanotic spells require palliation or complete surgical repair in the immediate neonatal period.[5] If palliation is completed in the neonatal period, a complete repair can be performed between 4 and 6 months of age. Neonates with TOF

Table 1
RVOTO manifestations and treatment

Degree of RVOTO	Mild RVOTO	Moderate RVOTO	Severe-Critical RVOTO	Hypercyanotic Spells
Symptoms	• Pink/acyanotic • Adequate oxygen saturations • + Systolic ejection murmur • At risk to develop CHF as PVR decreases	• Pink/acyanotic • Adequate oxygen saturations • + Systolic ejection murmur	• Cyanotic • Decreased oxygen saturations • ± Systolic ejection murmur • + Continuous murmur (PDA and/or MAPCAs)	• Crying/irritability • Hyperpnea • Very cyanotic • Pale • No murmur • Loss of consciousness • Metabolic acidosis
Systemic Blood Flow	Adequate	Balanced	Increased	Increased
Pulmonary Blood Flow	Increased	Balanced	Decreased to minimal	Minimal
Interventions and Treatment	• CHF symptoms managed with furosemide before surgery • Goal elective repair 3–6 mo • Unable to manage CHF repair <3 mo	• Elective repair 3–6 mo	• Severe RVOTO managed with propranolol before surgery • Critical RVOTO managed before surgery with PGE1 infusion • Repair <3 mo if severe RVOTO or neonatal repair if critical RVOTO	• Increase PBF with knee to chest position, oxygen, crystalloid fluid bolus, morphine, phenylephrine • May require urgent repair regardless of age

Abbreviations: CHF, congestive heart failure; PBF, pulmonary blood flow; PVR, pulmonary vascular resistance.

absent PV with severe airway compromise require surgical intervention in the neonatal period. Timing of surgical intervention is also based on the current practice and expertise of each surgical center. Some centers, based on their expertise, choose initial palliation followed by repair over early primary repair because of the low mortality associated with initial palliation.[5]

Morbidity and Mortality

Advances in cardiac surgery and postoperative intensive care have led to a significant improvement in outcomes for neonates with TOF. Before advances in corrective surgeries, the early mortality was about 25%, which has now been reduced to as little as 2%.[13,14] Overall survival rates into adulthood following TOF repair are now greater than 85%.[2,3,15] The diagnosis of TOF/PA has a worse late prognosis than other variants of TOF because of the associated branch PA stenosis and PV replacement in adulthood.[14] Children with the diagnosis of TOF with an associated genetic syndrome including 22q11 deletion syndrome and/or trisomy 21 have significantly increased morbidity and mortalities caused by PA hypoplasia, extracardiac anomalies requiring surgery, and immunodeficiency.[12] In-hospital mortality following initial palliation with a shunt in the neonatal period is 4% to 14%, with high morbidity rates of 9% to 18% attributed to shunt thrombosis.[16] The 30-day mortality in typical TOF repair is now approaching 0% at experienced centers.[12] Adults with TOF are at a higher risk of developing arrhythmias, progressive exercise intolerance, right heart failure, and sudden death.[17] Despite the improved short and intermediate outcomes, the long-term outcomes for patients with repaired TOF are still substantially worse than among the general population and these patients require close follow-up and long-term care.[17]

Neonatal Palliation

Approximately 25% of infants with TOF require early intervention in the neonatal period because of cyanosis or PGE1 dependence for PDA patency.[12] The initial management of symptomatic neonates remains an ongoing debate because of the adverse effects of bypass surgery on the neonatal brain, longer postoperative recovery and hospital stay following complete repair, and need for reoperations in childhood.[2,18] Neonatal repair is associated with low mortality; however, there is an association with increased morbidity and long-term impact on RV performance.[18] Options for surgical palliation include systemic-to-pulmonary arterial shunt (modified Blalock-Taussig [BT] shunt), balloon dilation, or stenting of the RVOT.[19]

The most common palliative procedure performed in the neonatal period is a modified BT shunt, a method that supplies a secure source of blood to the lungs by connecting the subclavian artery to the PA via a polytetrafluoroethylene graft.[3,20] Advantages of early palliation with a modified BT shunt include the potential to perform the procedure off bypass and that it allows for growth of the RVOT.[3] Shunted neonates also have shorter intensive care unit (ICU) and hospital stays postoperatively compared with neonates with primary surgical repair.[18] Surgical palliation does have disadvantages. Potential disadvantages following palliation include pressure overload of the RV, persistent hypoxemia, distortion of the branch PA, and shunt thrombosis.[3,21] Surgical palliation with a shunt predisposes these neonates to multiple surgical repairs over their lifetimes.

Complete Repair

Complete surgical repair also depends greatly on the individual infant's anatomy and element of RVOTO. In general, complete surgical repair of TOF entails closing the VSD, resecting muscle bundles within the RVOT with or without patch augmentation, augmenting the PA and branch PAs if indicated, and relieving severe obstruction at the PV annulus if indicated.[3]

Often, infants with mild RVOTO with well-developed PAs only require closure of the VSD and minimal muscle resection at the os infundibuli.[3] Closure of the VSD is performed via a transatrial approach. This approach allows the surgeon to minimize the length of the RV incision to only the necessary length to relieve RVOTO. The VSD is closed with a patch that is cut to size and sutured to the right side of the septum. The surgeon takes special care when suturing not to cause injury to the bundle of His-Purkinje system.[4]

In addition to VSD closure, infants with moderate to severe RVOTO require a ventriculotomy and resection of the hypertrophied muscle.[3] The PV annulus is measured and inspected intraoperatively for adequacy in size. The PV annulus is considered inadequate when the z score is more than 2 standard deviations less than normal.[3]

If the PV annulus is inadequate in size, the ventriculotomy incision is extended across the PV into the PA. This type of approach is called a transannular patch technique.[3,4] Transannular patch repair results in moderate to severe PI and volume loading of the RV. Transannular patch repair also increases the long-term risk of RV dysfunction and ventricular arrhythmias. Because of these risks, current surgical techniques focus on maintaining PV competency and tolerating mild RVOTO.[3]

If the PV annulus is adequate in size, a transatrial-transpulmonary valve-sparing technique is preferred. This technique spares the PV at the expense of tolerating mild RVOTO.[2,3,12] If the PA is hypoplastic, a patch can be used supravalvar and/or subvalvar into the RV if necessary. Current techniques also encourage avoidance of excessive right ventricular muscle resection to avoid associated RV diastolic dysfunction.[3]

Infants with TOF/PA or diffusely small PAs may require an RV-PA conduit. The type of conduit varies depending on surgeon expertise and preference. An RV-PA conduit commits an infant to multiple surgical repairs over a lifetime.[3]

Multiple Surgical Repairs Over the Lifetime

Some patients with TOF require multiple surgical interventions during their lifetimes. The most common reasons for reoperation include residual VSD, PS, RVOT aneurysm, PV replacement, and RV-PA conduit replacements.[22] Reconstruction of the RVOT can result in varying degrees of PI and PS based on the surgical technique used. Residual RVOTO may also be present after primary repair and/or degenerative changes after repair.[23] The use of an RV-PA conduit necessitates multiple surgical repairs over the lifetime because of conduit obstruction, degeneration, or failure.[22]

Indications for PV replacement continue to evolve.[15,23] Current guidelines exist from the American College of Cardiology and American Heart Association, Canadian Cardiovascular Society, and European Society of Cardiology with mild variations.[23] In general, current indications for PV replacement include moderate PS or RV-PA conduit obstruction, moderate to severe PI, mild shortness of breath, mild angina, slight limitation with ordinary activity, RV dysfunction and dilatation, decreased performance with exercise testing, sustained atrial or ventricular arrhythmias, and/or prolonged QRS interval.[15,22,23] Optimal timing of PV replacement can result in improved RV function and control of arrhythmias.[15]

In addition, the development of aortic root dilatation and aortic insufficiency is common in adults with TOF. The pathophysiology behind this development is not well understood. Guidelines for management of aortic root dilatation in TOF also continue to evolve but there are no specific recommendations.[7,23] Most providers recommend surgical interventions for more than a 0.5-cm increase in the aortic root dimension within 1 year.[23]

COMMON POSTOPERATIVE COMPLICATIONS AND MANAGEMENT STRATEGIES
Arrhythmias

Sustained or hemodynamically significant arrhythmias occur in up to 12% of patients following TOF repair, usually within the first 24 hours.[12] Atrial arrhythmias, ventricular arrhythmias, right bundle branch block (RBBB), junctional ectopic tachycardia (JET), and heart block (HB) are common arrhythmias experienced in the postoperative period.[3,12] Risk factors for developing postoperative arrhythmias include younger age, lower body weight, longer cardiopulmonary bypass time, longer aortic cross-clamp time, deep hypothermia, and cardiac arrest. The most common hemodynamically significant postoperative arrhythmias are JET, supraventricular tachycardia, and HB.[24] Typically, temporary atrial and ventricular pacing wires are placed for the diagnosis and management of postoperative arrhythmias.[4]

RBBB occurs in almost 100% of patients following TOF repair.[25–27] RBBB is an arrhythmia that occurs when the transmission of electrical impulse through the His-Purkinje system is interrupted or delayed. There are 3 potential sites for RBBB following surgical repair. RBBB can result from ventriculotomy caused by interruption of terminal right ventricular conduction, RV muscle resection caused by conduction inhibition within the moderator band, and VSD patch placement caused by disruption of the right bundle branch at the inferior border.[26] On electrocardiogram (ECG), a RBBB is shown by a widened QRS complex longer than 120 milliseconds with change in the directional vectors of the R and S waves, resulting in a bunny-ear appearance.[28] In general, RBBB is asymptomatic and does not require intervention. Resynchronization therapy is recommended later in the setting of low left ventricular ejection fraction and CHF.[29]

JET is a common postoperative arrhythmia experienced after TOF repair. After congenital heart surgery, JET is estimated to occur at a rate as high as 15% and more commonly occurs after TOF repair because of the close proximity of the repair to the atrioventricular (AV) node.[30] Additional risk factors for JET include younger age, longer cardiopulmonary bypass and aortic cross-clamp times, use of vasoactive agents postoperatively, and hypomagnesemia.[30,31] JET occurs when the AV node has increased automaticity and spontaneously depolarizes, resulting in dyssynchrony between the atria and ventricles. Clinically on ECG, JET is a tachycardic rate that manifests with the absence of p waves and a narrow QRS complex.[30,32] JET is associated with increased postoperative morbidity and mortality.[32] Incidence of JET is typically self-limited to the immediate postoperative period. Medical management of JET is designed to reduce heart rate and reestablish synchrony between the atria and ventricles via thermoregulation; correction of electrolyte imbalances; reducing catecholamine levels; temporary atrial overdrive pacing; and administration of pharmacotherapies such as dexmedetomidine, amiodarone, procainamide, and propranolol.[30,33,34]

HB develops as a result of damage to the cardiac conduction system following surgical repair of CHD. HB is a potential but uncommon risk, with occurrence ranging between 1% and 3%.[35] Repairs near or adjacent to the AV node have increased risk for HB. Studies have revealed that a longer surgery time is a risk factor for complete HB. Other risk factors for HB include morbidity in the immediate postsurgical period, moderate to severe hemodynamic compromise, mechanical ventilation longer than 5 days, and a cardiac reintervention within first 14 days after surgery.[36] Early postoperative HB can be transient or permanent. If HB persists after 2 weeks of temporary pacing, a permanent pacemaker is recommended. This condition is typically caused by damage to the bundle of His-Purkinje system or trifascicular damage associated with excessive bradycardia and risk of asystole.[37]

Right Ventricle Dysfunction

Almost 50% of patients after TOF repair experience restrictive RV physiology and RV diastolic dysfunction.[12,38] Advances in bedside echocardiogram (echo) technology provide detailed data regarding both RV and LV function. Initially, after TOF repair, the RV shows abnormal contractility, relaxation, wall motion, and loading conditions, while typically preserving LV function.[12,39] The hallmark echo finding consistent with severe restrictive RV physiology is the presence of antegrade flow to the PAs during diastole.[38] Because of the RV's inability to fill during diastole, the RV acts as a passive conduit, which explains the presence of antegrade flow to the PAs during diastole on echo.[3,38,40]

The precise cause and pathophysiology resulting in RV diastolic dysfunction is not well understood. Speculated causes include cardiopulmonary bypass, ventriculotomy, myocardial edema, and use of nonfunctional patches on the ventricular septum and RVOT.[38] Clinically, these patients experience increased central venous or right atrial pressures, decreased RV stroke volume, and prolonged inotropic support and chest tube drainage.[3,38,41]

RV diastolic dysfunction often responds to increases in end-diastolic pressures, which can be achieved with early extubation and minimization of positive pressure ventilation, optimization of venous return, volume support, and milrinone.[12,41,42] RV diastolic dysfunction is one of the main contributors to early postoperative low cardiac output syndrome (LCOS) because of inadequate RV filling and a reduction in the effective compliance of the LV.[3,12,42] The reduction in effective compliance of the LV results from the bowing of the ventricular septum into the LV as a result of RV hypertension.[42] Because of the risk for this phenomenon, surgeons may choose to leave a residual atrial septal defect (ASD) to allow for a small right-to-left shunt at the atrial level to maintain cardiac output during the early postoperative period.[3] RV diastolic dysfunction is transient and typically resolves within 72 hours.[2]

Low Cardiac Output Syndrome

LCOS is a common postoperative complication that occurs in approximately 25% of children.[43–45] LCOS is caused by an imbalance of oxygen supply and demand following cardiopulmonary bypass. Within 6 to 18 hours after cardiopulmonary bypass, children have the potential to experience a cardiac index of 2 L/min/m² or less.[43,45] Cardiopulmonary bypass contributes to postoperative myocardial injury and dysfunction because of the systemic inflammatory response and ischemic injury, increasing the risk for LCOS.[43,45,46] A milrinone infusion is frequently used for the prevention and treatment of LCOS following cardiopulmonary bypass. Milrinone is a type III phosphodiesterase inhibitor that provides inotropic support while reducing PVR and SVR with minimal impact on myocardial oxygen demand.[43,47] A double-blind study showed that a high-dose milrinone infusion postoperatively decreased occurrence of LCOS by 64% compared with placebo or low-moderate doses.[47]

The cause of postoperative LCOS is multifactorial and may be influenced by preload, afterload, myocardial contractility, heart rate, and rhythm.[43,46] LCOS after TOF repair is most likely to occur because of RV diastolic dysfunction or RV failure.[2,10,40] Early recognition of LCOS and timely intervention are essential for optimum outcomes. Frequent clinical assessments and continuous monitoring are essential for early recognition of LCOS.[10,46] Common signs of LCOS after TOF repair include tachycardia, increased right atrial pressure or central venous pressures, hypotension, poor peripheral perfusion, cool extremities, hepatomegaly, oliguria, decreased mixed venous oxygen saturation, and/or acidosis.[10,46] Management of LCOS varies depending on the source of dysfunction, because preload, afterload, myocardial contractility, heart rate, and/or rhythm can be altered. Maintenance of normal sinus rhythm, RV

Box 1
Management strategies for postoperative complications

Arrhythmias

- Temporary atrial and ventricular pacing wires
  - Use for all postoperative arrhythmias

- RBBB
  - Asymptomatic, no intervention required
  - Associated with low LV ejection fraction and CHF, resynchronization therapy indicated

- JET
  - Reestablish AV synchrony
  - Maintain normothermic status, prevent fevers
  - Correct electrolyte imbalance
  - Decrease catecholamine response
  - Temporary atrial overdrive pacing
  - Administer pharmacotherapies; dexmedetomidine, amiodarone, procainamide, propranolol

- HB
  - Temporary atrial and ventricular pacing
  - Persistent HB after 2 weeks, permanent pacemaker recommended

Right Ventricle Dysfunction

- Increase end diastolic pressures with early extubation and minimization of positive pressure ventilation

- Optimize venous return

- Volume support with crystalloids

- Optimize total cardiac output
  - Systemic vasodilation (afterload reduction)
    - Milrinone
  - Inotropic support (increase contractility)
    - Epinephrine

Low Cardiac Output Syndrome

- Maintain AV synchrony

- Optimize total cardiac output
  - Support RV preload
    - Administer volume replacement
  - Systemic vasodilation (afterload reduction)
    - Milrinone to reduce PVR and SVR with minimal impact on myocardial oxygen demand
  - Inotropic medications to assist contractility
    - Epinephrine
    - Milrinone

Residual Defects

- Awareness of residual defects assist in postoperative management

- Monitor with echo

preload, appropriate myocardial support, and ventilation are key in prevention of LCOS after repair of TOF.[40,43,46]

Residual Defects

Following TOF repair, a transesophageal echo is performed in the operating room to evaluate adequacy and residual defects.[48] Potential residual defects include PI, RVOTO, VSD, and/or ASD.[10] Awareness of residual defects is essential for adequate postoperative monitoring and management.[12] Residual PI is usually well tolerated in the immediate postoperative period but will require reintervention in the future. Presence of moderate residual RVOTO is also usually well tolerated and may require later reintervention.[10]

Knowledge of a residual ASD and/or VSD, with the potential to shunt deoxygenated blood from the RV to the LV, is crucial for determining goal oxygen saturation ranges in the postoperative period. A large residual VSD requiring surgical reintervention is rare. Significant residual VSDs are not well tolerated because of RV diastolic dysfunction and decreased RV compliance, which is exacerbated in the neonatal myocardium.[10] A residual ASD is typically well tolerated and on occasion intentionally left by cardiothoracic surgeons. A residual ASD ensures maintenance of preserved cardiac output at the expense of systemic oxygen desaturation.[3,10] Most residual ASDs and VSDs are not hemodynamically significant and close spontaneously over time. Residual defects should be closely monitored (**Box 1**).[10]

SUMMARY

With TOF being the most common cyanotic congenital heart defect, repair of TOF accounts for a considerable amount of the CHD population requiring postoperative care. Understanding the underlying anatomy and physiology is essential to postoperative ICU care. TOF includes a wide spectrum of RVOTO and multiple variants with surgical interventions and postoperative management tailored to each individual patient. Early recognition and intervention of postoperative complications are essential to improved patient outcomes. Continued advancements in knowledge, technology, surgical techniques, and postoperative management should lead to ongoing improvements in short-term, intermediate-term, and long-term outcomes for patients with TOF in the future.

REFERENCES

1. Triedman JK, Newburger JW. Trends in congenital heart disease: the next decade. Circulation 2016;133(25):2716–33.
2. Apitz C, Webb GD, Redington AN. Tetralogy of Fallot. Lancet 2009;374:1462–71.
3. Sharkey AM, Sharma A. Tetralogy of Fallot: anatomic variants and their impact on surgical management. Semin Cardiothorac Vasc Anesth 2012;16(2):88–96.
4. Bove EL, Hirsch JC. Tetralogy of Fallot. In: Stark J, deLeval M, Tsang VT, editors. Surgery for congenital heart defects. 3rd edition. West Sussex, United Kingdom: John Wiley and Sons, Ltd; 2006. p. 399–410.
5. Steiner MB, Tang X, Gossett JM, et al. Timing of complete repair of non-ductal-dependent tetralogy of Fallot and short-term postoperative outcomes, a multi-center analysis. J Thorac Cardiovasc Surg 2013;16(2):1–7.
6. Bailliard F, Anderson R. Tetralogy of Fallot. Orphanet J Rare Dis 2009;4:2.
7. Villafane J, Feinstein JA, Jenkins KJ, et al. Hot topics in tetralogy of Fallot. J Am Coll Cardiol 2013;62(23):2155–66.

8. Centers for Disease Control and Prevention. Facts about tetralogy of Fallot. 2018. Available at: https://www.cdc.gov/ncbddd/heartdefects/tetralogyoffallot.html. Accessed January 4, 2019.

9. Parker SE, Mai CT, Canfield MA, et al. Updated national birth prevalence estimates for selected birth defects in the United States, 2004-2006. Birth Defects Res A Clin Mol Teratol 2010;88:1008–16.

10. Davis S. Tetralogy of Fallot with and without pulmonary atresia. In: Critical heart disease in infants and children. 2nd edition. Philadelphia: Elsevier Mosby; 2006. p. 755–66.

11. Van Praagh R. The first Stella Van Praagh memorial lecture: the history and anatomy of tetralogy of Fallot. Semin Thorac Cardiovasc Surg Pediatr Card Surg Annu 2009;12(1):19–38.

12. Karl TF, Stocker C. Tetralogy of Fallot and its variants. Pediatr Crit Care Med 2016; 17(8):S330–6.

13. Hickey EJ, Veldtman G, Bradley TJ, et al. Functional health status in adult survivors of operative repair of tetralogy of Fallot. Am J Cardiol 2012;109(6):873–80.

14. Hickey E, Veldtman G, Bradley TJ, et al. Late risk of outcomes for adults with repaired tetralogy of Fallot from an inception cohort spanning four decades. Eur J Cardiothorac Surg 2009;35(1):156–64.

15. Martinez RM, Ringewald JM, Fontanet HL, et al. Management of adults with tetralogy of Fallot. Cardiol Young 2013;23(6):920–31.

16. Hobbes B, d'Udekem Y, Zannino D, et al. Determinants of adverse outcomes after systemic-to-pulmonary shunts in biventricular circulation. Ann Thorac Surg 2017;104(4):1365–70.

17. Dennis M, Moore B, Kotchetkova I, et al. Adults with repaired tetralogy: low mortality but high morbidity up to middle age. Open Heart 2017;4:e000564.

18. Kanter KR, Kogon BE, Kirshbom PM, et al. Symptomatic neonatal tetralogy of Fallot: repair or shunt? Ann Thorac Surg 2010;89:858–63.

19. Haas NA, Laser TK, Moysich A, et al. Stenting of the right ventricular outflow tract in symptomatic neonatal tetralogy of Fallot. Cardiol Young 2008;24(2):369–73.

20. Jo TK, Suh HR, Choi BG, et al. Outcome of neonatal palliative procedure for pulmonary atresia with ventricular septal defect or tetralogy of Fallot with severe pulmonary stenosis: experience in a single tertiary center. Korean J Pediatr 2018; 61(7):210–6.

21. Jonas R. Early primary repair of tetralogy of Fallot. Semin Thorac Cardiovasc Surg Pediatr Card Surg Annu 2009;12(1):39–47.

22. Tirilomis T, Friedrich M, Zenker D, et al. Indications for reoperation late after correction of tetralogy of Fallot. Cardiol Young 2010;20(4):396–401.

23. Downing TE, Kim YY. Tetralogy of Fallot. Cardiol Clin 2015;33(4):531–41.

24. Rekawek J, Kansy A, Miszczak-Knecht M, et al. Risk factors for cardiac arrhythmias in children with congenital heart disease after surgical intervention in the early postoperative period. J Thorac Cardiovasc Surg 2007;133(4):900–4.

25. Kuzevska-Maneva K, Kacarska R, Gurkova B. Arrhythmias and conduction abnormalities in children after repair of tetralogy of Fallot. Vojnosanit Pregl 2005; 62(2):97–102.

26. Hazan E, Bical O, Bex JP, et al. Is right bundle branch block avoidable in surgical correction of tetralogy of Fallot? Circulation 1980;62(4):852–4.

27. Horowitz LN, Simson MB, Spear JF, et al. The mechanism of apparent right bundle branch block after transatrial repair of tetralogy of Fallot. Circulation 1979;59(6):1241–52.

28. Udink Ten Cate FE, Sreeram N, Brockmeier K. The pathophysiologic aspects and clinical implications of electrocardiographic parameters of ventricular conduction delay in repaired tetralogy of Fallot. J Electrocardiol 2014;47(5):618–24.
29. Thambo JB, De Guillebon M, Dos Santos P, et al. Electrical dyssynchrony and re-synchronization in tetralogy of Fallot. Heart Rhythm 2011;8(6):909–14.
30. Smith AH. Arrhythmias in cardiac critical care. Pediatr Crit Care Med 2016;17(8 suppl 1):S146–54.
31. Abdelaziz O, Deraz S. Anticipation and management of junctional ectopic tachy-cardia in postoperative cardiac surgery: single center experience with high inci-dence. Ann Pediatr Cardiol 2014;7(1):19–24.
32. St.George-Hyslop C, Morton C, Daley E. Neonatal and pediatric guidelines for arrhythmia management. In: The Pediatric cardiac intensive care Society Web-site. 2014. Available at: https://www.pcics.org/wp-content/uploads/2014/12/Neo_Pedia_Guidelines_Arrhythmia.pdf. Accessed January 14, 2019.
33. El-Shmaa N, El Amrousy D, El Feky W. The efficacy of pre-emptive dexmedetomi-dine versus amiodarone in preventing postoperative junctional ectopic tachy-cardia in pediatric cardiac surgery. Ann Card Anaesth 2016;19(4):614–20.
34. Entenmann A, Michel M, Herberg U, et al. Management of postoperative junc-tional ectopic tachycardia in pediatric patients: a survey of 30 centers in Ger-many, Austria, and Switzerland. Eur J Pediatr 2017;176(9):1217–26.
35. Nasser BA, Mesned AR, Mohamad T, et al. Late-presenting complete heart block after pediatric cardiac surgery. J Saudi Heart Assoc 2015;28(1):59–62.
36. Corcia M, Salgado G, Moreno G, et al. Clinical predictors of permanent injury to the atrioventricular conduction system after congenital heart disease surgery. A new perspective on an old problem. Prog Pediatr Cardiol 2017;46:35–8.
37. Bonatti V, Agnetti A, Squarcia U. Early and late postoperative complete heart block in pediatric patients submitted to open-heart surgery for congenital heart disease. Pediatr Med Chir 2013;20(3):181–6.
38. Cullen S, Shore D, Redington A. Characterization of right ventricular diastolic per-formance after complete repair of tetralogy of Fallot. Restrictive physiology pre-dicts slow postoperative recovery. Circulation 1995;91(6):1782–9.
39. Peng E, Spooner R, Young D, et al. Acute b-type natriuretic peptide response and early postoperative right ventricular physiology following tetralogy of Fallot's repair. Interact Cardiovasc Thorac Surg 2012;15(3):335–9.
40. Redington A. Low cardiac output due to acute right ventricular dysfunction and cardiopulmonary interactions in congenital heart disease (2013 Grover Confer-ence series). Pulm Circ 2014;4(2):191–9.
41. Sachdev MS, Bhagyavathy A, Varghese R, et al. Right ventricular diastolic func-tion after repair of tetralogy of Fallot. Pediatr Cardiol 2006;27(2):250–5.
42. Bronicki R, Chang A. Management of the postoperative pediatric cardiac surgical patient. Crit Care Med 2011;39(8):1974–84.
43. Chandler HK, Kirsch R. Management of the low cardiac output syndrome following surgery for congenital heart disease. Curr Cardiol Rev 2016;12(2):107–11.
44. Parr GV, Blackstone EH, Kirklin JW. Cardiac performance and mortality early after intracardiac surgery in infants and young children. Circulation 1975;51(5):867–74.
45. Wernovsky G, Wypij D, Jonas RA, et al. Postoperative course and hemodynamic profile after the arterial switch operation in neonates and infants. A comparison of low-flow cardiopulmonary bypass and circulatory arrest. Circulation 1995;92(8):2226–35.

46. Sivarajan VB, Rotta AT. Critical care after surgery for congenital cardiac disease. In: Fuhrman B, Zimmerman J, Clark R, et al, editors. Pediatric critical care. 5th edition. Philadelphia: Elsevier; 2017. p. 447–79.
47. Hoffman TM, Wernovsky G, Atz AM, et al. Efficacy and safety of milrinone in preventing low cardiac output syndrome in infants and children after corrective surgery for congenital heart disease. Circulation 2003;107(7):996–1002.
48. Vaujois L, Gorincour G, Alison M, et al. Imaging of postoperative tetralogy of Fallot repair. Diagn Interv Imaging 2016;97(5):549–60.

Stroke Volume Optimization

Utilization of the Newest Cardiac Vital Sign: Considerations in Recovery from Cardiac Surgery

Alexander Johnson, MSN, RN, ACNP-BC, CCNS, CCRN*,
Jillian Stevenson, RN, BSN, CCRN, Hong Gu, RN, MSN, CCRN,
Jeffrey Huml, MD, FCCP, SCCM

KEYWORDS

- Stroke volume • Hemodynamics • Stroke volume optimization • Cardiac output
- Fluid management • Passive leg raise • Mean arterial pressure
- Pulmonary artery catheter

KEY POINTS

- Stroke volume (SV) is the most sensitive indicator to a change in volume or hemodynamic status.
- Many emerging minimally invasive cardiac output (CO) monitors on the market exist and no one device is perfect for all patients in all situations; however, the device supported by the most evidence is the esophageal Doppler.
- The central venous pressure (CVP) is a poor measure of preload and poor predictor of a response in cardiac output after a fluid challenge.
- The key threshold to determine fluid responsiveness after a fluid challenge is increase in SV by greater than 10%. All other hemodynamic parameters, such as systemic vascular resistance (SVR) and mean arterial pressure (MAP), are secondary parameters to trend.
- The stroke volume optimization (SVO) algorithm and the passive leg raise (PLR) are systematic, evidence-based strategies that are used to fluid-optimize patients.

In 1996, a pulmonologist Alfred Connors published a study suggesting that when pulmonary artery catheters (PAC) are used in critical care, there is a higher likelihood of patient death.[1] The following year, at the Pulmonary Artery Consensus Conference, the worldwide critical care thought leaders in attendance suggested that the PAC may be helpful; however, it was not mandatory for monitoring in cardiac surgery

Disclosure: The authors have nothing to disclose.
Northwestern Medicine-Central DuPage Hospital, Critical Care-Intensive Care Unit, 25 North Winfield Road, Winfield, IL 60190, USA
* Corresponding author.
E-mail address: apjccrn@hotmail.com

patients.[2] The most current best practice consensus guidelines for cardiac surgery by Stephens and Whitman[3] continue to reinforce PAC as an optional tool, stating that, "Routine placement of a pulmonary artery catheter is neither required nor helpful in the majority of patients." Meanwhile, the critical care landscape has been in search of an alternative to PAC for ongoing cardiac output (CO) monitoring at the bedside.

However, authors have maintained that the PAC is not in and of itself inherently harmful or dangerous. In fact, an Agency for Healthcare Research and Quality technology review and Cochrane Database systematic review of PAC suggested that clinician-to-clinician variability with PAC use is one of several reasons why studies have not consistently shown improved outcomes with use of the device.[4,5] Variability in how PAC values are acquired, interpreted, and treated have resulted in inconsistent results in studies of PAC impact on patient outcomes.

Many studies have been published regarding the limitations of physical assessment because of its subjective nature.[6–13] Thus, physical assessment, although perhaps helpful in trending perfusion status, should be coupled with objective data for evaluating adequacy of CO (**Fig. 1**).[3] As a result, bedside ultrasound has increased in popularity as a technique to couple with the physical examination to improve objectivity, reliability, and accuracy via imaging. Concurrently, many different minimally invasive hemodynamic monitoring techniques have also emerged to decrease subjectivity and improve ease of use and precision of ongoing CO assessments at the bedside.

EVOLUTION OF HEMODYNAMIC MONITORING

Additional factors influencing the trend away from the PAC toward more minimally invasive CO monitoring have been the transition from pressure-based (ie, static) to more flow-based (ie, dynamic) parameters. Pressure-based parameters, such as pulmonary artery occlusion pressure and central venous pressure, have been shown to be inconsistent measures of preload or predictors of changes in CO after a fluid challenge.[14–16] Several patient-specific factors decrease the ability of cardiac filling pressures to assess preload, including but not limited to: varying degrees of cardiac chamber compliance and resistance, juxtacardiac pressure (eg, pulmonary hypertension), alterations in intrathoracic pressure (eg, mechanical ventilation), changes in heart rate (HR), and various stages of cardiomyopathy (**Fig. 2**).

However, many authors have suggested that rather than the optimization of filling pressures, goals of hemodynamic monitoring should have always been the optimization of stroke volume (SV) and CO (eg, dynamic parameters).[17,18] In fact, 10 prospective randomized controlled trials (RCT) suggest that when SV is used as the primary end point for fluid optimization, patient outcomes are consistently improved.[19–28] The most recent of these RCTs and the largest of its kind (N = 450) was the FEDORA Trial.[28] **Fig. 3** illustrates the SV optimization (SVO) algorithm used in FEDORA, which is predicated on administering fluid challenges as long as the SV increases by greater than or equal to 10% or more in response. The greater than or equal to 10% SV increase threshold is the similar threshold used in the protocol for each of the other nine RCTs. A lack of protocolized use was cited as a reason for the lack of benefit in PAC patient outcome trials.[4,5,29]

MINIMALLY INVASIVE CARDIAC OUTPUT TECHNIQUES

Each of the previously mentioned 10 RCTs supporting SVO as the most evidence-based strategy for fluid optimization were all performed with esophageal Doppler.

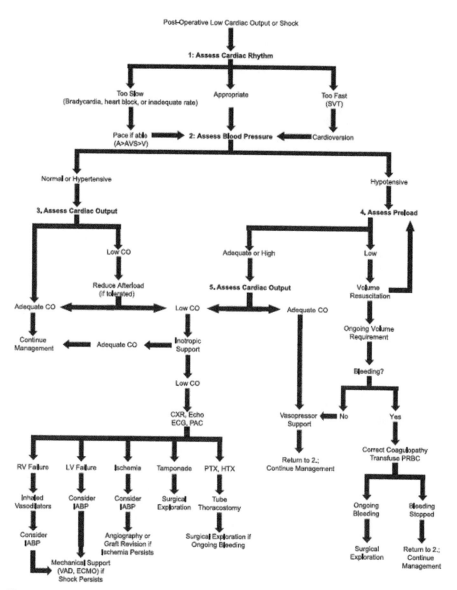

Fig. 1. Postoperative low CO or shock management algorithm from Cardiac Surgery Guidelines. CXR, chest radiograph; ECG, electrocardiogram; Echo, echocardiogram; ECMO, extracorporeal membrane oxygenation; LV, left ventricle; RV, right ventricle; VAD, ventricular-assist device; HTX, hemothorax; IABP, intra-aortic balloon pump; PRBC, packed red blood cells; PTX, pneumothorax; SVT, supra-ventricular tachycardia. (*From* Stephens RS, Whitman G. Postoperative critical care of the adult cardiac surgical patient. Part II: Procedure-specific considerations, management of complications, and quality improvement. Crit Care Med. 2015;43(9):1995-2014; with permission.)

However, several other minimally invasive cardiac devices are also available on the market. Accuracy and validity studies for most of these devices are still ongoing; however, four of the most commonly used devices are illustrated here according to principles of operation, advantages and disadvantages, and supporting evidence.

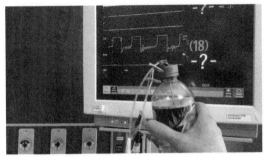

Fig. 2. Limitations of cardiac filling pressures, such as the central venous pressure (CVP). Limitations of cardiac filling pressures are illustrated by a transduced soda bottle exercise. After emptying the soda and filling with water, a hole is drilled through the bottle cap. A central line is inserted through the cap and the distal port is transduced. When the bottle is gently squeezed, pressure rises. However, when the bottle is released, the pressure wave on the monitor decreases. During this cycle of squeezing and releasing, the volume in the bottle never changes. These compliance and resistance factors, independent of volume, help explain factors that render pressures, such as the CVP, unreliable for measuring preload or response to fluid.

Pulse Contour Method

Principles of operation
The pulse contour method enables measurement of CO and SV from arterial lines. Values are obtained based on the greater than 100-year-old principle that pulse pressure is directly proportional to SV, and inversely proportional to arterial compliance. Blood flow measured from the arterial line allows CO and SV to be measured on a continuous basis at the bedside. Pulse pressure variation (PPV) and SV variation (SVV) are additional parameters often available to help identify and explain changes in CO.

When patients are mechanically ventilated and without spontaneous respiratory effort, SV may consistently fluctuate during the respiratory cycle. During inspiration in spontaneously breathing patients, the diaphragm drops, intrathoracic pressure decreases, and preload and SV increase. During exhalation, the diaphragm rises, intrathoracic pressure increases, and preload and SV decrease. Some degree of fluctuation of SV during this cycle is normal; however, increased fluctuation may be associated with volume depletion. Percent of fluctuation is measured by values, such as PPV and SVV. PPV[30] and SVV[30,31] are defined as follows:

$$PPV(\%) = \frac{PP_{max} - PP_{min} \times 100}{(PP_{max} + PP_{min})/2}$$

$$SVV(\%) = \frac{SV_{max} - SV_{min} \times 100}{(SV_{max} + SV_{min})/2}$$

PPV and SVV values greater than 10% to 13% may suggest that the patient is likely to be fluid responsive (ie, "If you're high, you may be dry"). Values less than 10% to 13% may suggest that the patient is less likely to be volume responsive and that alternatives to fluid replacement should be considered in hemodynamic optimization situations.

Advantages and disadvantages
A key advantage of the pulse contour method is convenience in patients when an arterial line is already in place. The physiologic principle for monitoring is also sound;

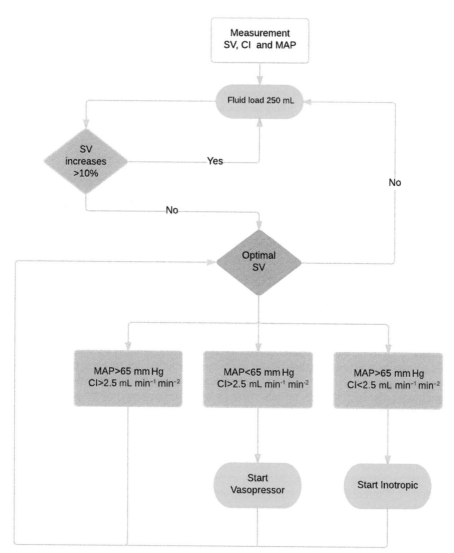

Fig. 3. SV optimization algorithm used in the FEDORA trial. CI, cardiac index; MAP, mean arterial pressure. (*From* Calvo-Vecino J, Ripolles-Melchor J, Mythen M, et al. Effect of goal-directed haemodynamic therapy on postoperative complications in low-moderate risk surgical patients: a multicenter randomized controlled trial (FEDORA trial). Br J Anaesth. 2018;120(4):737; with permission.)

however, several limitations exist that may interfere with the ability to obtain accurate readings. Such clinical conditions include, but are not limited to, spontaneous patient triggering on the mechanical ventilator, changes in vascular compliance or peripheral arterial resistance, atrial fibrillation, dysrhythmias, tidal volumes less than 8 mL/kg, abnormal chest wall compliance (accurate in closed chest conditions only), arteriosclerosis, and extremes in systemic vascular resistance (SVR) or CO (high or low).[16,32–34]

Supporting evidence

The body of supporting literature regarding the pulse contour method is still developing. Accuracy data are consistent in stable patients only when the proper patient conditions are met and factors impacting accuracy are controlled for (discussed previously).[35] Controlling for such factors is often challenging in the intensive care unit (ICU) setting. However, future considerations for further study include a focus on developing more large patient outcome studies, with data measuring impact on length of stay, complications, organ dysfunction, and mortality.[34,36]

Bioreactance

Principles of operation

This technique consists of electrodes on the neck and thorax, and impedance between the electrodes during the cardiac cycle enables derived estimates of CO and SV. Changes in electrical resistivity and amplitude caused by blood volume changes during systole and diastole elicit measured changes in frequency to allow for calculated estimates of preload, afterload, and contractility.[37]

Advantages and disadvantages

The noninvasive application of bioreactance make it a popular method to consider. However, several patient factors are important to be mindful of that could impact the accuracy of a bioreactance device. For example, patients with short necks, excessive secretions interfering with neck electrodes, fluid overloaded patients, pleural fluid, obese patients, movement-associated artifact, and electrode mal-positioning are all mitigating factors that have been shown to be influences limiting accuracy. Although this approach may pose challenges for implementation into critical care, the minimally invasive application may provide interesting opportunities for consideration in outpatient areas, step-down units, or care settings where resources may be limited.

Supporting evidence

Bioreactance is an interesting consideration for care areas that are not as well-positioned to initiate invasive monitoring; however, more studies regarding the accuracy of the device are needed in critical care to validate reliability. In a study of acute respiratory distress syndrome, cardiogenic, and septic shock patients by Fagnoul and colleagues[38] out of Belgium, the study was terminated early because of the CO of PAC and bioreactance actually trending opposite directions. Opportunities for future study include an increased focus on patient outcome studies (measuring impact on length of stay, mortality, complications, and so forth) and studies in critical care.

Esophageal Doppler

Principles of operation

The application of using Doppler to measure red blood cell velocity and flow has been available for more than 50 years. The esophageal Doppler monitor (EDM) is simple flow Doppler tube that is inserted into the esophagus by either the oral or nasal route (usually orally). After the tube is inserted to a depth of approximately T5-T7 (30–40 cm), the probe is then twisted until the beam of the ultrasound transducer at the end of the probe begins to measure descending thoracic aorta blood flow. The ability to capture and measure this flow allows for a beat-by-beat analysis of SV and CO.[39]

Advantages and disadvantages

Generally, any clinician trained to insert an orogastric or nasogastric tube can place an esophageal Doppler. Staff nurses can consistently be trained to be proficient on insertion, signal acquisition, and interpretation after somewhere between three to five esophageal Doppler insertions. However, disadvantages include that often a patient must be intubated and sedated for ease of use. This is because increased patient movement may obscure the signal such that the bedside clinician may need to slightly adjust the depth or rotation of the probe to reacquire the waveform (however, increased patient movement may increase risk of inaccuracy no matter which CO monitor used). More than 43 studies have validated that EDM-measured CO is as accurate as PAC.[39] Advantages include accuracy, the ability to continuously monitor patients, and ease of use.

Supporting evidence

The esophageal Doppler is associated with the most supporting evidence in comparison with any of the currently available minimally invasive CO monitors. Patient outcome data supporting the EDM are also noteworthy. Ten RCTs suggest that when the EDM is used according to the SVO algorithm, patient outcomes are consistently improved with respect to control subjects.[19–28] In each of the 10 RCTs studying SVO, improved patient outcomes include, but were not limited to, complication rates (eg, reduced ileus and postoperative nausea), decreased blood lactate values, decreased vasopressor use, improved time to tolerating oral intake, lower length of stay, and even reduced mortality. A caveat, however, is that most of the literature supporting SVO focuses on the perioperative population. However, research has focused specifically on the area of postoperative cardiac surgery and with similarly improved outcomes.[22] Opportunities for future study include patient populations, such as sepsis and the medical-surgical population.

Capnometry

Ongoing waveform capnometry (measurement of end-tidal CO_2 [$EtCO_2$]) is also a key consideration for any SVO program or any patient being measured with hemodynamic monitoring. Because gas exchange is contingent on adequate right ventricular CO to the lungs, $EtCO_2$ may serve as an indicator of changes in CO. In addition to being able to confirm securement of an advanced airway, hemodynamic reasons supporting continuous $EtCO_2$ monitoring in critical care include, but are not limited to: (1) Capnography trends similarly with CO (increasing or decreasing) as long as minute ventilation remains unchanged. This helps provide CO correlation, trending, and can add confidence in comparison with other minimally invasive CO values. (2) Capnography waveforms also provide indicators of end-expiration, which is helpful when determining respiratory variation on CO or acquiring pulmonary artery occlusion pressure. (3) Changes in the capnometry value can also provide an early indication of when to troubleshoot or investigate a potential change in CO (**Fig. 4**). For example, if minute ventilation remains constant, abrupt drops in $EtCO_2$ may indicate a decreased CO or bleeding to investigate.[40,41]

Devices Summary

Any minimally invasive CO monitor on the market has its own inherent advantages and disadvantages, and no one device is perfect for all patients in all situations. However, all devices generally have metrics to measure preload, afterload, and contractility and should trend similarly. The device that is supported by the most evidence is esophageal Doppler.[42]

END POINTS TO OPTIMIZE STROKE VOLUME
Preload

Generally speaking, all minimally invasive CO monitors available today provide some measurement of preload. For example, bioreactance calculates thoracic fluid content

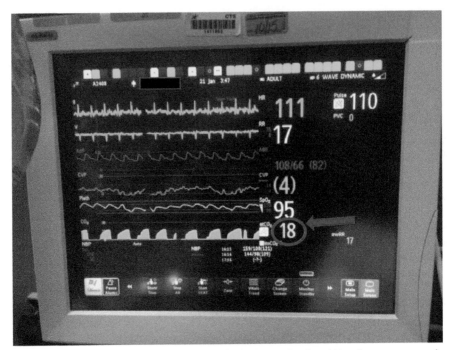

Fig. 4. Waveform capnometry use in hemodynamic monitoring. Waveform capnography EtCO$_2$ is a key component to complement hemodynamic monitoring because of (1) the ability of EtCO$_2$ to provide an early sign of a change in CO, (2) trending similarly to CO to validate additional CO measurements (as long as minute ventilation remains unchanged), and (3) to provide an indicator for end-expiration for hemodynamic measurements.

based on the electrical conductivity through the water and blood content of the chest cavity. Bioreactance, the pulse contour method, and esophageal Doppler all measure SVV and/or PPV. The esophageal Doppler can also display a metric called systolic flow time corrected (FTc). The FTc measures the time spent in systole in milliseconds (corrected for a HR of 60) and is an indication of ventricular filling (**Fig. 5**). The FTc also corresponds to the width of the aortic pulse wave. The waveform narrows (and FTc decreases) as volume depletion worsens (eg, in bleeding), and the wave widens (while FTc increases) as fluid replacement is given.

However, the key tenet, no matter which minimally invasive CO monitor is being used, is the response of SV to fluid challenges. The improvement of SV by greater than or equal to 10% after a fluid challenge is the key indication of fluid responsiveness. Preload, afterload, and contractility metrics are all secondary parameters that are intended to help inform how to best optimize SV.

Contractility

The measurement of contractility has historically been limited with PAC. However, esophageal Doppler provides a more direct reflection of contractility with the measurement of peak velocity (PV). PV corresponds with the amplitude of the aortic pulse wave. When a positive response to inotropes is observed, waveform amplitude and PV increase, often accompanied by an increase in SV. The availability of PV provides a distinct advantage of identifying patients in need of inotropic support, especially in patient situations involving vasopressor up-titration (**Fig. 6**).

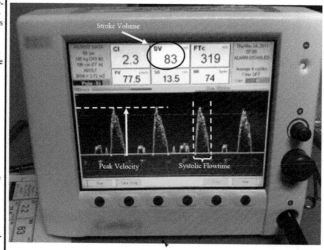

The acronym "SHAG" enables clinicians to observe for key aortic waveform criteria in order to confirm accuracy of values. This stands for:

- **S: Sound**— Confirm whether or not an aortic pulse wave is audible with a doppler "swoosh." Volume depleted patients often have a short, quicker-pitched sound. Hypervolemic patients often have a more prolonged "swoosh" due to the LV attempting to accommodate more volume and flow.

- **H: Heart Rate**— Confirm whether or not the HR on the doppler correlates with the EKG HR.

- **A: Arrows**—Are there arrows on the screen denoting the beginning and end of systole?

- **G: Green Follower**—A thin, green line should also appear covering the top of the wave.

Fig. 5. Esophageal Doppler waveform analysis and signal acquisition. EKG, electrocardiography; LV, left ventricle.

Other minimally invasive CO techniques provide contractility metrics. For example, bioreactance provides a parameter called ventricular ejection time. However, the influence of contractility is usually estimated by deduction in the pulse contour method after evaluating the other hemodynamic data and response to treatment.

Afterload

The measurement of SVR is typically considered a secondary parameter in SVO. Tracking and trending SVR may still provide helpful information that aids in characterizing the hemodynamic profile; however, the primary value of SVR is to monitor for any impact the SVR may have on the SV. All minimally invasive CO monitors generally calculate and display SVR, including esophageal Doppler, bioreactance, and pulse contour devices.

Limitations of Mean Arterial Pressure

The primary objective of administering a fluid challenge is to optimize SV[16] and CO to optimize tissue oxygenation (eg, saturation of mixed-venous oxyhemoglobin [SvO_2]). Although preload, afterload, and contractility parameters allow clinicians insight into how to best optimize SV, the mean arterial pressure (MAP) is still commonly used as a first-line monitoring parameter and resuscitation end point in operating rooms and ICUs. However, many compensatory mechanisms exist to keep MAP normal (**Fig. 7**). This is a reason why MAP is such a late sign of patient changes. Yet, MAP is still often identified as one of the most important and first-line monitoring parameters. Although CO and SV may trend similarly with MAP, changes in pressure are often secondary to changes in blood flow. For example, in bleeding patients, SV decreases first as the left ventricle (LV) begins to fill with less blood. If the blood loss is not

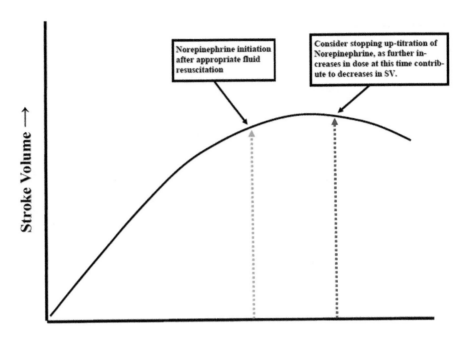

Fig. 6. SV response to vasopressor titration. This figure illustrates how SV may often increase when vasopressors are initiated. However, in this example, if norepinephrine is repeatedly uptitrated without regard to SV, a "point of diminishing returns" along the curve may exist and the increased norepinephrine dose may actually exacerbate afterload and resistance to left ventricular ejection to the point that SV and CO are impeded.

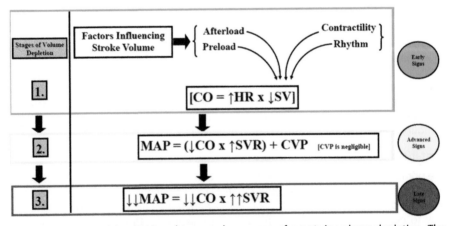

Fig. 7. Factors comprising MAP and temporal sequence of events in volume depletion. The stages of volume depletion may illustrate why SV is an earlier and more sensitive indicator of volume responsiveness, whereas MAP is a late sign of volume depletion. In stage 1, SV decreases because of low ventricular filling. Heart increases to compensate. In stage 2, SVR increases to shunt blood centrally to the vital organs and compensate for the decreased CO. Finally, in stage 3, after the tissues have exhausted consuming an increased amount of oxygen off of the hemoglobin, MAP falls as a final step once all compensatory mechanisms have failed. CVP, central venous pressure.

corrected soon enough or aggressively enough, MAP drops eventually as a late sign because blood flow decreases before pressures decrease. Initially in this scenario, SV continues to decrease while MAP stays the same, and compensatory mechanisms must fail in order for MAP to finally decrease. Vasoactive infusions and fluid replacement are ultimately designed to improve SV first and the rest of the hemodynamic variables secondarily as a result of improved SV. This is a key reason why hemodynamic monitoring has shifted from pressure-based monitoring to flow-based monitoring.

Epicardial Pacing to Optimize Cardiac Output

Epicardial pacing has traditionally been a commonly used strategy to optimize CO postcardiac surgery. The influence of pacing on the CO is largely caused by either the pacemaker-mediated increase in HR or an assumed change in the SV. However, at times pacing may actually decrease the SV by creating a more inefficient ventricular contraction. Without an accurate assessment of the SV response to pacing, clinicians may be compelled to overcompensate and increase the paced rate even further to achieve the desired CO. Clinicians may assume that the SV remains constant during the pacemaker initiation process when it likely does not. However, thankfully minimally invasive CO technology has advanced such that now the HR and SV response can be accurately assessed to determine the collective influence on the CO.

Many clinicians have observed CO and blood pressure (BP) either improve or worsen after the initiation of epicardial pacing (eg, hypotension immediately after VVI pacing). This normally occurs because of three main reasons: (1) ventricular filling has increased or decreased, (2) the velocity of blood ejected from the LV is increased or decreased, or (3) the observed change is HR-induced. In many minimally invasive CO techniques, these preload or contractility parameters can be calculated; however the Doppler techniques can directly measure them with FTc and PV. The systolic flow time (FTc) (ie, the time spent in systole) measures ventricular filling and the PV (ie, amplitude of the aortic pulse wave) can measure velocity of blood ejected from the LV. PV is also a reflection of the strength of LV contraction.

SV response can also be assessed in other situations involving pacemaker adjustment in addition to basic adjustments in HR. For example, SV can be assessed in response to changes in the A-V interval, and with the impact of changing modes from A-pacing versus V-pacing versus A-V pacing, and situations involving weaning of pacemaker therapy. Advanced heart failure (HF) care has set a great precedent for the more sophisticated and advanced assessment of CO and SV response to pacing. Advances in minimally invasive CO monitoring have now positioned clinicians to apply what was learned in biventricular pacing for HF to the way they optimize temporary pacemaker therapy postcardiac surgery. The cardiac surgery guidelines identify the type and location of epicardial pacing wires postcardiac surgery to be according to surgeon discretion.[3] However, a cardiac surgery study by Straka and colleagues[43] showed statistically significant greater CO and cardiac index (CI) with DDD biventricular pacing over DDD right ventricle pacing with corrected LV dyssynchrony and better hemodynamic results, indicating opportunities for further study in this area.

CASE STUDIES
Low Preload

A 56-year-old man underwent two-vessel coronary artery bypass grafting (CABG) with aortic valve replacement 2 hours ago (**Table 1**). In this case, the PV greater than 50 suggests that the LV contractility and strength is adequate, ruling out the need for

Table 1
Low preload case study

Time	BP (mm Hg)	HR	CI (L/m²)	SV (mL)	PV (cm/s)	FTc (ms)	SVR (dyne/ s/cm⁵)	SvO₂ (%)	
0800	79/48	106	1.9	42	75	255	1103	49	250 mL 5% albumin bolus initiated x1
0810	84/54	98	2.0	66	76	295	1097	56	After 250 mL 5% albumin bolus
0820	97/61	92	2.5	68	74	332	1112	68	After second 250 mL 5% albumin bolus

inotropes at this time. As volume is administered, the aortic waveform widens (and FTc increases) because of the improvement of ventricular filling. The increase in flow can also be identified and confirmed via the Doppler auditory signal. SV increases by greater than or equal to 10% (the determination of fluid responsiveness) until fluid challenges are appropriately stopped because of SV improvements less than or equal to 10% from 66 mL to 68 mL.

Low Cardiac Index

A 72-year-old woman with a preoperative ejection fraction of 35% underwent a four-vessel CABG 4 hours ago (**Table 2**). The immediate postoperative warming protocol is complete and core temperature from the PAC is 98.5°F. A total of 500 mL of 5% albumin has been administered to increase the CI and SV only improved from 48 mL to 49 mL after the last bolus, suggesting that no further volume administration is needed. However, the PV of 38 suggests the LV is still weak and unable to meet the oxygen demand of the tissues based on an SvO₂ of 54%. Dobutamine is initiated at 5 μg/kg/min and CI, SV, and PV all increase as expected, bringing the SV from 49 mL to 62 mL and SvO₂ to 67%.

Cardiac Tamponade

A 67-year-old man underwent a four-vessel CABG with MAZE procedure for atrial fibrillation 7 hours ago (**Table 3**). Chest tube output has been consistently observed to be 200 mL to 225 mL per hour since the patient has been out of surgery. Two units

Table 2
Low CI case study

Time	BP (mm Hg)	HR	CI (L/m²)	SV (mL)	PV (cm/s)	FTc (ms)	SVR (dyne/ s/cm⁵)	SvO₂ (%)	
1000	86/44	111	1.8	47	38	296	1103	49	Warmed to 98.5°
1010	89/53	92	2.0	48	39	334	1097	53	After 500 mL 5% albumin bolus
1020	91/56	91	2.1	49	38	337	1112	54	Previous albumin bolus finished Initiation of dobutamine 5 μg/kg/min
1030	110/66	97	2.6	62	59	344	1009	67	Dobutamine at 5 μg/kg/min

Table 3								
Cardiac tamponade case study								
Time	BP (mm Hg)	HR	CI (L/m²)	SV (mL)	PV (cm/s)	FTc (ms)	SVR (dyne/ s/cm⁵)	SvO₂ (%)	
1400	96/55	94	2.2	42	43	301	1097	46	Hgb 6.7, Hct 21%
1410	90/49	97	2.0	44	41	381	1103	49	After 2 unit PRBCs transfused
1420	85/44	103	1.8	41	44	369	1112	42	After epinephrine initiated at 2.5 μg/min
1430	81/39	110	1.7	40	39	390	997	39	Taken back to OR

Abbreviations: Hct, hematocrit; Hg, hemoglobin; OR, operating room; PRBCs, packed red blood cells.

of packed red blood cells are transfused to replace the blood loss; however, this only improved SV from 42 mL to 44 mL. Because of decreasing BP, CI, SvO₂, and PV, an epinephrine drip is initiated. However, all of the previously mentioned parameters do not respond to the epinephrine drip and the FTc continues to increase to 390 ms. Increased FTc in this case suggests the LV is failing and unable to keep up with increasing intrathoracic and juxtacardiac pressure demands. The patient is then taken back to the operating room for mediastinal exploration.

Low Afterload

An 81-year-old woman is being recovered postoperatively in the cardiac ICU following a one-vessel CABG with aortic valve replacement (**Table 4**). Approximately 20 minutes after transfer from the operating room to the ICU, the arterial BP drifts down to 79/48. Because of an SvO₂ of 49%, tachycardia, SV of 61 mL, and a FTc of 255 ms suggesting volume depletion, a 250-mL fluid challenge of 5% albumin is initiated. SV increases from 61 mL to 79 mL (>10%) after the albumin. Because the SV increased greater than 10% and the FTc increased from 255 ms to 296 ms suggesting the patient is fluid-responsive, another bottle of albumin is administered according to the SVO algorithm. After the second bottle of albumin is finished, the SV is observed to only have improved from 79 mL to 81 mL (<10% improvement), suggesting no more fluid is necessary and a point of diminishing returns has been achieved along the Starling curve. Because the SV has now been optimized with volume replacement and the

Table 4								
Low afterload case study								
Time	BP (mm Hg)	HR	CI (L/m²)	SV (mL)	PV (cm/s)	FTc (ms)	SVR (dyne/ s/cm⁵)	SvO₂	
2100	79/48	109	2.4	61	81	255	812	49%	250 mL 5% albumin bolus given
2110	83/54	98	2.6	79	78	296	789	56%	Another 250 mL 5% albumin bolus given
2120	81/55	94	2.5	81	79	342	798	57%	Albumin bolus finished Levophed initiated at 5 μg/min
2140	99/59	87	2.6	82	78	344	1089	67%	Levophed infusing

PV is 79, preload and contractility, respectively, have been addressed. Treatment is still required because of an arterial BP of 81/55 and an SvO_2 of 57%. Preload and contractility have been optimized, which leaves afterload as the third and last component of SV to focus on. Levophed 5 μg/min is initiated and BP, SVR, and SvO_2 improve to target levels.

Use of SVO can guide the clinician regarding when to initiate vasopressors, when to titrate them, and by how much to titrate them. For example, after preload and contractility have been optimized, the initiation of vasopressors will likely yield additional and measurable improvement in SV. However, if vasopressors are up-titrated without attention to the impact on SV, there is risk of increasing afterload to a point such that the resistance to LV ejection is more impeded than it is improved by the vasopressor. This reinforces why SV is a key resuscitation end point for any vasoactive infusion and why inherent dangers exist in using a BP or MAP target as a primary end point for titration independent of SV, which may lead to a potential overuse or misuse of vasopressors (see **Fig. 6**).

NURSING CONSIDERATIONS
Signal Acquisition

Although advancements have been made with signal acquisition in many of the minimally invasive hemodynamic monitors on the market, a trained clinician is always required to validate the accuracy of signal acquisition and that risk of artifact and false readings are minimized. Hemodynamic monitors are only as valuable as the clinician's ability to acquire, interpret, and appropriately incorporate the data into a treatment plan.

In pulse contour techniques, inaccurate, positional, or dampened arterial lines may obscure results. These devices also require regular recalibration because of highly derived algorithms in the software to correct for physiologic factors to maintain accuracy. Bioreactance devices are also influenced by poor electrode adherence, and patient situations including, but not limited to, patients with oily skin, diaphoresis, excessive hair, or oral secretions that may drip down affecting neck electrodes. Pleural effusions or obese patients also influence bioreactance readings because of the increased electrical resistivity created by water and soft tissue through which to conduct the signal between electrodes.

Doppler is a long-standing technique used for measuring blood flow, such as in carotid Dopplers, cranial Dopplers, venous Dopplers, and echocardiograms. Accuracy studies also support Doppler use in hemodynamic monitoring, because 43 studies suggest that esophageal Doppler is as accurate as PAC for measuring CO and SV.[39] In fact, Doppler has also been found to be as accurate and consistent as an aortic flow probe in patients undergoing cardiac surgery.[44] Maintaining accuracy with esophageal Doppler can also be aided with the use of a simple acronym (SHAG), which reminds clinicians to evaluate for four key waveform analysis criteria first before measurements could be considered valid (see **Fig. 5**).

Additional Monitoring, Treatment, and Surveillance Considerations

Treating decreased stroke volume post–initial fluid resuscitation
According to the SVO algorithm, most fluid challenges and treatment occur early in the resuscitation (eg, within the first 3–6 hours postoperatively). However, SVO can still guide hemodynamic optimization 12 hours postoperatively, 24 hours postoperatively,

or beyond. Any time after the initial fluid loading, if the SV decreases greater than 10%, the patient can be reentered into the fluid challenge loop of the algorithm (see **Fig. 3**).

Doppler as conservative measurement

Another advantage of Doppler monitoring is that Doppler never overestimates blood flow. Doppler-based parameters, such as stroke distance (ie, the distance the column of fluid moves during systole) and PV, are directly measured parameters and not calculated or derived. Therefore, any accurate values obtained from Doppler-based devices provide at the least, a conservative estimate of blood flow, enabling the clinician to be confident in measurements and that the physiologic flow will never be lower than what the Doppler indicates.

Application of reference ranges

Reference ranges are necessary whenever initially becoming familiar with a new device for minimally invasive CO monitoring (**Table 5**). However, reference ranges are limited because of they may not apply to all patients. What is considered normal, expected, or baseline values for every patient varies. In fact, what is considered normal for a patient may vary day-to-day or even hour-to-hour depending on changes in underlying condition, HR, ventilator settings, core temperature, changes in medications or drips, and so forth. Rather, it is how values respond to changes in treatment or condition according to a trend over time that dictates what is considered normal for that patient at any moment in time.

Fluid challenge administration

The rate at which fluid challenges are administered cannot be overemphasized. Blood flow often decreases before BP decreases, creating what some authors call occult hypovolemia. Hypovolemia is also a time-sensitive condition because tissues become deprived of oxygen and nutrients. This may often necessitate fluid replacement to be administered rapidly, faster than the 999 mL per hour that is the maximum infusion rate of most commercially available intravenous (IV) pumps. Instead, fluid boluses should be administered via pressure bags or rapid infusion tubing whenever appropriate. Administering fluid challenges via two lines wide open simultaneously is another consideration. Gauge of vascular access is an additional consideration for rapid fluid administration. For example, a large-gauge peripheral IV catheter in the upper arm or introducer sheath allows for more rapid

Table 5	
Hemodynamic reference ranges	
Parameter	**Reference Range**
Stroke volume	50–100 mL
Stroke index	25–45 mL/m^2
Stroke volume variation	<10%–13%
Pulse pressure variation	<10%–13%
Cardiac output	5–10 L/min
Cardiac index	2.5–4 L/m^2
Peak velocity	50–120 cm/s
Systolic flow time	330–360 ms
SvO$_2$ (mixed venous oxyhemoglobin)	60%–75%
Systemic vascular resistance	900–1300 dyne/s/cm^5

fluid administration than any lumen of most conventional triple-lumen catheter central lines. These more rapid infusion considerations also yield a more dramatic increase in SV.

Administration of fluid challenges in patients with heart failure

Using response to fluid challenges as the criteria for subsequent fluid challenges according to the SVO algorithm guides clinicians to individualize or customize the amount of fluid administered based on that specific patient's physiology. The dose-based-response framework in the algorithm can help safeguard against fluid overloading or underloading. This can help avoid complications of occult hypovolemia and fluid overload complications, such as pulmonary edema and third spacing. This is particularly helpful in patients with HF or delicate fluid-volume balances. A stigma or fear is often associated with administering IV fluid to patients with HF because of a hyperavoidance of fluid overload. However, the SVO algorithm can increase the likelihood that patients with HF will receive as much fluid as they truly need while avoiding fluid overload. Although patients with HF have a pressure-volume curve that is shifted downward and to the right (**Fig. 8**), the SVO process for patients with HF is the same. As a result, the SVO algorithm can thereby help decrease the likelihood of

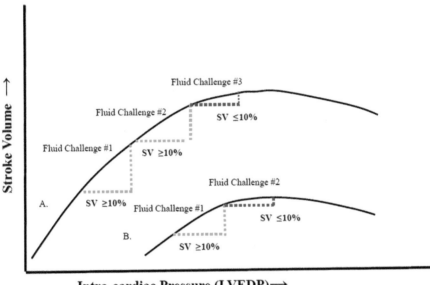

Fig. 8. SV optimization along pressure-volume curve. This figure depicts the cardiac pressure-volume curve in which SV increases as left ventricular end-diastolic pressure increases. *Example A* is a normally functioning and compliant left ventricle. Fluid challenges are repeated appropriately as the SV improves by ≥10% (ie, "recruitable" cardiac output). However, IV boluses are stopped after Fluid Challenge #3 because the SV has stopped improving by ≥10%. *Example B* illustrates a pressure-volume curve of a patient with HF, which is shifted downward and to the right. The fluid challenge is repeated and then stopped appropriately using the same methodology as *Example A*. However, *Example B* illustrates how the SVO algorithm can enable clinicians to give fluid with confidence in patients with HF. SVO can guide clinicians to adequately fluid resuscitate patients with HF with less fear of pulmonary edema or fluid overload. LVEDP, left ventricular end-diastolic pressure.

end-organ damage in patients with HF, a particularly vulnerable patient population that is already at risk for end-organ damage because of decreased CO. In fact, in a multicenter study (N = 18,122) of patients with sepsis with intermediate lactate values, patients in the sepsis bundle intervention group with a history of HF or kidney disease had a more significant (P<.01) decreased mortality compared with patients without this history.[45]

FUTURE CONSIDERATIONS
Implications for Future Research

Despite the increased amount of research already in support of SVO, more research is needed. Most of the studies validating SVO for fluid optimization have been performed in the perioperative population. Further study is needed in medical surgical populations, such as sepsis, and in at-risk populations, such as HF.

Passive Leg Raise

One limitation of SVO is that to predict fluid-responsiveness, one must administer fluid to determine if the patient will respond to the fluid. This can pose challenges in patients with an already tenuous fluid balance, or patients where the initial "test dose" fluid challenge of the SVO algorithm may already be considered too much. Patients with capillary leak may also be at increased risk for this reason. As a result, the passive leg raise (PLR) maneuver may be used to provide predictive value for fluid-responsiveness without requiring fluid to be administered to make the determination.

The PLR maneuver to determine fluid responsiveness is simple. Stage one involves acquiring SV and CO baseline measurements in a supine patient with the head of bed at 30° to 45°. In stage two, SV and CO are repeated with the trunk of the patient flat with legs elevated 45°. Stage two essentially provides an endogenous fluid challenge of 200 mL to 250 mL of blood to the central circulation. Any potential SV or CO response at this time would only require 90 seconds to manifest. Next, a final set of CO and SV measurements may be taken with the patient again supine with head of bed at 45°. However, the key fundamental determinant of fluid responsiveness remains the same: evaluation centers around the evaluation of whether or not SV is greater than or equal to 10% after the PLR in stage 2. If the SV is greater than or equal to 10% in stage 2 compared with stage 1, then the patient is considered likely fluid responsive with a sensitivity of 85% and a specificity of 91%.[46]

SUMMARY

The hemodynamic monitoring landscape is rapidly evolving from pressure-based and static parameters to more blood flow–based and dynamic parameters. Even in the realm of cardiac surgery, PAC is no longer considered a standard of care as more minimally invasive CO monitoring techniques are considered. However, in addition to technical considerations of new devices, resuscitation strategies by which these devices would be used are also evolving. Regardless of the CO monitor used, SVO is the resuscitation algorithm supported by the most evidence. Each emerging minimally invasive CO monitor has unique advantages and disadvantages and no one device is perfect for all patients in all situations. However, the device supported by the most evidence is esophageal Doppler. Further research is needed regarding SVO patient outcomes studies in populations, such as medical-surgical and sepsis. However, SVO for fluid optimization in the perioperative population is supported by the equivalent of level 1A evidence. Until a standard of care for hemodynamic monitoring in cardiac surgery is more clearly established, best available evidence suggests the use of dynamic parameters as appropriate and the avoidance of cardiac filling pressures, such as central venous pressure, to be used as primary end points for fluid resuscitation.

REFERENCES

1. Connors A, Speroff T, Dawson N, et al. The effectiveness of right heart catheterization in the initial care of critically ill patients. SUPPORT Investigators. JAMA 1996;276(11):889–97.
2. Pulmonary Artery Catheter Consensus Conference Participants Pulmonary artery catheter consensus conference: consensus statement. Crit Care Med 1997; 25(6):910.
3. Stephens RS, Whitman G. Postoperative critical care of the adult cardiac surgical patient. Part I: routine postoperative care. Crit Care Med 2015;43(7):1477–97.
4. Balk E, Raman G, Chung M, et al. Evaluation of the evidence on benefits and harms of pulmonary artery catheter use in critical care settings. Rockville (MD): Agency for Healthcare Research and Quality; 2008. Available at: http://www.cms.gov/determinationprocess/downloads/id55TA.pdf. Accessed October 29, 2014.
5. Rajaram SS, Desai NK, Kalra A, et al. Pulmonary artery catheters for adult patients in intensive care. Cochrane Database Syst Rev 2013;(2):CD003408.
6. Connors AF Jr, Dawson NV, Shaw PK, et al. Hemodynamic status in critically ill patients with and without acute heart disease. Chest 1990;98(5):1200–6.
7. Dawson NV, Connors AF Jr, Speroff T, et al. Hemodynamic assessment in managing the critically ill: is physician confidence warranted? Med Decis Making 1993; 13(3):258–66.
8. Eisenberg PR, Jaffe AS, Schuster DP. Clinical evaluation compared to pulmonary artery catheterization in the hemodynamic assessment of critically ill patients. Crit Care Med 1984;12(7):549–53.
9. Hoeft A, Schorn B, Weyland A, et al. Bedside assessment of intravascular volume status in patients undergoing coronary bypass surgery. Anesthesiology 1994; 81(1):76–86.
10. Iregui MG, Prentice D, Sherman G, et al. Physicians' estimates of cardiac index and intravascular volume based on clinical assessment versus transesophageal Doppler measurements obtained by critical care nurses. Am J Crit Care 2003; 12(4):336–42.
11. Neath SX, Lazio L, Guss DA. Utility of impedance cardiography to improve physician estimation of hemodynamic parameters in the emergency department. Congest Heart Fail 2005;11(1):17–20.
12. Staudinger T, Locker GJ, Laczika K, et al. Diagnostic validity of pulmonary artery catheterization for residents at an intensive care unit. J Trauma 1998;44(5):902–6.
13. Celoria G, Steingrub J, Vickers-Lahti M, et al. Clinical assessment of hemodynamic values in two surgical intensive care units: effects of therapy. Arch Surg 1990;125(8):1036–9.
14. Marik P, Cavallazzi R. Does the central venous pressure predict fluid responsiveness? An updated meta-analysis and a plea for some common sense. Crit Care Med 2013;41(7):1774–81.
15. Benington S, Ferris P, Nirmalan M. Emerging trends in minimally invasive haemodynamic monitoring and optimization of fluid therapy. Eur J Anaesthesiol 2009; 26(11):893–905.

16. Marik P, Monnet X, Teboul JL. Hemodynamic parameters to guide fluid therapy. Ann Intensive Care 2011;1(1):1–9.

17. Marik P, Baram M, Vahid B. Does central venous pressure predict fluid responsiveness? A systematic review of the literature and the tale of seven mares. Chest 2008;134(1):172–8.

18. Marik P. Surviving sepsis: going beyond the guidelines. Ann Intensive Care 2011; 1(17):1–6.

19. Chytra I, Pradl R, Bosman R, et al. Esophageal Doppler-guided fluid management decreases blood lactate levels in multiple-trauma patients: a randomized controlled trial. Crit Care 2007;11(1):R24.

20. Conway DH, Mayall R, Abdul-Latif MS, et al. Randomized controlled trial investigating the influence of intravenous fluid titration using esophageal Doppler monitoring during bowel surgery. Anaesthesia 2002;57(9):845–9.

21. Gan TJ, Soppitt A, Maroof M, et al. Goal-directed intraoperative fluid administration reduces length of hospital stay after major surgery. Anesthesiology 2002; 97(4):820–6.

22. McKendry M, McGloin H, Saberi D, et al. Randomised controlled trial assessing the impact of a nurse delivered, flow monitored protocol for optimisation of circulatory status after cardiac surgery. BMJ 2004;329(7460):258–61.

23. Mythen MG, Webb AR. Perioperative plasma volume expansion reduces the incidence of gut mucosal hypoperfusion during cardiac surgery. Arch Surg 1995; 130(4):423–9.

24. Sinclair S, James S, Singer M. Intraoperative intravascular volume optimization and length of hospital stay after repair of proximal femoral fracture: randomised controlled trial. BMJ 1997;315(7113):909–12.

25. Venn R, Steele A, Richardson P, et al. Randomized controlled trial to investigate influence of the fluid challenge on duration of hospital stay and perioperative morbidity in patients with hip fractures. Br J Anaesth 2002;88(1):65–71.

26. Wakeling HG, McFall MR, Jenkins CS, et al. Intraoperative oesophageal Doppler guided fluid management shortens postoperative hospital stay after major bowel surgery. Br J Anaesth 2005;95(5):634–42.

27. Noblett S, Snowden C, Shenton B, et al. Randomized clinical trial assessing the effect of Doppler-optimized fluid management on outcome after elective colorectal resection. Br J Surg 2006;93(9):1069–76.

28. Calvo-Vecino J, Ripolles-Melchor J, Mythen M, et al. Effect of goal-directed haemodynamic therapy on postoperative complications in low-moderate risk surgical patients: a multicenter randomized controlled trial (FEDORA trial). Br J Anaesth 2018;120(4):734–44.

29. Hadian M, Pinsky M. Evidence-based review of the use of the pulmonary artery catheter: impact data and complications. Crit Care 2006;10(Suppl 3):S8.

30. Arimanickam G, Manikandan S. Correlation of systolic pressure variation, pulse pressure variation and stroke volume variation in different preload conditions following a single dose mannitol infusion in elective neurosurgical patients. J Neuroanaesth Crit Care 2016;3:219–26.

31. Li C, Lin F, Fu S, et al. Stroke volume variation for prediction of fluid responsiveness in patients undergoing gastrointestinal surgery. Int J Med Sci 2013;10(2): 148–55.

32. Mehta Y, Arora D. Newer methods of cardiac output monitoring. World J Cardiol 2014;6(9):1022–9.

33. Greenfield N, Balk R. Evaluating the adequacy of fluid resuscitation in patients with septic shock: controversies and future directions. Hosp Pract 2012;40(2): 147–57.

34. Critchley L. Pulse contour analysis: is it able to reliably detect changes in cardiac output in the haemodynamically unstable patient? Crit Care 2011;15:106.

35. Slagt C, Malagon I, Groeneveld A. Systematic review of uncalibrated arterial pressure waveform analysis to determine cardiac output and stroke volume variation. Br J Anaesth 2014;112(4):626–37.

36. Reisner A. Academic assessment of arterial pulse contour analysis: missing the forest for the trees? Br J Anaesth 2016;116(6):733–6.

37. Mohammed I, Phillips C. Techniques for determining cardiac output in the intensive care unit. Crit Care Clin 2010;26:355–64.

38. Fagnoul D, Vincent JL, De Backer D. Cardiac output measurements using the bioreactance technique in critically ill patients. Crit Care 2012;16:460.

39. Schober P, Loer S, Schwarte L. Perioperative hemodynamic monitoring with transesophageal Doppler technology. Anesth Analg 2009;109:340–53.

40. Johnson A, Schweitzer D, Ahrens T. Time to throw away your stethoscope? Capnography: evidence-based patient monitoring technology. J Radiol Nurs 2011;30: 25–34.

41. Johnson A, Mohajer-Esfahani M. Exploring hemodynamics: a review of current and emerging noninvasive monitoring techniques. Crit Care Nurs Clin North Am 2014;26(3):357–75.

42. Johnson A, Ahrens T. Stroke volume optimization: the new hemodynamic algorithm. Crit Care Nurse 2015;35(1):11–27.

43. Straka F, Pirk J, Pindak M, et al. Biventricular pacing in the early postoperative period after cardiac surgery. Physiol Res 2011;60:877–85.

44. DiCorte C, Latham P, Greilich P, et al. Esophageal Doppler monitor determinations of cardiac output and preload during cardiac operations. Ann Thorac Surg 2000;69:1782–6.

45. Liu V, Morehouse J, Marelich G, et al. Multicenter implementation of a treatment bundle for patients with sepsis and intermediate lactate values. Am J Respir Crit Care Med 2016;193(11):1264–70.

46. Monnet X, Marik P, Teboul JL. Passive leg raising for predicting fluid responsiveness: a systematic review and meta-analysis. Intensive Care Med 2016;42(12): 1935–47.

Managing Vasoactive Medications Following Cardiothoracic Surgery

Michael Petty, PhD, RN, APRN, CNS, CCNS*,
Kathleen Kopp, BSN, MAOL, RN, CCRN

KEYWORDS

- Vasoactive medications • Cardiac output • Blood pressure • Preload • Contractility
- Afterload • Heart rate

KEY POINTS

- Nurses use invasive and noninvasive strategies to evaluate the patient's condition and physiologic derangements contributing to inadequate cardiac output and/or blood pressure.
- Selection and titration of vasoactive medications is driven by patient physiology.
- Balancing cardiac output and blood pressure while minimizing the impact on myocardial oxygen demand is an important component of titration of vasoactive medications.

INTRODUCTION

Since the 1950s, open heart surgery has saved countless lives. Individuals limited by defects of cardiac structures and/or great vessels, blocked coronary arteries, and defective cardiac valves, among other disorders, have undergone surgical correction (eg, repair of congenital anomalies) or restoration of function (eg, valve repair, valve replacement, and coronary artery bypass grafting). The goal of those procedures is to relieve symptoms, improve cardiac function, and improve the duration and quality of life.

However, in the short term the surgery itself can have a profound negative effect on cardiovascular physiology. The combined impact of induced hypothermia, cardioplegia, cardiopulmonary bypass, kaliuresis, and cardiac reperfusion contribute to depression of cardiac function; the associated release of cytokines often stimulates a systemic inflammatory response.[1] In addition, cardiac surgery is associated with a hypermetabolic state that can persist for up to 48 hours.[2] Ineffectively managed, these

Disclosure: The authors have nothing to disclose.
Cardiovascular ICU (Unit 4E), University of Minnesota Medical Center, 500 Harvard Street Southeast, Minneapolis, MN 55455, USA
* Corresponding author.
E-mail address: Mpetty1@fairview.org

Crit Care Nurs Clin N Am 31 (2019) 349–366
https://doi.org/10.1016/j.cnc.2019.05.005
0899-5885/19/© 2019 Elsevier Inc. All rights reserved.

negative effects can result in low cardiac output syndrome and associated hypotension. The resultant inadequate perfusion of end organs is associated with anaerobic metabolism, which can contribute to metabolic acidosis, increased morbidity and mortality, and significantly prolonged length of stay in the intensive care unit (ICU) and hospital.

Patient management in the early period following cardiothoracic surgery frequently includes titration of vasoactive medications to support hemodynamic function and end-organ perfusion. Caregivers' understanding of postoperative physiology along with the pharmacology and associated physiology of those drugs helps them to recognize the rationale for drug selection and initiation as well as strategies associated with drug titration. Applying this knowledge will facilitate adequate cardiac output and blood pressure to support organ function; delivery of oxygenated, nutrient-rich blood supports the patient's rapid recovery from the rigors of cardiac surgery, promotes candidacy for early extubation and early mobility, and reduces length of stay in the ICU.

The purpose of this article is to focus on continuous vasoactive infusions commonly prescribed following cardiothoracic surgery and their role in supporting recovery from a cardiovascular surgical procedure.

IMPORTANCE OF ASSOCIATING CARDIAC OUTPUT AND BLOOD PRESSURE TO ACHIEVE ADEQUATE ORGAN PERFUSION

It is crucial to integrate the importance of forward flow (cardiac output/cardiac index) with organ perfusion. Organ perfusion depends on adequate blood pressure (systolic blood pressure 100–120 mm Hg, mean arterial pressure 60–70 mm Hg),[3] the result of the intersection of cardiac output and peripheral vascular resistance (**Table 1**). Cardiac output is the product of the volume of blood ejected with each beat of the heart (stroke volume) and the number of beats per minute (heart rate). Cardiac index relates cardiac output to body size and is derived by dividing cardiac output by body surface area (BSA) (see **Table 1**). Stroke volume (**Table 2**) has 3 contributing elements: preload (the volume of blood in the ventricle at the end of diastole); contractility (the force exerted by the ventricle against that blood volume); and afterload (the resistance which the ventricle must overcome for blood to move into the aorta and to the systemic circulation). The analysis of hemodynamics (see related Alexander Johnson and colleagues' article, "Stroke Volume Optimization: Utilization of the Newest Cardiac Vital Sign: Considerations in Recovery from Cardiac Surgery," in this issue) can assist the clinician to understand which element of cardiac output (stroke volume or heart rate) and/or blood pressure needs to be treated to optimize flow and perfusion.[4]

While blood pressure directly depends on cardiac output, it is also affected by peripheral vascular resistance generated by systemic arterioles (see **Table 1**). In the setting of vasoplegia, the peripheral arterioles are incapable of constricting; even supranormal cardiac output may not generate adequate pressure to overcome the lack of peripheral resistance. In this setting a cardiac output of greater than 5 to 6 L/min may not be adequate to generate a minimum mean arterial blood pressure

Table 1	
Mathematics of blood flow and blood pressure	
Cardiac output (CO) (L/min) =	Stroke volume (SV) × heart rate (HR)
Cardiac index (CI) (L/min/m^2) =	Cardiac output ÷ body surface area (BSA)
Blood pressure (BP) (mm Hg) =	Cardiac output (CO) × peripheral vascular resistance (PVR)

Table 2	
Determinants of stroke volume	
Preload	Volume in the ventricle at the end of diastole
Contractility	Force exerted against ventricular volume to expel blood from the ventricle and into the great vessels
Afterload	Resistance the ventricle must overcome to eject blood into the great vessels, created by arterioles

of 60 to 70 mm Hg. Thus, although hypotension following cardiac surgery most often is correctly attributed to decreased cardiac output, effective management requires that the clinician gather enough information to validate this conclusion and treat inadequate peripheral vascular resistance when indicated.

Patient assessment is the first step in determining the necessity, appropriateness, and effectiveness of vasoactive medication administration. The caregiver should integrate invasive and noninvasive signals of adequate or inadequate cardiac output and organ perfusion in that evaluation. Commonly, cardiac output measurements through continuous cardiac output technology, thermodilution cardiac output evaluation, or derived cardiac output using the Fick equation are the first tools at the clinician's disposal. However, other physiologic measures such as heart rate and mixed venous oxygen saturation can also provide indications that cardiac output is inadequate to meet the patient's metabolic needs. Blood pressure, urine output, and assessment of peripheral perfusion such as skin temperature are additional data points available to be integrated into the comprehensive analysis of the patient's cardiac output and organ perfusion. Laboratory values such as pH, bicarbonate, and lactate round out the picture of the adequacy of organ perfusion.

Vasoactive medications can play a role in affecting any of the 4 components of cardiac output. Venodilators can reduce excessive preload, decreasing demand on the right ventricle and permitting more effective cardiac function; inotropic agents can increase the contractile force of the myocardium, augmenting stroke volume; vasoconstrictors can increase peripheral vascular resistance, raising blood pressure to desired levels; and arterial vasodilators can decrease the peripheral resistance to ejection, resulting in greater blood volume ejected with a similar myocardial oxygen demand. Finally, chronotropic agents can be used to optimize heart rate such that the heart has time to fill yet ejects frequently enough to support adequate cardiac output.

Reduced cardiac output may generate a response of arteriolar vasoconstriction to increase blood pressure and associated end-organ perfusion. This elevation of the afterload may further decrease cardiac output as the weakened ventricle must overcome increasing resistance to eject blood into the systemic circulation. However, as already noted, "normal" cardiac output does not always yield adequate blood pressure to support end-organ perfusion and function either.

These 2 summary elements (cardiac output and blood pressure) create the foundation of goal-directed therapy using vasoactive infusions following cardiovascular surgery. The knowledgeable clinician will keep these competing priorities in mind while titrating vasoactive medications.

ACHIEVING GOALS OF THERAPY

As noted earlier, blood supply to organs depends on adequate flow (cardiac output) and resistance (peripheral vascular resistance) to generate a blood pressure

(pressure = flow × resistance), which supports perfusion of organs and tissues (see **Table 1**). The following sections address the use of vasoactive medications to affect the specific components of cardiac output and blood pressure, which will guide the clinician's decisions regarding medication management.

Optimizing Heart Rate (Chronotropy)

Chronotropy describes the effect on rate or timing of a physiologic process such as heart rate. Chronotropic medications (**Table 3**) are commonly used in patients undergoing cardiac surgery. Although temporary or permanent pacemakers are also commonly seen in cardiac surgery populations, for this discussion medications remain the focus.

Heart rate response to various stressors (including open heart surgery) enhances cardiac output and associated delivery of oxygen to the tissues. It is important to remember that oxygen delivery to the heart muscle itself occurs mostly during the diastolic phase of the cardiac cycle.[5] The diastolic component of the cardiac cycle decreases as heart rate increases; therefore, reduction of heart rate or controlling the heart rate allows for an optimal diastolic period, prolonging coronary perfusion time and improved performance of myocardial contraction.[5]

Positive chronotropic medications increase heart rate whereas conversely, negative chronotropic medications decrease heart rate (see **Table 3**). Many inotropes discussed in **Table 3** have chronotropic effects as well, affecting both heart rate and contractility. Increasing the heart rate to achieve greater cardiac output through the use of various catecholamines or inotropes such as epinephrine, dopamine, or norepinephrine may be necessary to meet tissue oxygen demands. Milrinone, glucagon, and atropine also exhibit positive chronotropic effects in post–cardiac surgery patients; however, their mechanisms of action differ from inotropes. When increasing the heart rate, it is important to keep in mind that such a change will concurrently increase myocardial oxygen consumption and decrease diastolic duration. Balancing these seemingly competing aspects of heart rate adjustment is important to achieving therapeutic goals.

Conversely, reducing the heart rate by administering negative chronotropic medications will also affect cardiac output and, ultimately, myocardial oxygen supply. Although their mechanisms of action differ, medications such as β-blockers, calcium-channel blockers, acetylcholine, and some antiarrhythmics such as amiodarone demonstrate a negative chronotropic effect along with a negative inotropic impact. Treating heart rate variations in the postoperative setting using these various

Table 3	
Chronotropic medications	
Positive Chronotropic Effects (Increased Heart Rate)	**Negative Chronotropic Effects (Decreased Heart Rate)**
Atropine	β-Blockers (eg, metoprolol, sotalol)
Dopamine	Acetylcholine
Epinephrine	Digoxin
Isoproterenol	Nondihydropyridine calcium-channel
Milrinone	blockers (eg, diltiazem, verapamil)

Adapted from Alboni P, Menozzi C, Brignole M, et al. Effects of permanent pacemaker and oral theophylline in sick sinus syndrome: the THEOPACE study: a randomized controlled trial. Circulation. 96(1):260–6; with permission.

agents is critical to patient optimization, but their potential impact on the other elements of cardiac output must be considered.

In the setting of cardiovascular surgery, before initiating rate-modifying medications it is important for the clinician to determine and treat the likely cause of the abnormal heart rate. For example, tachycardia in a patient who is hypovolemic should be treated with fluid resuscitation by administering colloid or crystalloid volume replacement. Similarly, bradycardia may be better addressed by determining its cause before initiating positive chronotropic agents.

Optimizing Preload

Preload depends on the interaction between circulating blood volume and venous tone. Surrogate markers of preload used for assessing fluid status in post–cardiac surgery patients include central venous pressure, pulmonary artery occlusion pressure or wedge pressure, and pulmonary diastolic pressure.[6] Fluid resuscitation is considered the first line of therapy for managing postoperative instability. Four predominant reasons drive fluid resuscitation in postoperative cardiac surgery patients: blood loss; cardiopulmonary bypass–induced inflammatory response resulting in third-spacing of fluid; increased vascular capacitance experienced with rewarming; and increased preload needs secondary to reperfusion injury, myocardial stunning, and decreased ventricular compliance.[6] Inadequate preload is generally treated with infusions of crystalloid or colloid solutions.

Excessive preload is associated with heart failure, acute kidney injury,[6] and increased mortality.[7] Excessive preload can be reduced with diuretics and/or venodilators, specifically nitroglycerin.[6] Nitroglycerin is often the first line of defense in managing excessive preload in postoperative patients because it is relatively inexpensive, moderately effective, and has a short half-life allowing for easy titration in the setting of postoperative instability.[8] With the use of nitroglycerin, myocardial wall tension is reduced as a result of a decrease in ventricular end diastolic pressure, resulting in decreased myocardial oxygen consumption and enhanced oxygen supply.[6]

Enhancing Contractility (Inotropy)

As mentioned earlier, a decrease in cardiac contractility can be attributed to the exogenous chemicals associated with cardioplegia and cardiopulmonary bypass. Routinely used in postoperative management of cardiac surgery patients, inotropes increase tissue oxygen delivery by improving the pumping function of the heart.[9] Inotropes strengthen cardiac contractility, resulting in increased cardiac output, an associated increase in mean arterial pressure, and ultimately improved end-organ perfusion.[10] For most inotropes, the primary mechanism of action involves increasing intracellular calcium either by facilitating its release from the sarcoplasmic reticulum or increasing the cellular influx during the action potential.[10] Inotropic medications increase myocardial oxygen demand; arrhythmogenicity is a known side effect of inotropic use.[6]

Catecholamines, endogenous or synthetic, are the most commonly used types of inotropes. Catecholamines act on the sympathetic nervous system. Cardiac effects associated with catecholamine use are primarily attributed to α-adrenergic and β-adrenergic receptor stimulation.[10] The beta one (β_1) receptor is the primary receptor in cardiac muscle affecting rate and force of contraction. Catecholamines bind to β_1 receptors resulting in an increase of calcium flowing into the cell, released from the sarcoplasmic reticulum. Additional calcium is then available to bind to troponin-C, resulting in enhanced myocardial contractility.[10]

Most inotropes are administered as continuous infusions because of their short medication half-life. Catecholamines are estimated to have a 2-minute half-life and most stable-state blood concentrations of inotropes are achieved within 10 minutes of infusion initiation.[10] A detailed description of inotropic medications and their effects is presented in **Table 4**.

Calcium is required for normal contraction in cardiac, skeletal, and smooth muscle. It is unclear how supplemental calcium administration is useful in the setting of cardiac surgery patients. When extracellular calcium levels are elevated by supplemental administration, systolic function may improve temporarily; however, a negative effect can be seen through reduced diastolic relaxation and enhanced afterload.[8] Exogenous calcium administration has a short effect after administration. The impact of calcium administration may be related to anesthetic processes, blood administration, or solutions used during cardiopulmonary bypass.[8]

Managing Afterload

Various physiologic factors contribute to afterload (eg, aortic stenosis, hypertension, increased peripheral vascular resistance, hypertrophic cardiomyopathy), which creates resistance to ventricular ejection, in turn increasing total myocardial wall stress (or tension) during systole and impeding coronary blood flow during diastole. Increased left ventricular output impedance requires a greater ventricular contractile force to be generated during systole to achieve forward flow of blood, and will result in an increase in myocardial oxygen demand.[13] Because myocardial reserve is already compromised owing to the stresses of the surgical intervention, excessive afterload can significantly reduce cardiac output.

The majority of afterload is contributed by peripheral vascular resistance (PVR). Managing increased PVR can be more complicated because it can be either the cause of decreased cardiac output or the result of it. When cardiac output is inadequate to support blood pressure, the peripheral vasculature responds to signals from baroreceptors in the aortic arch and carotid bodies to increase blood pressure by constricting peripheral arterioles. Although this response will augment blood pressure, the increased afterload can cause a downward spiral of reduced cardiac output.

Afterload can also be increased by the α-adrenergic agents associated with higher doses of inotropes such as epinephrine, norepinephrine, or dopamine being used to increase both cardiac output and blood pressure. In settings of vasodilatory shock or septic shock, norepinephrine has been identified as a drug of choice to increase blood pressure through arterial constriction. Recognizing they are being used to elevate blood pressure, increasing cardiac output and vasoconstriction concurrently requires the clinician to consider again the balance of afterload with organ perfusion.

On the other hand, hypertension is a common occurrence in post–cardiac surgery patients. Increased afterload associated with hypertension also can compromise cardiac function, potentiate bleeding, and jeopardize new anastomoses.[6] Afterload reduction, balanced against maintaining adequate mean arterial pressure, can increase cardiac output significantly, decreasing left ventricular filling volume/pressure.[6,14]

Vasodilators such as nitroglycerin or nitroprusside are short-acting and effective medications for managing hypertension in the immediate postoperative phase. However, because of their vasodilatory effect on both veins and arteries, flow to the right ventricle and pulmonary vasculature may be reduced as a result of peripheral venous pooling of blood volume as well as being associated with instances of hypoxemia.[6,14] Nicardipine, a calcium-channel blocker, is an alternative vasodilating agent that can

Table 4
Inotropic medications

Drug	Classification	Mechanism of Action	Response	Receptor	Dosing	Adverse Effects
Epinephrine	Inotrope (sympathomimetic catecholamine)	Acts at all adrenergic receptor sites, predominately β-agonist	Increased MAP and SVR, CI, HR, blood pressure	Combined α- and β-receptor agonist; higher doses stimulate α receptors	0.01–3 μg/kg/min	Tachycardia, dysrhythmia, mesenteric hypoperfusion
Dobutamine	Inotrope (synthetic catecholamine)	Stimulates β receptors of the heart	Decrease in SVR, increased contractility[3]	α1, β1, and β2	2–20 μg/kg/min	Tachycardia, dysrhythmia, hypotension
Dopamine	Inotropic and chronotropic effects (natural catecholamine and a neurotransmitter)	Low-dose dopaminergic response; medium dose acts at β1 inotropic, high dose acts at α1 vasoconstrictor	Increased HR, cardiac contractility, increased CI, higher doses increase afterload affecting CI	α1, β1, and dopaminergic	1–20 μg/kg/min	Tachycardia, dysrhythmia, mesenteric hypoperfusion
Norepinephrine	Inotropic (sympathomimetic amine)	α-Adrenergic and β-adrenergic	Increased SVR, no or minimal change in CO, coronary artery vasodilation	α- and β-agonist, acts at α1 receptor	0.02–3 μg/kg/min	Peripheral ischemia, mixed effects of myocardial performance, mesenteric hypoperfusion

(continued on next page)

Table 4
(continued)

Drug	Classification	Mechanism of Action	Response	Receptor	Dosing	Adverse Effects
Phenylephrine	synthetic sympathomimetic agent	α-Receptor agonist, minimal β-receptors	Increases BP through vasoconstriction, possible decreased CO	Pure α-agonist	0.5–9 µg/kg/min	Peripheral ischemia, mixed effects of myocardial performance
Vasopressin	Vasoconstrictor (antidiuretic hormone [ADH])	Stimulates the release of vasoconstrictive Ca^{2+} causing contraction of vascular smooth muscle	Increases smooth muscle contraction	V1 receptor coupled with phospholipase C; V2 receptors are stimulated at lower doses resulting in an antidiuretic effect	0–4 units/h	Mixed effects on myocardial performance, mesenteric hypoperfusion, peripheral ischemia, hyponatremia, thrombocytopenia
Milrinone	Bipyridine inotrope/vasodilator	Selectively inhibits peak III cyclic adenosine monophosphate (cAMP) phosphodiesterase isozyme in cardiac and vascular muscle resulting in increased intracellular Ca^{2+}	Positive inotropic and vasodilating effects, increased SV and CO, potential decreased BP, increased HR, decreased PCWP	None	0.1–0.75 µg/kg/min	Arrhythmia, hypotension, thrombocytopenia Use with caution in patients with renal failure

Abbreviations: BP, blood pressure; CI, cardiac index; CO, cardiac output; CVP, central venous pressure; HR, heart rate; MAP, mean arterial pressure; PCWP, pulmonary capillary wedge pressure; PVR, pulmonary vascular resistance; SV, stroke volume; SVR, systemic vascular resistance.
Data from Refs.[9–12]

be used to reduce afterload and lower blood pressure; however, the half-life is longer than that of the other vasodilators.[6] **Table 5** presents medications that affect afterload.

Phosphodiesterase inhibitors such as milrinone, while used to enhance cardiac output, also have a vasodilatory effect on the pulmonary vasculature, reducing right ventricular afterload.[10] Inhaled nitric oxide, an endothelium-derived vascular relaxing factor, and inhaled epoprostenol are newer therapies that can be used to reduce right ventricular afterload postoperatively. In the setting of postoperative cardiac surgery patients, both are best administered via endotracheal tube in a ventilated patient, limiting their utility.[8,15]

Considering Myocardial Oxygen Demand in the Titration of Vasoactive Medications

Finally, it is important to balance achieving adequate cardiac output and blood pressure against myocardial oxygen supply and demand. Given that the heart has undergone a surgical disruption of its normal function, increasing heart rate, contractility, and/or afterload will increase myocardial oxygen demand. As the myocardium likely received reduced oxygen supply during surgery, it is reasonable to conclude that the heart may be unable to respond to significant demands because of reduced oxygen reserve from the operation.

TITRATION PEARLS

The key to successful management of vasoactive medications in the postoperative period following cardiac surgery is to focus on the condition(s) that led to their selection.

1. Begin by confirming that there is adequate preload (normal central venous pressure). If not, consider orders for fluid resuscitation with crystalloid or colloid solutions.
2. If preload is determined to be adequate, reduced cardiac output may be secondary to reduced contractility (commonly seen after a cardiopulmonary bypass run). In this case, orders for inotropes to enhance contractility is an obvious selection. As the heart recovers and contractility and cardiac output increase, weaning of those inotropes is the logical approach.
3. If the administration of sympathetic agents such as dopamine or dobutamine results in an increased heart rate, the observant clinician must consider the possibility that the patient's intravascular volume is inadequate, leading to consideration of additional intravenous volume.
4. If cardiac output is reduced and afterload is increased, careful titration of vasodilators may achieve an increase in cardiac output. Assessing the patient's peripheral perfusion and skin temperature is a useful guide to the degree of peripheral vasodilation present. Furthermore, the increase in cardiac output (flow) offsets the vasodilator's reduction in afterload (resistance), resulting in a minimal net change in blood pressure (see **Table 1**).
5. Continued hypotension in the setting of normal cardiac output often reflects decreased afterload. Uptitrating medications to increase vasoconstriction such as norepinephrine or phenylephrine can help to increase blood pressure and organ perfusion. Norepinephrine does so by stimulating both β and α receptors; phenylephrine by activating α receptors. Determining which to reduce first is based on provider preference and the need to enhance contractility. If contractility is adequate, norepinephrine often would be the first drug to wean; if contractility remains an issue, phenylephrine commonly would be the first medication to reduce.

Table 5
Infusion medications affecting afterload

Drug	Classification	Mechanism of Action	Response	Receptor	Dosing	Adverse Effects
Hydralazine	Vasodilator		Decreased BP, PAWP, left ventricular volume			
Nitroglycerin	Lusitropic vasodilator	Increases guanosine 3′,5′-monophosphate (GMP) in smooth muscle by stimulating guanylate cyclase through formation of free radical nitric oxide = dephosphorylation of the myosin light chain	Decreased CVP, PCWP, left ventricular volume, BP		Infusion 0.1–3 μg/kg/min	Hypotension
Nitroprusside	Lusitropic vasodilator	Increases synthesis of nitric oxide in vascular smooth muscle; creates balanced arterial and venous dilation	Increased CI by reducing afterload; decreased venous pressure, PCWP, LV volume, SVR, BP	Interacts with oxyhemoglobin to produce methemoglobin, cyanide, and nitric oxide; nitric oxide reacts with guanylate cyclase to produce vascular smooth muscle relaxation through cyclic GMP-mediated reduction in intracellular Ca^{2+}	Continuous IV infusion 0.5–3 μg/kg/min	Hypotension, flushing, headaches, tachycardia; cyanide toxicity with prolonged administration Use with caution in patients with renal failure or insufficiency

Abbreviations: BP, blood pressure; CI, cardiac index; CVP, central venous pressure; IV, intravenous; LV, left ventricular; PAWP, pulmonary artery wedge pressure; PCWP, pulmonary capillary wedge pressure; SVR, systemic vascular resistance.
Data from DiPiro J, Talbert R, Yee G, et al. Pharmacotherapy: a pathophysiologic approach. 9th ed. New York: McGraw Hill Education; 2014.

Table 6
Hemodynamic measurements on arrival at ICU through extubation

Hemodynamic Metric	13:00	14:00	15:00	16:00	17:00	18:00	19:00
Temp. (°F)	98.0	97.9	98.2	98.8	99.0	99.5	99.7
HR	81	80	80	80	80	80	80
BP	107/43	94/50	99/53	101/50	107/53	110/55	106/55
MAP	71	67	68	69	72	75	75
RR	16	16	16	16	16	18	23
Spo$_2$	100	100	100	100	100	98	98
CVP	8	—	—	13	—	16	—
PAP	28/16	—	—	30/16	—	29/13	—
PAD	—	—	—	—	—	—	—
SVR	774	—	—	848	—	746	—
CI	2.7	—	—	2.5	—	2.9	—
CO	5.9	—	—	5.5	—	6.4	—
Svo$_2$	72	—	—	71	—	74	—
O$_2$ device	Vent 40%	Vent 40%	Vent 40%	Vent 40%	Vent 40%	Vent 40%	Vent 40%
Rhythm	Paced	Paced	Paced	Paced	Paced	Paced	Paced

CASE STUDIES

The following case studies are provided to demonstrate application of the principles of vasoactive medication administration described in this article.

Case Study #1: Mitral Valve Replacement with Tricuspid Valve Repair and Patent Foramen Ovale Repair

This patient was an 84-year old man with a medical history positive for chronic atrial fibrillation, tobacco use, patent foramen ovale, mitral valve regurgitation, and tricuspid valve insufficiency. He underwent a biological mitral valve replacement, tricuspid valve ring repair, and closure of a patent foramen ovale. The patient's operative course was unremarkable. He was transferred to the ICU on completion of surgery at 13:00 h. His postoperative course through extubation is reported in **Tables 6–9**.

Discussion of postoperative hemodynamic stabilization

On arrival at the ICU the patient was sedated and mechanically ventilated, requiring 2 vasoactive infusions (epinephrine and norepinephrine) to support cardiac output and blood pressure. On initial assessment, the patient's pH was slightly acidotic and his lactate slightly elevated (normal <1). The central venous pressure (CVP) measurement

Table 7
Infusions on arrival at ICU through extubation

Medication	13:00	14:00	15:00	16:00	17:00	18:00	19:00
Dexmedetomidine (μg/kg/h)	0.4	0.4	0.4	0	0	0	0
Epinephrine (μg/kg/min)	0.04	0.04	0.04	0.04	0.04	0.04	0.03
Insulin (units/h)	2	2	3	5	5	5	1.5
Norepinephrine (μg/kg/min)	0.06	0.06	0.03	0	0	0	0
Propofol (μg/kg/min)	30	20	20	0	0	0	0

Table 8
Intake and output on arrival at ICU through extubation

Intake	13:00	14:00	15:00	16:00	17:00	18:00	19:00
Crystalloid	300	10	10	10	250	10	10
Colloid	—	250	—	—	—	—	—
Output	—	—	—	—	—	—	—
Chest tube	70	70	40	20	0	35	50
Urine	0	100	50	60	35	50	75

was normal; however, in the setting of altered chamber pressure as is often the case in the presence of mitral and tricuspid regurgitation, the CVP may be relatively low for this patient. Urine output in the first hour was 0 mL. Initially, a 250-mL crystalloid bolus was given and 250 mL of 5% albumin was administered 1 hour later (Pearl #1: ensure adequate preload). Sedation was decreased slightly and the norepinephrine infusion was weaned off as the patient's BP, mean arterial pressure (MAP), CVP, and urine output responded appropriately after completion of the fluid boluses, leaving only epinephrine for its inotropic contribution.

After obtaining a repeat ABG at 16:00, the patient's sedation was stopped in attempts to liberate him from the ventilator as per institutional protocol. The patient was placed on pressure support via the ventilator at approximately 17:00. The ABG results at 18:00 demonstrated correction of the initial acidosis. The patient was extubated. The patient's lactate level continued to increase at 16:00 and urine output decreased at 17:00, so an additional 250 mL of crystalloid was administered (Pearl #1: ensure adequate preload). The patient's urine output increased after the additional fluid bolus and the lactate level began to normalize. The patient's hemoglobin was stable postoperatively and the chest tube output was unremarkable.

Based on postoperative assessment, the major treatment interventions in this case included low-dose inotropes to enhance contractility, along with fluid administration to ensure that preload was sustained in the postoperative period.

Case Study #2: Coronary Artery Bypass Grafting of 4 Vessels with Left Atrial Appendage Ligation

This patient was a 67-year old man who underwent coronary artery bypass grafting of 4 vessels with a left atrial appendage ligation. The patient's medical history is

Table 9
Laboratory tests on arrival at ICU through extubation

Arterial Blood Gas	13:00	14:00	15:00	16:00	17:00	18:00	19:00
pH	—	7.31	—	7.35	—	7.41	—
Pao$_2$	—	109	—	120	—	118	—
Paco$_2$	—	47	—	40	—	37	—
HCO$_3$	—	24	—	22	—	24	—
Base	—	2.4	—	3.0	—	0.9	—
Oxyhemoglobin	—	94	—	95	—	97	—
Additional Labs							
Lactate	2.5	—	—	3.1	—	—	1.7
Hemoglobin	—	13.2	—	13.1	—	—	11.6

Table 10
Hemodynamic measurements on arrival at ICU through extubation

Metric	15:00	16:00	17:00	18:00	19:00	20:00	21:00	22:00	23:00	00:00	01:00	02:00	03:00	04:00	05:00	06:00	07:00
Temp. (°F)	96.4	97.1	—	—	—	98.3	—	—	100.9	99.9	—	—	—	100.5	—	—	98.6
HR	74	67	72	78	67	113	86	71	77	85	80	82	76	69	73	75	77
BP	79/45	101/64	111/62	98/56	100/48	96/56	94/55	95/54	72/51	89/51	97/54	131/82	91/49	90/49	98/50	98/49	118/63
MAP	57	77	80	73	66	69	70	68	62	66	69	98	63	62	66	64	80
RR	18	18	18	18	18	18	18	18	18	18	18	18	18	19	20	17	21
Spo$_2$	95	97	97	96	97	97	97	97	98	97	97	98	98	97	98	97	96
CVP	9	—	—	—	—	16	—	—	—	13	—	—	—	13	—	—	6
PAP	38/24	—	—	—	—	52/28	—	—	—	44/22	—	—	—	52/22	—	—	42/20
SVR	685	—	—	—	—	333	—	—	—	539	—	—	—	500	—	—	794
CI	3.9	2	2.7	2.6	2.6	2.3	2.7	3.9	2.6	2.8	—	—	—	2.6	—	—	2.9
CO	8.1	—	—	—	—	6.5	7.9	8.5	7.6	8	—	—	—	8	—	—	7.5
Svo$_2$	68	67	68	68	68	70	72	73	73	67	73	75	76	66	67	68	62
Airway	Vent 50%	Vent 50%	Vent 50%	Vent 50%	Vent 50%	Vent 50%	Vent 50%	Vent 50%	Vent 45%	Vent 45%	Vent 45%	Vent 45%	Vent 45%	Vent 40%	Vent 40%	Vent 40%	Bipap 40%
Rhythm	NSR	PACs	PACs	PACs	PACs	PACs	PACs	PACs	PACs	PACs	PACs	PACs	PACs	PACs	PACs	PACs	PACs

Abbreviations: NSR, normal sinus rhythm; PACs, premature atrial contractions.

Table 11
Infusions on arrival at ICU through extubation

Medication	15:00	16:00	17:00	18:00	19:00	20:00	21:00	22:00	23:00	00:00	01:00	02:00	03:00	04:00	05:00	06:00	07:00
Amiodarone (mg/min)	0	0.5	0.5	0.5	0.5	0.5	0.5	0.5	0.5	0.5	0.5	0.5	0.5	0.5	0.5	0.5	0.5
Dexmedetomidine (µg/kg/h)	0.3	0.3	0.3	0.3	0.3	0.3	0.2	0	0	0	0	0	0	0	0	0	0
Epinephrine (µg/kg/min)	0.01	0.02	0.02	0.03	0.03	0.03	0.01	0.01	0.01	0.01	0.01	0.01	0.01	0.01	0.02	0.02	0.02
Fentanyl (µg/h)	—	—	—	—	—	—	50	50	50	50	50	50	50	50	50	50	50
Insulin (units/h)	2	3	3	3	3	3	3	2	2	2.5	2.5	2.5	2.5	2.5	3	3	3
Norepinephrine (µg/kg/min)	0	0	0	0	0	0.02	0.03	0.03	0.04	0.04	0.05	0.06	0.06	0.06	0.07	0.07	0.05
Propofol (µg/kg/min)	0	0	0	0	0	0	20	25	35	40	40	30	25	25	25	0	0

Table 12
Intake and output on arrival at ICU through extubation

Intake	15:00	16:00	17:00	18:00	19:00	20:00	21:00	22:00	23:00	00:00	01:00	02:00	03:00	04:00	05:00	06:00	07:00
Crystalloid (mL/h)	10	10	10	10	10	10	10	10	10	10	50	10	10	10	100	75	75
Colloid (mL/h)	—	250	250	—	500	—	—	—	—	—	—	—	—	—	—	—	—
Output																	
Chest tube (mL/h)	13	82	25	35	25	7	10	55	55	20	10	20	10	10	20	10	20
Urine (mL/h)	—	—	245	85	90	45	60	40	40	33	38	40	30	30	35	25	35

Table 13
Laboratory tests on arrival at ICU through extubation

ABG	15:00	16:00	17:00	18:00	19:00	20:00	21:00	22:00	23:00	00:00	01:00	02:00	03:00	04:00	05:00	06:00	07:00
pH	7.35	—	7.36	—	—	—	7.37	—	—	—	—	—	—	7.40	—	—	7.37
Pao_2	71	—	79	—	—	—	86	—	—	—	—	—	—	84	—	—	83
$Paco_2$	38	—	35	—	—	—	35	—	—	—	—	—	—	35	—	—	35
HCO_3	21	—	20	—	—	—	20	—	—	—	—	—	—	22	—	—	20
Base	4.6	—	5.1	—	—	—	5.1	—	—	—	—	—	—	2.7	—	—	4.6
Oxyhemoglobin	92	—	94	—	—	—	94	—	—	—	—	—	—	95	—	—	94
Additional Labs																	
Lactate	0.9	—	—	—	—	1.0	—	—	—	—	—	—	—	0.8	—	—	—
Hemoglobin	10.8	—	—	—	—	10.7	—	—	—	—	—	—	—	10.9	—	—	—

significant for coronary artery disease, obstructive sleep apnea, chronic atrial fibrillation, hyperlipidemia, hypertension, diabetes mellitus type II, recent deep vein thrombosis, and recent bilateral cellulitis progressing to profound sepsis and acute kidney injury requiring long-term hospitalization with significant deconditioning. His postoperative course through extubation is reported in **Tables 10–13**.

Discussion of postoperative hemodynamic stabilization

The patient arrived in the ICU after completion of a 4-vessel coronary artery bypass graft with left atrial appendage ligation. The initial vital signs on arrival indicated hypotension with an MAP of 57. The patient's PaO$_2$, although normal, was suboptimal after cardiac surgery. The patient was given 250 mL of 5% albumin for decreased blood pressure (Pearl #1: ensure adequate preload).

The patient's blood pressure, MAP, CVP, and cardiac index improved, reflecting the additional preload; however, again at 18:00, the patient's urine output and MAP began declining. The epinephrine drip was increased (Pearl #2: preload is adequate, attempt to increase contractility by increasing inotropes) at this time without resolution. At approximately 19:00, an additional 500 mL of 5% albumin was administered. On reassessing his hemodynamic status at 20:00, the patient's decreased systemic vascular resistance indicated vasoplegia postoperatively, requiring vasoconstriction and additional inotropic support with norepinephrine (Pearl #5: normal cardiac output however hypotensive, add vasoconstrictor such as norepinephrine).

The patient did respond to the various interventions; however, the additional inotropic support was more arrhythmogenic despite amiodarone 0.5 mg/min already infusing for rate control related to the patient's history of chronic atrial fibrillation. Around 23:00, the decision was made to decrease the epinephrine drip to 0.01 µg/kg/min to support cardiac output, and increase norepinephrine to compensate inotropic support and maintain afterload while reducing arrhythmogenic effects.

The patient's temperature increased to 100.9°F (38.3°C) from 96.4°F (35.8°C) on ICU admission. Warming interventions (such as warm blankets and heat lamps) were removed. The patient's sedation was decreased in the early hours as his hemodynamic status began to stabilize. His lactate and hemoglobin were normal and stable throughout the recovery process. After weaning off sedation, he was successfully extubated and placed on home Bipap settings.

SUMMARY

The administration of vasoactive medications to optimize cardiac output and blood pressure in patients following cardiac surgery is an important tool in facilitating recovery and promoting recovery to hospital discharge. To achieve this goal, the clinician needs to understand the physiologic disruptions that are hindering the patient's recovery from surgery, then use the appropriate medications to support cardiac output and blood pressure to achieve effective organ perfusion. In this way, the nurse achieves one of Florence Nightingale's most important objectives for nursing:

…What nursing has to do…is to put the patient in the best condition for nature to act on him.[12(p75)]

REFERENCES

1. Kouchoukos NT, Blackstone EH, Hanley FL, et al. Postoperative care. In: Kouchoukos NT, Blackstone EH, Hanley FL, et al, editors. Cardiac surgery, vol. 1, 4th edition. Philadelphia: Elsevier Saunders; 2013. p. 189–250.

2. Aneman A, Brechot N, Brodie D, et al. Advances in critical care management of patients undergoing cardiac surgery. Intensive Care Med 2018;44(6):799–810.
3. Lemmer JH, Vlahakes GJ. Handbook of patient care in cardiac surgery. 7th edition. Philadelphia: Wolters Kluwer Health/Lippincott Williams & Wilkins; 2010.
4. Manual of perioperative care in adult cardiac surgery. In: Bojar RM, editor. 4th edition. Malden (MA): Blackwell Publishing Ltd; 2005.
5. Orso F, Baldasseroni S, Maggioni A. Heart rate in coronary syndromes and heart failure. Prog Cardiovasc Dis 2009;52:38–45.
6. Stephens RS, Whitman GJR. Postoperative critical care of the adult cardiac surgical patient. Part I: routine postoperative care. Crit Care Med 2015;43(7): 1477–97.
7. Scheeren TWL, Wiesenack C, Gerlach H, et al. Goal-directed intraoperative fluid therapy guided by stroke volume and its variation in high-risk surgical patients: a prospective randomized multicentre study. J Clin Monit Comput 2013;27(3): 225–33.
8. Liu LL, Gropper MA. Respiratory and hemodynamic management after cardiac surgery. Curr Treat Options Cardiovasc Med 2002;4(2):161–9.
9. Zaloga GP, Prielipp RC, Butterworth J F 4th, et al. Pharmacologic cardiovascular support. Crit Care Clin 1993;9(2):335–62.
10. Berry, W, McKenzie, C, Use of inotropes in critical care. Clin Pharmacist, 2, 395–396.
11. Inotropes. Drug information online: Micromedex. 2019. Available at: https://securegateway.fairview.org/Citrix/sgstoreWeb/. Accessed December 12, 2018.
12. Nightingale F. Notes on nursing: what it and what it is not. New York: D.Appleton and Company; 1860.
13. Norton JM. Toward consistent definitions for preload and afterload. Adv Physiol Educ 2001;25(1–4):53–61.
14. Gillies B, Bellomo R, Doolan L, et al. Bench-to-bedside review: inotropic drug therapy after adult cardiac surgery—a systematic literature review. Crit Care 2005;9(3):266–79.
15. Piette JD, Striplin D, Marinec N, et al. A mobile health intervention supporting heart failure patients and their informal caregivers: a randomized comparative effectiveness trial. J Med Internet Res 2015;17(6):e142.

Common Postcardiothoracic Surgery Arrhythmias

Kirstan Clay-Weinfeld, MSN, CRNP, AGACNP-BC, CCRN-CSC-CMC[a],*,
Melissa Callans, MSN, CRNP, CCDS, FHRS[a,b]

KEYWORDS

- Cardiac surgery • Postoperative arrhythmia • Atrial fibrillation
- Coronary artery bypass graft • Valvular surgery • Ventricular tachycardia
- Atrioventricular block

KEY POINTS

- Cardiac arrhythmias are a major source of complications after cardiac surgery and can increase patient morbidity, extend hospital stays, and increase health care costs.
- Mechanisms responsible for most arrhythmias after cardiac surgery include automaticity and reentry; triggered activity is less common.
- Bradycardias are common after cardiac surgery and are typically transient. Permanent pacemaker implant may be indicated after 5 to 7 days of persistent bradycardia.
- Atrial fibrillation is the most common postoperative arrhythmia and is associated with increased risk of long-term morbidity and mortality.
- Sustained ventricular arrhythmias are not common; however, they are associated with high long-term mortality rates; therefore, patients should be evaluated for implantable cardioverter-defibrillators.

INTRODUCTION

The development of arrhythmias after cardiac surgery is a common phenomenon, and were once believed to be clinically irrelevant.[1] Most of these arrhythmias are transient and often benign; however, many have long-term and lasting sequelae. Depending on risk factors, postoperative arrhythmias (POAs) can contribute to a protracted course of illness known to increase hospital costs and lengthen hospital stays.[2] Furthermore, POAs may be predictors for recurrent arrhythmias and long-term mortality.[3,4] Treating

Disclosure Statement: K. Clay-Weinfeld has nothing to disclose. M. Callans has received honoraria for lectures provided by Medtronic in the area of implantable cardiac devices.
[a] Department of Cardiac Electrophysiology, Pennsylvania Hospital, University of Pennsylvania Health System, Philadelphia, PA, USA; [b] AGACNP Program, University of Pennsylvania School of Nursing, Philadelphia, 418 Curie Boulevard, Philadelphia, PA 19104, USA
* Corresponding author. 800 Spruce Street, Philadelphia, PA 19107.
E-mail address: kirstan.clay-weinfeld@pennmedicine.upenn.edu

Crit Care Nurs Clin N Am 31 (2019) 367–388
https://doi.org/10.1016/j.cnc.2019.05.006
0899-5885/19/© 2019 Elsevier Inc. All rights reserved.

arrhythmias early in the postoperative period can limit postoperative morbidity and mortality and reduce intensive care unit and hospital stays. This article describes mechanisms, pathogenesis, and treatment modalities for the arrhythmias encountered after cardiac surgery.

MECHANISMS FOR ARRHYTHMIAS

Arrhythmias are the result of failed, altered, or enhanced impulse formation or impulse conduction. Mechanisms responsible for arrhythmogenesis are classified based on shared electrophysiologic properties on a cellular level and are identified as automaticity, triggered activity, and reentry. Comprehension of these mechanisms provides a basis for proper diagnosis and treatment of the arrhythmia.

Abnormal Impulse Formation

Automaticity
Automaticity is the property of spontaneous impulse generation by cardiac myocytes, particularly in the sinoatrial (SA) node, the atrioventricular (AV) node, and the His-Purkinje system. Normal automaticity can be enhanced, such as when SA node stimulation results in sinus tachycardia; it also can be enhanced in subsidiary sites, such as in the pulmonary veins, and cause atrial fibrillation (AF). Enhanced normal automaticity can also occur in the AV node, particularly in acute myocardial infarction, digitalis toxicity, and after cardiac surgery, with a resultant accelerated junctional rhythm or junctional tachycardia.[5]

Abnormal automaticity occurs in nonpacemaker cells that typically do not normally display spontaneous activity. A pathologic process partially depolarizes these cells; high levels of extracellular potassium, low intracellular pH, and catecholamine release are common pathologies known to trigger abnormal automaticity following cardiac surgery.[6] Premature depolarizations, atrial tachycardia, idioventricular rhythm, and ventricular tachycardia (VT) are a result of this mechanism.

Triggered activity
Triggered activity is an abnormal impulse generation of myocardial cells, called after-depolarization (AD), which occurs when repolarization of the previous action potential has not completed. If the AD reaches the threshold membrane potential, a triggered response may occur, which may then lead to a self-sustaining triggered activity or arrhythmia. The timing of the AD within the previous action potential determines the type of arrhythmia. Delayed after-depolarizations (DADs) occur during phase 4 of the action potential; these are caused by digitalis toxicity, catecholamine surge, ischemia, some electrolyte abnormalities, hypertrophy, heart failure, and class IA antiarrhythmic drugs. Examples of DAD-triggered arrhythmias are atrial tachycardia, accelerated ventricular rhythms, and some forms of VT.[5,6]

Early after-depolarizations (EADs) occur during phase 2 or phase 3 of the previous action potential and occur only in the setting of a prolonged action potential, demonstrated on the surface electrocardiogram (ECG) as QT prolongation. EAD-triggered arrhythmias are rate-dependent, typically provoked by bradycardia or compensatory pauses. Class IA and III antiarrhythmic drugs can become proarrhythmic by prolonging the action potential. Other agents implicated in action potential prolongation include some tricyclic and tetracyclic antidepressants, phenothiazine antipsychotics, antiemetics, and macrolide antibiotics. Torsades de pointes is an example of an EAD-triggered arrhythmia.[5,6]

Abnormal Impulse Conduction

Reentry

Normal conduction is dependent on methodical homogeneous impulse propagation in an organized sequence from the SA node through distal fibers of the Purkinje system and ventricular tissue. The impulse terminates when all cells have been activated and are refractory, or unable to propagate further activation. If a group of abnormal cells is not activated during the initial wave of depolarization, they can recover excitability in time to be depolarized before the impulse dies. When this occurs, it initiates a repetitive reactivation process termed "reentry." The group of abnormal cells creates an "obstacle" for the wavefront to travel around; the obstacle can be either anatomic or functional.[7,8]

When an anatomic obstacle is present, an impulse must propagate down one side and back up the other side in a circular fashion, forming a circuit for reentry. Examples of anatomic reentry tachycardias include AV reentrant tachycardia (AVRT) associated with a bypass tract, AV nodal reentrant tachycardia (AVNRT), atrial flutter, and postinfarction VTs. A functional obstacle with heterogeneous electrophysiological properties can be responsible for more complex conduction problems. Ventricular fibrillation (VF) and polymorphic VT are examples of functional reentrant arrhythmias.[5,6] Reentry is clinically relevant because it is the most common mechanism for tachyarrhythmias following cardiac surgery.[9]

Block

A block occurs when a propagating potential fails to follow its normal path. At high rates, cardiac tissue can block because it remains refractory, that is, not fully repolarized and able to accept a potential. Physiologic and pathophysiological blocks can occur when conduction is altered, as with degenerative processes, drugs (such as beta blockers, calcium channel blockers, digitalis, and adenosine), enhanced vagal tone, or direct surgical trauma.

PATHOPHYSIOLOGY

Arrhythmias develop due to mechanisms of either altered automaticity or altered conductivity, regardless of the setting. In the context of cardiac surgery, they are most notably a manifestation of underlying pathology, either cardiac or extracardiac, and can be the result of a combination of factors. Perioperative elements contributing to the to the development of POAs may differ substantially, but follow common proarrhythmic themes, including cardiac factors, respiratory factors, electrolyte imbalances, sympathetic stimulation, mechanical irritation, and therapeutic drugs.[9] Treatment should be directed toward the correction of the underlying pathology, with concomitant therapy to correct the arrhythmia.

BRADYARRHYTHMIAS
Epidemiology

After cardiac surgery, up to 25% of patients may experience transient AV conduction disturbances; they occur more commonly in the setting of compromised left ventricular (LV) function, severe coronary artery disease, hypertension (HTN), long aortic cross-clamp times, and use of cold cardioplegia for myocardial protection. Predisposing factors for persistent high-degree AV blocks include older age, perivalvular calcification, preexisting left bundle branch block (LBBB), LV aneurysmectomy, left coronary artery main disease, a higher number of bypassed arteries, and extended cardiopulmonary bypass pump time.[10]

Bradycardias resulting from sinus node dysfunction (SND) are not as common after cardiac surgery, and usually have a preexisting component, although SND following orthotopic heart transplantation may lead to pacemaker implantation rates as high as 21%, particularly in patients affected by older donor age, longer donor ischemic time, and longer aortic cross-clamp time.[10,11]

Pathogenesis

Disease of the sinus node is failure of impulse generation, occurring most commonly as a result of degeneration. Ischemia, inflammation, and fibrosis can also contribute and compound the degeneration. Hypothermia, hypothyroidism, increased vagal tone from surgery or anesthesia, and drugs such as beta blockers or narcotics also can cause SND, resulting in sinus bradycardia (**Fig. 1**), sinus pauses or arrest (**Fig. 2**), or sinus exit block.[8,11,12] After cardiac surgery, SND may be transient yet still cause considerable hemodynamic instability. It is especially challenging to manage when it is caused by medications for prevention or treatment of AF.

AV block is a failure of impulse propagation with abnormal conduction velocity and refractoriness of the AV node or His-Purkinje system.[12] AV block is much more common after valvular surgery than coronary artery bypass graft surgery (CABG), and is often a result of direct surgical trauma and localized edema. Most cases resolve within 24 to 48 hours, with resolution of edema and inflammation and increased perfusion to the AV node.[13] AV block is classified based on the level of the block, which also determines the severity.

Postoperatively, a new right bundle branch block (RBBB) can appear suddenly with rapid elevations of right-sided filling pressures, as would occur with pulmonary embolism. It also can transiently occur during placement of a pulmonary artery (PA) catheter due to local trauma to the right bundle branch. The left bundle branch has 2 fascicles, and either or both branches may be blocked. A blockage of the left anterior branch is associated with myocardial infarction (MI), left ventricular hypertrophy (LVH), and certain cardiomyopathies. A block of the left posterior fascicle has an ominous prognostic value because it is uncommon in the absence of underlying cardiac disease. A persistent new LBBB suggests a possible perioperative infarction; following transcatheter aortic valve replacement (TAVR), a new LBBB is a prognostic indicator for all-cause mortality.[14]

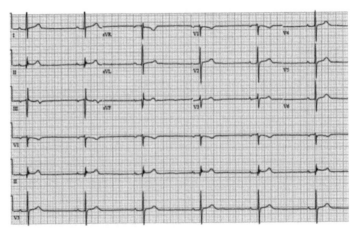

Fig. 1. SND presenting as marked sinus bradycardia with a rate of just more than 30 beats per minute.

Fig. 2. AF with sinus arrest/conversion pause, a junctional escape beat, and then resumption of AF.

Diagnosis

Diagnosis is made via bedside telemetry, 12-lead ECG, and atrial electrogram (AEG) if atrial epicardial leads are present. First-degree block is a relatively benign condition and rarely causes symptoms, or is it likely to progress to a life-threatening heart block.[12] It is manifested on the surface ECG as a prolonged PR interval, greater than 200 ms. A rare finding is a rapidly lengthening PR interval that occurs over days; in the context of an aortic root abscess this may signal impending progression to third-degree heart block.[7]

Second-degree AV block is intermittent conduction to the ventricles. Depending on the location of the block, it can be benign or more serious. Disease below the AV node tends to progress to a more severe condition, whereas Mobitz I or Wenckebach is disease within the AV node and is benign. Mobitz I is characterized by a beat-to-beat prolongation of the PR interval until eventual failure of P wave to conduct for 1 cycle. The following PR interval is shorter than the one immediately preceding the blocked P wave **(Fig. 3)**. It is reflective of increased or delayed refractoriness within the AV node and is generally benign and nonprogressive; however, if it first appears following cardiac surgery with accompanying bradycardia, it is more likely disease or damage distal to the AV node, and implantation of a permanent pacemaker (PPM) should be considered if it persists.[7]

Second-degree AV block type II, or Mobitz II block presents as an intermittently dropped QRS complex with constant PR intervals **(Fig. 4)**. It always represents disease below the AV node and may be accompanied by a newly acquired bundle branch block (BBB). A 2:1 block is a special classification of Mobitz II in which every other P wave fails to conduct to the ventricle. A 2:1 block requires closer examination to distinguish between Mobitz I and a higher-degree block and the level of the block **(Figs. 5 and 6)**. A 12-lead ECG, atropine, exercise, and vagal maneuvers can assist in the

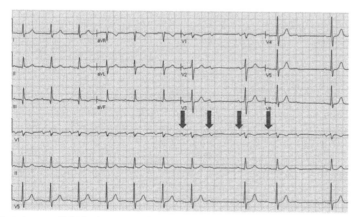

Fig. 3. First-degree AV block progressing to second-degree AV block Mobitz I (Wenckebach). The red arrows identify *P waves*.

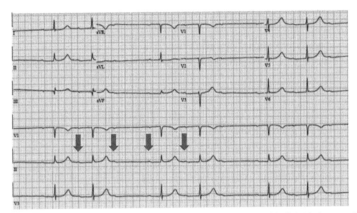

Fig. 4. Mobitz II AV block with constant PR interval, and every third QRS dropped. The red arrows identify *P waves.*

diagnosis (**Table 1**). High-grade AV block is represented by a constant PR interval, but 2 or more consecutive P waves fail to conduct (**Fig. 7**).

Third-degree AV block, or complete heart block, occurs when there is absence of AV conduction, and ventricular activity is completely dependent on subsidiary escape pacemakers below the level of block (**Fig. 8**). AV nodal block tends to have relatively stable pacemakers; however, more distal blocks can be unreliable and slow.[9]

Junctional rhythm is an escape rhythm when there is failure of a higher pacemaker (**Fig. 9**). It can be caused by hypokalemia, inferior MI, SND, either acute or chronic, or antiarrhythmic drugs (AAD). Postoperative treatment mimics that of other postoperative bradyarrhythmias. Untreated, it tends to be self-limiting. If it is not transient and the patient is symptomatic, it may indicate an underlying sick sinus syndrome (SSS) and PPM should be considered.

Treatment

Benign and asymptomatic bradycardias and low-degree AV blocks with stable escape rhythms are best left untreated. Temporary measures may be necessary following

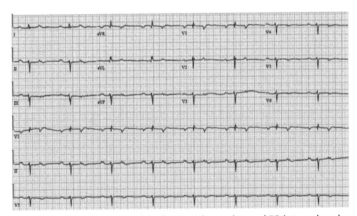

Fig. 5. Wenckebach presenting as 2.1 block; note the prolonged PR interval and narrow QRS complex. This is a stable and benign rhythm.

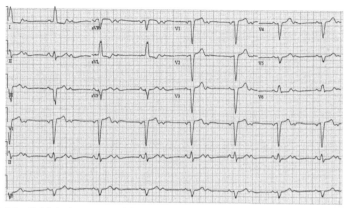

Fig. 6. Mobitz II high-degree AV block presenting as 2.1 block; note the constant and normal PR interval and wide QRS complex with LBBB pattern. The underlying escape rhythm is infranodal and can progress to complete heart block.

cardiac surgery to optimize low cardiac output states in patients with static stroke volumes. Profound SND may compromise hemodynamic stability. Conservative treatment, involving temporary withdrawal of AADs, temporary epicardial pacing, and watchful waiting is best, as SSS has a lower propensity for asystole than AV block.[7] If AV conduction is preserved, atrial pacing is preferred, especially in the setting of reduced left ventricular ejection fraction (LVEF).[7] Atrial pacing can provide a 20% to 30% increase in stroke volume as a result of atrial filling or "kick," particularly in patients with LVH and systemic HTN.[9]

Catecholamine infusion can stimulate the sinus mechanism in the absence or failure of atrial epicardial pacing wires. Epinephrine at lower doses acts predominantly on beta receptors, resulting in an increase in heart rate and contractility. Dopamine infusion at mid-range doses also exerts beta effects. Caution is advised in using catecholamines, as they can contribute to metabolic derangement, particularly hyperglycemia, hypokalemia, and lactic acidosis.[7] Ventricular pacing is an option in the absence or failure of atrial wires or inadequate response to pharmacologic modalities; however, hemodynamic response is less pronounced because of the loss of atrial kick, and may not be tolerated.

Table 1
Differentiation of AV nodal and infranodal block

Measurement/ Intervention	AV Nodal	Infranodal
PR interval	Usually prolonged (>200 ms)	Usually normal or short
QRS duration	Usually narrow (<120 ms)	Usually wide (>120 ms)
Exercise	Improves	Conduction ratio may worsen
Isoproterenol	Improves	Conduction ratio may worsen
Atropine	Improves	Conduction ratio may worsen
Vagal maneuvers (CSM)	Worsens	No change or improves conduction ratio

Abbreviations: AV, atrioventricular; CSM, carotid sinus massage.
    Data from Fogoros RN. Electrophysiologic testing. 5th ed. Chichester: John Wiley & Sons; 2013.

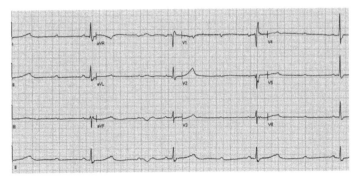

Fig. 7. High-grade AV block with intermittent conduction; note constant PR of conducted beats.

As advanced AV blocks are usually transient, they are also best treated with temporary pacing via epicardial wires. If the sinus rate is adequate, DDD pacing is preferred for atrial tracking. If the sinus rate is slow, either DVI or DDD may be used. Temporary withdrawal of offending medications also may be necessary (**Table 2**).

Permanent pacing is indicated for SND or AV block in up to 3.4% of patients following CABG surgery.[15] Valvular surgery has a much higher incidence of permanent pacing, cited as up to 24% following some types of operations, particularly tricuspid valve replacement and aortic valve replacement for calcified aortic stenosis.[10,11] Patients undergoing mitral valve (MV) repair and replacement have similar instances of defects of AV conduction requiring intervention.[16] Repeat valve surgery poses a nearly fourfold increase in incidence of permanent pacing over initial valve surgery.[15] The higher risks for PPM implant following valvular surgery are largely due to the geographic location of the AV node and infranodal conduction system. These structures are in close proximity, bordered by the commissure between the noncoronary and right coronary sinuses of the aortic valve, the anterior mitral leaflet, and the septal tricuspid leaflet, making them particularly susceptible to direct injury or ischemia.[13]

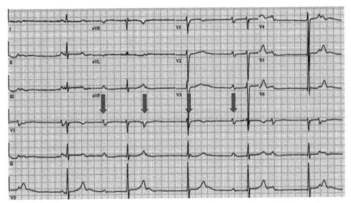

Fig. 8. Third-degree AV block, or complete heart block; note the AV dyssynchrony with sinus rate just more than 50, indicating a concomitant SSS. The escape rhythm is nodal and is stable. The red arrows identify *P waves*.

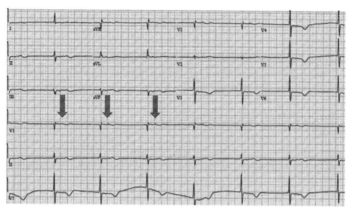

Fig. 9. Junctional rhythm with retrograde P waves following the QRS complex. The red arrows identify *P waves*.

Over time, there has been an overall increase in PPM implantation following cardiac surgery, with the greatest increase following aortic valve surgery. TAVR surgery carries PPM rates up to 30%.[13] A preexisting RBBB is a known risk factor for PPM following TAVR.[17,18] A new LBBB has been considered a prognostic indicator for PPM implant following surgical aortic valve replacement; however, new incidence after TAVR may be device-specific and not prognostic of PPM.[14,17]

Table 2		
Common bradyarrhythmia causes and treatments		
Arrhythmia	**Causes and Contributing Factors**	**Treatment**

SND
• Sinus bradycardia
• Sinus pauses/arrest
	• Underlying SSS
	• Hypothermia
	• Ischemia
	• Edema
	• Inflammation
	• Increased vagal tone
	• Beta blockers
	• Narcotics
	• Orthotopic heart transplant
		• Correct treatable causes
		• Pacing
		  ○ AAI if intact AV conduction
		  ○ DDD if abnormal AV conduction or profound bradycardia
		• Medications
		  ○ Epinephrine 1–2 μg/min
		  ○ Dopamine 3–10 μg/min
		  ○ Isoproterenol 1–2 μg/min
		• VVI if failure of other modalities and medications
		• PPM if persistent

AV block: • Mobitz II • High-degree 2:1 block • 3rd-degree AV block	• Surgical trauma • Edema • Inflammation • Beta blockers	• DDD if atrial rate is adequate for atrial tracking • DDD or DVI if atrial rate inadequate • PPM if persistent
Junctional rhythm	• See SND	• Correct treatable causes • See SND

Abbreviations: AAI/DDD/VVI/DVI, North American Society of Pacing and Electrophysiology and British Pacing and Electrophysiology Group Generic pacemaker code settings; AV, atrioventricular; BB, beta blocker; PPM, permanent pacemaker; SND, sinus node dysfunction; SSS, sick sinus syndrome.

Data from Bojar RM. Manual of perioperative care in adult cardiac surgery. Hoboken: John Wiley & Sons; 2011; and Smith W, Hood M. Arrhythmias. In: Sidebotham D, McKee A, Gillham M, Levy J, editors. Cardiothoracic critical care. Philadelphia: Butterworth Heinemann Elsevier; 2007:316-341.

Timing of PPM remains a challenge, as studies have shown recovery is common with long-term follow-up; however, recovery may take months.[13,15,19] The American College of Cardiology/American Heart Association/Heart Rhythm Society device-based therapy guidelines recommend PPM implantation after 5 to 7 days of persistent SND or AV block.[20] Earlier implants may be indicated in the setting of absent intrinsic rhythm or failed epicardial leads.[15]

SUPRAVENTRICULAR TACHYARRHYTHMIAS
Sinus Tachycardia

Sinus tachycardia following cardiovascular surgery is multifactorial and not patho-logic. Autonomic modification, blood and volume loss, use of vasoactive agents, and postoperative confounding factors contribute. Attention should be paid to treating and supporting the underlying cause.

Atrial Flutter

Typical atrial flutter is a macro-reentrant circuit that propagates in a counterclockwise direction around the right atrium. On 12-lead ECG, the distinctive sawtooth flutter waves are negative in II, III, and aVF and positive in V1. The ventricular response can be regular or irregular (**Fig. 10**). Atypical atrial flutter is a sawtooth pattern with any presentation differing from that described previously and can represent activation either around the right atrium, left atrium, or around scar tissue formed after previous surgery. The mechanisms of atrial flutter and AF are quite different; however, treatment in this patient population is the same.

Atrial Fibrillation

Epidemiology
As the most common adverse event following cardiac surgery, AF is associated with increased morbidity and mortality, along with prolonged hospital stay and increased cost. The incidence ranges from 30% to 50% with lowest risk after CABG, highest with combined CABG/valvular surgery, and solitary valve surgery falling in the mid-dle.[21] Given that the risk of postoperative AF (POAF) increases with age, the increasing age of the population portends a further increased prevalence over time. Although POAF typically resolves in 4 to 6 weeks, it also increases the risk of stroke and hemo-dynamic compromise.[22]

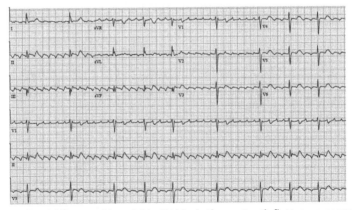

Fig. 10. Typical atrial flutter with variable AV block; the sawtooth flutter waves are negative in II, III, and aVF, and positive in V1.

Pathogenesis

There are multiple contributing factors to the initiation and maintenance of AF, specifically POAF, although the exact mechanisms remain elusive. Inflammation, oxidative stress, and adrenergic stimulation confound already understood properties of left atrial enlargement, fibrosis, and arrhythmogenesis of the pulmonary veins.[23]

Diagnosis

AF is characterized by rapid atrial activity, often 300 to 400 beats per minute, with an irregularly irregular ventricular response, and is diagnosed on telemetry, AEG, and 12-lead ECG (**Fig. 11**).

Risk stratification

The CHA_2DS_2VASc score is a standard in clinical practice for determining stroke risk in patients with AF. There is also recent evidence to support use of CHA_2DS_2VASc score as an independent predictor for the development of POAF[24]; however, evidence-based guidelines to differentiate patients at normal versus high risk for POAF are still needed. The Society of Cardiovascular Anesthesiologists and European Association of Cardiothoracic Anaesthetists working group recently designated a list of risk factors for POAF, using expert opinion and published POAF risk score models. They postulated that the development of risk stratification would facilitate adherence to a set of evidence-based recommendations and current best practices (**Fig. 12**). They reported the following as relevant risk factors to help delineate normal versus high risk of developing POAF: age, history of AF, renal failure, MV surgery/disease, heart failure, and chronic obstructive pulmonary disease.[21]

Prophylaxis

Although there are many pharmacologic options for reducing POAF, the most commonly studied are beta blockers and amiodarone. The Beta blocker Length of Stay (BLOS) trial demonstrated a 20% reduction in the risk of POAF on a dosage of 100 to 150 mg daily of metoprolol, although a length of stay reduction benefit remained elusive.[25] Subsequently, various clinical guidelines have come to recommend continuing beta blockers perioperatively to prevent withdrawal, as well as for POAF prophylaxis.[21,26–28] Numerous guidelines also suggest amiodarone should be considered for prophylaxis against POAF in patients who present in sinus rhythm but are deemed high risk, although without dose recommendations.[21,27–30] Long-term risks

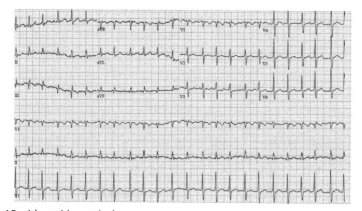

Fig. 11. AF with rapid ventricular response.

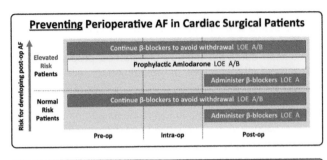

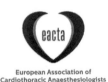

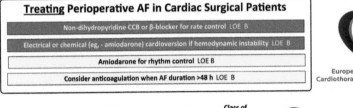

Fig. 12. Risk factors, prophylaxis, and treatment of perioperative AF. CCB, calcium channel blocker; COPD, chronic obstructive pulmonary disease; intra-op, intraoperative; LOE, level of evidence; post-op, postoperative; pre-op, preoperative. (*From* O'Brien B, Burrage PS, Ngai JY, et al. Society of Cardiovascular Anesthesiologists/European Association of Cardiothoracic Anaesthetists practice advisory for the management of perioperative atrial fibrillation in patients undergoing cardiac surgery. J Cardiothorac Vasc Anesth. 2019;33(1):12-26; with permission.)

and side effects of amiodarone are not as relevant with short-term administration; however, providers remain hesitant to administer given concern for such.[21] There are some data to suggest prophylaxis with sotalol should be considered as well in patients at risk for developing POAF.[26,29]

Statin therapy may prove efficacious as a POAF prophylactic: The Atorvastatin for Reduction in Myocardial Dysrhythmia After cardiac surgery (ARMYDA) trial reports that atorvastatin 40 mg daily, started 7 days before elective CABG, significantly reduced incidence of POAF and reduced duration of hospital stay.[31] That said, statin use is considered overall equivocal in prevention of POAF. Colchicine also has shown some benefit; however long-hailed digoxin has not been shown to reduce POAF.[21,29,32]

Treatment

The treatment of POAF is aimed at rate control, rhythm control, and thromboembolic risk reduction. A comparison of rate versus rhythm control in POAF validated similar complication rates, length of hospital stay, and freedom from AF at 60 days with both strategies.[33] Guidelines adhere to the recommendation that new-onset asymptomatic POAF should be managed initially with rate control and anticoagulation if indicated.[21,27,32] For rate control, a beta blocker or nondihydropyridine calcium channel blocker should be administered in the absence of contraindications.[21,28,29,32] For hemodynamically unstable POAF, restoration of sinus rhythm either by antiarrhythmic drug or cardioversion is indicated and also should be considered for hemodynamically stable but symptomatic patients (**Table 3**).[21,27,29]

Although the estimated risk of thromboembolic events in the setting of AF is well-documented in the CHA_2DS_2VASc score, it remains less clear what the long-term risk of thromboembolism is in patients who develop new POAF. A recently published cohort study of patients with first-time CABG surgery who developed POAF were matched with patients with nonvalvular AF (NVAF); thromboembolism in the POAF population was significantly lower than the patients with NVAF patients (18.3% vs

Table 3 Common supraventricular arrhythmia causes and treatments		
Arrhythmia	**Causes and Contributing Factors**	**Treatment**
Sinus tachycardia	• Fever • Pain • BB withdrawal • Hypovolemia • Tamponade • Increased sympathetic tone • Inotropes • Catecholamines • Acute decompensated heart failure	• Treat underlying cause • Antipyretics • Pain relief • Fluids, colloids, blood products if necessary • BB • Diuresis
MAT	• Hypoxia • Hypercapnea • Acidosis	• Correct underlying cause
AVRT/AVNRT	• Abnormal AV node architecture • Accessory pathway • Initiated by PAC, PVC • BB withdrawal • Catecholamines	• Paroxysmal in nature, usually self-limiting • Adenosine • Atrial overdrive pacing • BB, CCB
Atrial fibrillation	• Stretched atrial myocardium • Pericardial effusion • Inflammatory processes • BB withdrawal • Catecholamines	• Rate control: ○ BB or CCB • DCCV for hemodynamic instability • Consider amiodarone for rhythm control • Consider anticoagulation if persists > 24 h
Atrial flutter	• BB withdrawal • See atrial fibrillation	• See atrial fibrillation
Junctional tachycardia/ Accelerated junctional rhythm	• Increased sympathetic tone • BB withdrawal	• Usually self-limiting • BB if treatment needed

Abbreviations: AV, atrioventricular; AVNRT, atrioventricular nodal reentrant tachycardia; AVRT, atrioventricular reentrant tachycardia; BB, beta blocker; CCB, calcium channel blocker; DCCV, direct current cardioversion; MAT, multifocal atrial tachycardia; PAC, premature atrial contraction; PVC, premature ventricular contraction.

Data from Smith W, Hood M. Arrhythmias. In: Sidebotham D, McKee A, Gillham M, Levy J, editors. Cardiothoracic critical care. Philadelphia: Butterworth Heinemann Elsevier; 2007:316-341; and O'Brien B, Burrage PS, Ngai JY, et al. Society of Cardiovascular Anesthesiologists/European Association of Cardiothoracic Anaesthetists practice advisory for the management of perioperative atrial fibrillation in patients undergoing cardiac surgery. J Cardiothorac Vasc Anesth. 2019;33(1):12-26.

42.9%).[34] Patients who were anticoagulated had a lower risk of thromboembolic events compared with those who were not anticoagulated. Interestingly, the thromboembolism risk was not found to be significantly higher in the POAF population as compared with those who did not develop post-CABG POAF. Overall, this suggests patients with de novo POAF should not be considered in the same realm of risk as patients with NVAF.[34]

VENTRICULAR TACHYARRHYTHMIAS
Epidemiology

Although nonsustained ventricular arrhythmias (VAs) are quite common following cardiac surgery, VT and VF occur in only 1% to 3% of patients.[4,35] Despite these seemingly low numbers, sustained VAs carry an in-hospital mortality rate as high as 25% and poor long-term prognosis.[4,36] Patients with postoperative VT are more likely to have prior MI, depressed LVEF (<40%), and severe congestive heart failure.[4] Additional factors predisposing to the development of postoperative VAs include older age and emergent nature of surgery, whereas off-pump procedures have been found to offer some protection from VA occurrence.[35,36]

Occurring much more frequently postoperatively are nonsustained VT (NSVT) and premature ventricular contractions (PVCs). These VAs are of an automatic mechanism usually occurring in the setting of acute illness. However, recurrent de novo NSVT or PVCs occurring more than 30 per hour, especially in the setting of compromised LVEF, should prompt aggressive treatment, as they may precipitate malignant arrhythmias, particularly if intraoperative myocardial protection was inadequate.[9,10] Triggered VAs, such as pause-dependent or bradycardia-dependent VAs are less common after cardiac surgery; however, they can occur with congenital or medication-induced prolongation of the QT interval. For an extensive list of medications known for QT prolongation, view the following: https://crediblemeds.org/pdftemp/pdf/CombinedList.pdf.

Pathogenesis

VAs occurring in the immediate postoperative period are often provoked by predisposing conditions, such as hypokalemia, metabolic acidosis, hypoxia, hypovolemia, AADs with proarrhythmic features used for treatment of AF, or increased sympathetic tone. Perioperative ischemia can provoke automatic VAs, as can hemodynamic instability and catecholamine infusions.[7,37] PA catheter irritation can induce nonsustained VAs as well.

Reentry accounts for most sustained VAs, particularly monomorphic VT (MMVT), and are associated with scar from previous infarction or chronic heart disease. Revascularization of a chronically occluded vessel, particularly a noncollateralized vessel feeding an infarct zone, imparts an additional 22-fold risk of postoperative sustained VT/VF, suggesting reperfusion plays a critical role in the development of reentrant VT circuits.[4]

Diagnosis

VAs are wide-complex arrhythmias easily recognized on bedside telemetry. NSVT is a series of 3 or more PVCs in succession, lasting less than 30 seconds.[38] AEG can assist with differentiating between SVT with aberrancy and stable VT; however, AEG should not replace a surface 12-lead ECG (**Fig. 13**A, B). Clues suggesting VT include AV dissociation, ventricular concordance across precordial leads, QRS duration greater than 140 ms, or presence of capture or fusion beats (**Table 4**).[7,12] It is prudent to

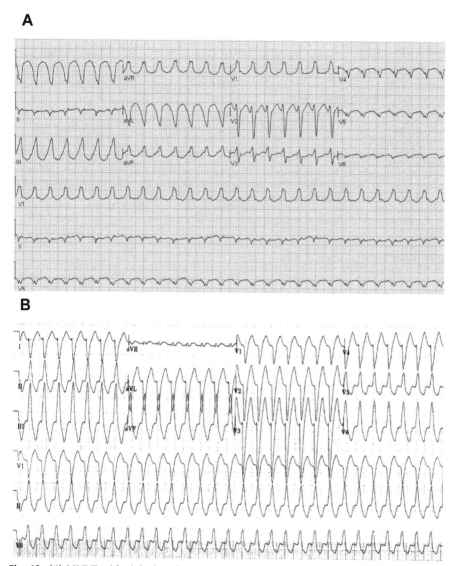

Fig. 13. (*A*) MMVT with right bundle branch morphology. (*B*) Supraventricular tachycardia with aberrancy in a patient with Wolff-Parkinson-White; the wide complex makes it indistinguishable from monomorphic tachycardia on surface ECG.

assume that a wide-complex tachycardia in a patient with prior MI or cardiomyopathy is VT, unless it can be proven otherwise.[12] VT can be monomorphic in which all the complexes are of similar amplitude, or polymorphic (PMVT), in which complexes are of variable amplitude (**Fig. 14**). PMVT tends to be faster and less stable than MMVT. VF is a disorganized tachyarrhythmia without discrete QRS complexes (**Fig. 15**).[12] Torsades de pointe is a specific form of PMVT recognized by its signature "twisting" around the ECG isoelectric baseline (**Fig. 16**). Torsades de pointe can occur in short bursts, or it can persist to cause sudden death.[12]

Table 4 Differentiation of SVT and VT		
ECG Feature	**VT**	**SVT with Aberrancy**
AV dissociation	Often	No
QRS duration	>140 ms	Often <140 ms
Morphology same as SR with BBB	Never	Likely
Concordance	Likely	Not likely
Morphology	More likely RBBB	Indeterminate
Delta wave in SR	No	Likely
Capture or fusion beats	Often	Not likely

Abbreviations: AV, atrioventricular; BBB, bundle branch block; RBBB: right bundle branch block; SR, sinus rhythm; SVT, supraventricular dissociation; VT, ventricular tachycardia.

Data from Smith W, Hood M. Arrhythmias. In: Sidebotham D, McKee A, Gillham M, Levy J, editors. Cardiothoracic critical care. Philadelphia: Butterworth Heinemann Elsevier; 2007:316-341.

Prophylaxis

An empiric strategy with vigilance to acid-base, electrolyte, and fluid balance correction, and measures that reduce myocardial demand and increase myocardial perfusion, will provide some prophylaxis against correctable and reversible automatic arrhythmias. Patients with CAD should be given empiric beta blockers, although efficacy of this practice in cardiac surgery patients is not well established.[39] Statin use has been shown to offer some protection against perioperative cardiac events.[40] Patient selection and appropriate revascularization strategy is critical to mitigating appropriate risk.[35,36]

Treatment

PVCs and NSVT are often temporary and corrected with treatment of the underlying cause. Potassium, magnesium, and fluid repletion should be pursued accordingly; otherwise, empiric treatment with AADs or overdrive pacing in asymptomatic patients with preserved LVEF is of limited benefit in the immediate postoperative period.[41] If they persists after correction of underlying cause, consider acute ischemia, MI, or ventricular dysfunction. If recurrent NSVT persists in the setting of low LVEF, electrophysiology study (EPS) should be considered to determine inducibility. If sustained VA is inducible, an implantable cardioverter-defibrillator (ICD) should be placed before hospital discharge for secondary prevention of sudden cardiac death (SCD). The Multicenter Automatic Defibrillator Implantation Trial (MADIT) and Multicenter Unsustained Tachycardia Trial (MUSTT) demonstrated significant reduction of SCD with ICDs versus conventional medical therapy or no therapy in patients with CAD, LVEF up to 40%, NSVT, and inducibility in EPS.[42,43] The Coronary Bypass Graft Patch Trial (CABG-Patch) demonstrated applicability in the immediate postoperative period following cardiac surgery is not well established.[44]

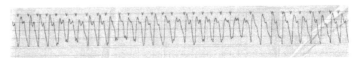

Fig. 14. Rhythm strip showing variable morphology of the QRS complex characteristic of polymorphic VT.

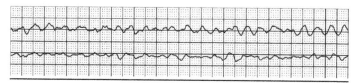

Fig. 15. Rhythm strip showing chaotic and amorphous appearance of VF.

Emergency measures including early defibrillation should be instituted in situations of sustained VT/VF and hemodynamic collapse, or VT refractory to AAD. The 2018 American Heart Association–focused update does not give preference to either amiodarone or lidocaine as AADs of choice; neither have shown superiority in long-term survival or survival with good neurologic outcome.[45] Likewise, the Society of Thoracic Surgeons acknowledges similar efficacy; however, they recommend amiodarone after 3 failed defibrillation attempts.[46] As PMVT is more indicative of ischemia, graft closure or other sources of ischemia should be ruled out. MMVT is a more organized rhythm, typically slower than PMVT, and is generally more tolerated; however, in the postoperative state, a stable VT rhythm can quickly deteriorate to one of hemodynamic instability and collapse and should be chemically or electrically cardioverted promptly.

Amiodarone and lidocaine are recommended options for chemical cardioversion of stable sustained MMVT. If ventricular epicardial wires are in place, overdrive pacing at a rate faster than the tachycardia may terminate the arrhythmia; emergency equipment should be present as acceleration of the VT and deterioration to VF can occur. If less invasive options of chemical conversion and pace-termination are not successful, synchronized cardioversion should be performed.

For PMVT, chemical cardioversion can be attempted with amiodarone or lidocaine. If AAD conversion is not successful, cardioversion should be performed due to the unstable nature of these arrhythmias. Magnesium may be considered in episodes of PMVT associated with prolonged QT interval (torsades de pointe); the benefit of magnesium is limited to this arrhythmia and actually prevents reinitiation of the arrhythmia rather than conversion (**Table 5**).[45]

Because of the high risk of SCD in and outside the hospital following a sustained VA, any patient experiencing a sustained VA, particularly in the absence of a correctable cause, should be evaluated for ICD implantation by way of EPS, as it is the only treatment to reliably reduce the risk of SCD from VAs in most patients.[12] Patients with

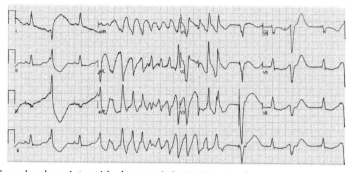

Fig. 16. Torsades de pointe with characteristic "twisting" of axis.

Table 5
Common ventricular arrhythmia causes and treatments

Arrhythmia	Causes and Contributing Factors	Treatment
PVC/NSVT	• Electrolyte disturbances • Underlying CAD • Myocardial ischemia • MI • Reperfusion • Inotropes • PDE inhibitors • Catecholamines • Inadequate myocardial protection • PA catheter manipulation	• Treat electrolyte disturbances • BB • Amiodarone 150 mg IV bolus (may repeat)[a] OR • Lidocaine 1–1.5 mg/kg IV bolus ○ May repeat 0.5–0.75 mg/kg[a] • Atrial overdrive pacing of PVCs with relative bradycardia

MMVT (stable)	• Underlying CAD
	• Myocardial ischemia
	• MI
	• Scar from prior MI
	• Hyperkalemia
	• Reperfusion
	• AAD
		• Amiodarone 150 mg IV bolus (may repeat)[a]
		OR
		• Lidocaine 1–1.5 mg/kg IV bolus
		  ○ May repeat 0.5–0.75 mg/kg IV bolus[a]
		• Ventricular overdrive pacing[b]
		• DCCV
		• Be prepared to institute emergency measures:
		  ○ Defibrillation

PMVT/TdP (stable)	• Ischemia
	• Hyperkalemia
	• Hypothermia
	• Reperfusion
	• QT prolongation
	• Inadequate myocardial protection
		• Amiodarone 150 mg IV bolus (may repeat)[a]
		OR
		• Lidocaine 1–1.5 mg/kg IV bolus
		  ○ May repeat 0.5–0.75 mg/kg IV bolus[a]
		• Magnesium sulfate for prolonged QT
		  ○ 1–2 g IV bolus
		• Be prepared to institute emergency measures:
		  ○ Defibrillation

Pulseless VT/VF	• Ischemia • Rewarming • Reperfusion • Inadequate myocardial protection	• Defibrillation • Amiodarone 300 mg IV bolus ○ May repeat 150 mg IV bolus[a] OR • Lidocaine 1 mg/kg (may repeat)[a]

Abbreviations: AAD, antiarrhythmic drugs; BB, beta blocker; CAD, coronary artery disease; DCCV, direct current cardioversion; IV, intravenous; MI, myocardial infarction; MMVT, monomorphic ventricular tachycardia; NSVT, nonsustained ventricular tachycardia; PA, pulmonary artery; PDE, phosphodiesterase; PMVT, polymorphic ventricular tachycardia; PVC, premature ventricular contraction; TdP, torsades de pointe; VF, ventricular fibrillation; VT, ventricular tachycardia.
[a] Follow with infusion.
[b] May accelerate to VF.
Data from Panchal AR, Berg KM, Kudenchuk PJ, et al. 2018 American Heart Association focused update on advanced cardiovascular life support use of antiarrhythmic drugs during and immediately after cardiac arrest: An update to the American Heart Association guidelines for cardiopulmonary resuscitation and emergency cardiovascular care. Circulation. 2018;138(23):e740; and Dunning J, Levine A, Ley J, et al. The Society of Thoracic Surgeons expert consensus for the resuscitation of patients who arrest after cardiac surgery. Ann Thorac Surg. 2017;103(3):1005-1020.

newly diagnosed reduced LVEF should be initiated on guideline-directed medical therapy, including beta-blockade and angiotensin-converting enzyme inhibition or angiotensin receptor blockade, and consideration should be given to a wearable external defibrillator.

SUMMARY

Postoperative arrhythmias are common after cardiac surgery. Bradyarrhythmias are usually transient, with initial treatment aimed at supportive care; bradycardias that do not recover spontaneously after 5 to 7 days are more likely permanent, and consideration should be given to permanent pacemaker implantation. SVTs, particularly AF, are the most commonly occurring arrhythmia after cardiac surgery. Treatment of POAF is similar to treatment in any other setting: rate control, rhythm control, and minimizing thromboembolic risk. Sustained VAs have an ominous prognosis and may be indicative of ischemia or infarction; consideration should be given to ICD implantation. Treatment of all POAs should be directed at treating the underlying cause, with concurrent arrhythmia treatment, activating emergency measures as necessary.

REFERENCES

1. Angelini P, Feldman MI, Lufschanowski R, et al. Cardiac arrhythmias during and after heart surgery: diagnosis and management. Prog Cardiovasc Dis 1974; 16(5):469–95.
2. Mathew JP, Fontes ML, Tudor IC, et al. A multicenter risk index for atrial fibrillation after cardiac surgery. JAMA 2004;291(14):1720–9.
3. Batra G, Ahlsson A, Lindahl B, et al. Atrial fibrillation in patients undergoing coronary artery surgery is associated with adverse outcome. Ups J Med Sci 2018;1–8. https://doi.org/10.1080/03009734.2018.1504148. Available at: https://www.ncbi.nlm.nih.gov/pubmed/30265179.
4. Steinberg JS, Gaur A, Sciacca R, et al. New-onset sustained ventricular tachycardia after cardiac surgery. Circulation 1999;99(7):903. Available at: http://circ.ahajournals.org/cgi/content/abstract/99/7/903.
5. Tse G. Mechanisms of cardiac arrhythmias. J Arrhythm 2016;32:75–81. Available at: https://www.ncbi.nlm.nih.gov/pmc/journals/2797/.
6. Gaztañaga L, Marchlinski FE, Betensky BP. Mechanisms of cardiac arrhythmias. Rev Esp Cardiol (Engl Ed) 2012;65(2):174–85. Available at: https://www.sciencedirect.com/science/article/pii/S1885585711006086.
7. Smith W, Hood M. Arrhythmias. In: Sidebotham D, McKee A, Gillham M, et al, editors. Cardiothoracic critical care. Philadelphia: Butterworth Heinemann Elsevier; 2007. p. 316–41.
8. Holt AW. Cardiac arrhythmias. In: Berstein AD, Handy JM, editors. Oh's intensive care manual. 8th edition. Philadelphia: Elsevier; 2018. p. 277.e4. Available at: https://www.clinicalkey.es/playcontent/3-s2.0-B9780702072215000225.
9. Bojar RM. Manual of perioperative care in adult cardiac surgery. Hoboken (NJ): John Wiley & Sons, Incorporated; 2011.
10. Peretto G, Durante A, Limite LR, et al. Postoperative arrhythmias after cardiac surgery: incidence, risk factors, and therapeutic management. Cardiol Res Pract 2014. https://doi.org/10.1155/2014/615987.
11. Chung M. Cardiac surgery: postoperative arrhythmias. Crit Care Med 2000;28(10 Suppl):N144. Available at: http://ovidsp.ovid.com/ovidweb.cgi?T=JS&NEWS=n&CSC=Y&PAGE=fulltext&D=ovft&AN=00003246-200010001-00005.
12. Fogoros RN. Electrophysiologic testing. 5th edition. Chichester (West Sussex): John Wiley & Sons; 2013.
13. Raza SS, Li JM, John R, et al. Long-term mortality and pacing outcomes of patients with permanent pacemaker implantation after cardiac surgery. Pacing Clin Electrophysiol 2011;34(3):331–8. Available at: https://onlinelibrary.wiley.com/doi/abs/10.1111/j.1540-8159.2010.02972.x.

14. Houthuizen P, Van Garsse, Leen AFM, et al. Left bundle-branch block induced by transcatheter aortic valve implantation increases risk of death. Circulation 2012; 126(6):720–8. Available at: https://www.narcis.nl/publication/RecordID/oai:cris. maastrichtuniversity.nl:publications%2F87726161-7444-4656-a10f-c2fb2ac1856f.

15. Jaeger FJ, Trohman RG, Brener S, et al. Permanent pacing following repeat cardiac valve surgery. Am J Cardiol 1994;74(5):505–7. Available at: https://www.sciencedirect.com/science/article/pii/0002914994909164.

16. Brodell GK, Cosgrove D, Schiavone W, et al. Cardiac rhythm and conduction disturbances in patients undergoing mitral valve surgery. Cleve Clin J Med 1991; 58(5):397–9.

17. Siontis G, Juni P, Pilgrim T, et al. Predictors of permanent pacemaker implantation in patients with severe aortic stenosis undergoing TAVR. J Am Coll Cardiol 2014;64(2):129–40. Available at: https://www.clinicalkey.es/playcontent/1-s2.0-S073510971402436X.

18. Auffret V, Webb JG, Eltchaninoff H, et al. Clinical impact of baseline right bundle branch block in patients undergoing transcatheter aortic valve replacement. JACC Cardiovasc Interv 2017;10(15):1564–74. Available at: https://www.sciencedirect.com/science/article/pii/S1936879817309937.

19. Socie P, Nicot F, Baudinaud P, et al. Frequency of recovery from complete atrioventricular block after cardiac surgery. Am J Cardiol 2017;120(10):1841–6. Available at: https://www.sciencedirect.com/science/article/pii/S0002914917312961.

20. Epstein AE, DiMarco JP, Ellenbogen KA, et al. ACC/AHA/HRS 2008 guidelines for device-based therapy of cardiac rhythm abnormalities: a report of the American College of Cardiology/American Heart Association task force on practice guidelines (writing committee to revise the ACC/AHA/NASPE 2002 guideline update for implantation of cardiac pacemakers and antiarrhythmia devices): developed in collaboration with the American Association for Thoracic Surgery and Society of Thoracic Surgeons. Circulation 2008;117(21):e350. Available at: http://circ.ahajournals.org/cgi/content/extract/117/21/e350.

21. O'Brien B, Burrage PS, Ngai JY, et al. Society of Cardiovascular Anesthesiologists/European Association of Cardiothoracic Anaesthetists practice advisory for the management of perioperative atrial fibrillation in patients undergoing cardiac surgery. J Cardiothorac Vasc Anesth 2019;33(1):12–26. Available at: https://www.sciencedirect.com/science/article/pii/S1053077018309248.

22. Li R, White CM, Mehmeti J, et al. Impact of a perioperative prophylaxis guideline on post–cardiothoracic surgery atrial fibrillation. Ann Pharmacother 2017; 51(9):743–50. Available at: https://journals.sagepub.com/doi/full/10.1177/1060028017709290.

23. Maesen B, Nijs J, Maessen J, et al. Post-operative atrial fibrillation: a maze of mechanisms. Europace 2012;14(2):159–74. Available at: https://www.narcis.nl/publication/RecordID/oai:cris.maastrichtuniversity.nl:publications%2F48d0027b-7933-421f-9a3f-dab3f9c0cd52.

24. Baker WL, Coleman CI, White CM, et al. Use of preoperative CHA2DS2-VASc score to predict the risk of atrial fibrillation after cardiothoracic surgery: a nested case-control study from the atrial fibrillation suppression trials (AFIST) I, II, and III. Pharmacotherapy 2013;33(5):489–95.

25. Connolly SJ, Cybulsky I, Lamy A, et al. Double-blind, placebo-controlled, randomized trial of prophylactic metoprolol for reduction of hospital length of stay after heart surgery: the β-blocker length of stay (BLOS) study. Am Heart J 2003; 145(2):226–32. Available at: https://www.sciencedirect.com/science/article/pii/S0002870302948374.

26. Koniari I, Apostolakis E, Rogkakou C, et al. Pharmacologic prophylaxis for atrial fibrillation following cardiac surgery: a systematic review. J Cardiothorac Surg 2010;5(1):121.

27. Kirchhof P, Benussi S, Kotecha D, et al. 2016 ESC guidelines for the management of atrial fibrillation developed in collaboration with EACTS. Eur Heart J 2016;37(38): 2893–962. Available at: https://www.narcis.nl/publication/RecordID/oai:cris. maastrichtuniversity.nl:publications%2F21a1ca79-6b6f-437b-8e3a-dcee75afe83d.

28. Hillis LD, Smith P, Anderson J, et al. 2011 ACCF/AHA guideline for coronary artery bypass graft surgery. J Am Coll Cardiol 2011;58(24):e210. Available at: https:// www.ncbi.nlm.nih.gov/pubmed/22070836.

29. January CT, Wann LS, Alpert JS, et al. 2014 AHA/ACC/HRS guideline for the management of patients with atrial fibrillation: executive summary. J Am Coll Cardiol 2014;64(21):2246–80. Available at: https://www.clinicalkey.es/playcontent/1-s2.0-S0735109714017392.

30. Kolh P, Windecker S, Alfonso F, et al. 2014 ESC/EACTS guidelines on myocardial revascularization. Eur J Cardiothorac Surg 2014;46(4):517–92.

31. Patti G, Chello M, Candura D, et al. Randomized trial of atorvastatin for reduction of postoperative atrial fibrillation in patients undergoing cardiac surgery: results of the ARMYDA-3 (atorvastatin for reduction of MYocardial dysrhythmia after cardiac surgery) study. Circulation 2006;114(14):1455–61. Available at: http://circ. ahajournals.org/cgi/content/abstract/114/14/1455.

32. Jones C, Pollit V, Fitzmaurice D, et al. The management of atrial fibrillation: summary of updated NICE guidance. BMJ 2014;348(jun19 1):g3655. Available at:.

33. Gillinov AM, Bagiella E, Moskowitz AJ, et al. Rate control versus rhythm control for atrial fibrillation after cardiac surgery. N Engl J Med 2016;374(20):1911–21.

34. Butt JH, Xian Y, Peterson ED, et al. Long-term thromboembolic risk in patients with postoperative atrial fibrillation after coronary artery bypass graft surgery and patients with nonvalvular atrial fibrillation. JAMA Cardiol 2018;3(5):417.

35. El-Chami MF, Sawaya FJ, Kilgo P, et al. Ventricular arrhythmia after cardiac surgery: incidence, predictors, and outcomes. J Am Coll Cardiol 2012;60(25): 2664–71.

36. Ascione R, Reeves BC, Santo K, et al. Predictors of new malignant ventricular arrhythmias after coronary surgery: a case-control study. J Am Coll Cardiol 2004; 43(9):1630. Available at: http://content.onlinejacc.org/cgi/content/abstract/43/9/ 1630.

37. Rho RW, Bridges CR, Kocovic D. Management of postoperative arrhythmias. Semin Thorac Cardiovasc Surg 2000;12(4):349–61. Available at: https://www. sciencedirect.com/science/article/pii/S1043067900700426.

38. Buxton AE, Calkins H, Callans DJ, et al. ACC/AHA/HRS 2006 key data elements and definitions for electrophysiological studies and procedures. J Am Coll Cardiol 2006;48(11):2360–96. Available at: https://www.sciencedirect.com/science/ article/pii/S0735109706024454.

39. Bouri S, Shun-Shin MJ, Cole GD, et al. Meta-analysis of secure randomised controlled trials of beta-blockade to prevent perioperative death in non-cardiac surgery. Heart 2014;100(6):456–64. Available at: https://www.ncbi.nlm.nih.gov/ pubmed/23904357.

40. Mitchell LB, Powell JL, Gillis AM, AVID Investigators, et al. Are lipid-lowering drugs also antiarrhythmic drugs?: an analysis of the antiarrhythmics versus implantable defibrillators (AVID) trial. J Am Coll Cardiol 2003;42(1):81. Available at: http://content.onlinejacc.org/cgi/content/abstract/42/1/81.

41. Pinto RP, Romerill DB, Nasser WK, et al. Prognosis of patients with frequent premature ventricular complexes and nonsustained ventricular tachycardia after coronary artery bypass graft surgery. Clin Cardiol 1996;19(4):321–4. Available at: https://www.ncbi.nlm.nih.gov/pubmed/8706373.

42. Moss AJ, Hall WJ, Cannom DS, et al. Improved survival with an implanted defibrillator in patients with coronary disease at high risk for ventricular arrhythmia. N Engl J Med 1996;335(26):1933–40. Available at: http://content.nejm.org/cgi/content/abstract/335/26/1933.

43. Buxton AE, Lee KL, Fisher JD, et al. A randomized study of the prevention of sudden death in patients with coronary artery disease. multicenter unsustained tachycardia trial investigators. N Engl J Med 1999;341(25):1882. Available at: https://www.ncbi.nlm.nih.gov/pubmed/10601507.

44. Bigger J JT. Prophylactic use of implanted cardiac defibrillators in patients at high risk for ventricular arrhythmias after coronary-artery bypass graft surgery. coronary artery bypass graft (CABG) patch trial investigators. N Engl J Med 1997;337(22):1569. Available at: https://www.ncbi.nlm.nih.gov/pubmed/9371853.

45. Panchal AR, Berg KM, Kudenchuk PJ, et al. 2018 American Heart Association focused update on advanced cardiovascular life support use of antiarrhythmic drugs during and immediately after cardiac arrest: an update to the American Heart Association guidelines for cardiopulmonary resuscitation and emergency cardiovascular care. Circulation 2018;138(23):e740. Available at: https://www.ncbi.nlm.nih.gov/pubmed/30571262.

46. Dunning J, Levine A, Ley J, et al. The Society of Thoracic Surgeons expert consensus for the resuscitation of patients who arrest after cardiac surgery. Ann Thorac Surg 2017;103(3):1005–20. Available at: https://www.clinicalkey.es/playcontent/1-s2.0-S0003497516314825.

Pain Control in the Cardiothoracic Surgery Patient

Kelly A. Thompson-Brazill, DNP, ACNP-BC, CCRN-CSC, FCCM[a,b]

KEYWORDS

- Enhanced recovery after surgery • Opioid analgesics • Liposomal bupivacaine
- Ketamine • Multimodal pain control • Epidural analgesia • Nonopioid adjuncts
- Postoperative pain management

KEY POINTS

- Opioids remain the cornerstone of postoperative cardiothoracic surgery pain management.
- Clinicians are responsible for safely prescribing opioids as well as preventing and managing their untoward effects, including respiratory depression, hyperalgesia, tolerance, withdrawal, and dependence.
- Central and peripheral nerve blocks are effective methods of pain control.
- Multimodal pain control and enhanced recovery programs decrease postoperative opioid consumption.

INTRODUCTION

Postoperative pain is ubiquitous after cardiothoracic surgery. Opioids are the traditional mainstay for treatment of postoperative pain in the cardiothoracic surgical population.[1] Despite their efficacy, opioids pose significant patient safety risks. Incorporating patient-specific characteristics, such as level of sedation, existence of renal or hepatic dysfunction, and the presence of opioid tolerance are critical components of avoiding adverse events.[2] Concerns regarding patient safety combined with potential risks of addiction and overdose have sparked a national trend toward using nonopioid analgesics, multimodal treatment regimens, neuraxial analgesia, and regional nerve blocks with extended-release liposomal bupivacaine, to reduce patients' postsurgical opioid consumption.[3–7] This article evaluates the efficacy of

Disclosure Statement: The author has nothing to disclose.
a Adult-Gerontology Acute Care Nurse Practitioner Program, Georgetown University School of Nursing and Health Studies, 3700 Reservoir Road Northwest, Washington, DC 20057, USA;
b Wake Med Heart and Vascular Cardiothoracic Surgery, 3000 New Bern Avenue, Suite 1100, Raleigh, NC 27616, USA
E-mail address: kelly.thompsonbrazill@georgetown.edu

Crit Care Nurs Clin N Am 31 (2019) 389–405
https://doi.org/10.1016/j.cnc.2019.05.007

contemporary perioperative pain management strategies and makes therapeutic recommendations based on national guidelines and current evidence.

Surgical trauma causes local release of inflammatory mediators, including cytokines, leukotrienes, prostanoids, and histamine, increasing sensitivity at afferent nerve terminals.[8] The level of pain experienced is usually proportional to the extent of the surgery and the amount of tissue involved.[8] In postoperative patients, pain occurs at the surgical site, organ, and/or tissue levels (skin, subcutaneous fat, fascia, muscle, bone), and is occasionally referred to more distal locations.[8,9] Pain characteristics and severity vary depending on the extent of surgical manipulation and the structures involved.[9]

The ability to sense pain (nociception) is present in various parts of the body, including organs and muscles. Types of postsurgical pain include neuropathic, somatic, and visceral.[9] Neuropathic and somatic pain are more common after chest surgery than visceral pain.[9] Nerve roots located in the thoracic spine form intercostal nerves that innervate the bony thorax and surrounding tissues.[9] Phrenic nerve fibers are located in the parietal pericardium and vagal nerve fibers are located in the visceral pericardium.[9] A multitude of nerve fibers in the parietal pleura are sensitive to both chemical and mechanical irritation.[9]

Iatrogenic neuropathic pain results from nerve injury or inflammation. It may be localized or diffuse depending on the nerve(s) involved. It is typically characterized as "pins and needles," "burning," "shooting," or "sharp."[10] Reports of peripheral nerve injury in the cardiac surgery literature range from 2.7% to 13%.[11] The brachial plexus is the most commonly injured structure, followed by the ulnar nerve.[11,12] Diabetic individuals and patients with a history of peripheral neuropathy or peripheral arterial disease are at higher risk of developing postoperative neuropathy.[11,12]

The brachial plexus is a large group of nerves on either side of the body, arising from cervical spine nerve roots C5 to C8.[13] The plexus innervates the muscles of the chest and upper arm, enabling both motion and sensation.[13] Damage typically results from either stretch or compression of a portion of the nerve network due to patient positioning in the operating room (OR) or from sternal retractors.[12] Brachial plexus injury (BPI) is associated with the degree of sternal retraction (distance between the sternal halves), the location of retraction (less common with caudal retraction), and the type of retractor used (more common with asymmetrical retractors).[12] Nerve stretch induces ischemia by altering the microvasculature blood supply.[11] In cases of more severe trauma, connective tissue may provoke hemorrhage or necrosis of the involved nerve cells, worsening the risk of developing neuropathy.[11]

The ulnar nerve innervates the sensory portion of half of the fourth digit, all of the fifth digit, and the medial portion of the hand.[14] Ulnar injury is more common in the left upper extremity.[15] Clinical examples of stretch-induced BPI in median sternotomy patients include paresthesias and anesthesia of the ipsilateral median and radial nerves.[12] Ulnar nerve compression can occur at the upper arm, forearm, and wrist, but is most common at the elbow.[14] Pressure at the elbow causes paresthesia and anesthesia in the ipsilateral fourth and fifth digits, in addition to the lateral portion of the hand. It does not affect forearm sensation.[14] These sensory changes occur with or without impaired motor function and weakness. Ipsilateral vascular cannulation may lead to right upper extremity mononeuropathies.[15] If the involved nerve is not completely severed, regeneration is possible.[11] Nerve restoration is a slow process with repair of only 1 mm of nerve tissue in a 24-hour period.[11]

Rehabilitation, including occupational therapy, is an important part of the recovery process for both BPI and ulnar nerve injury.[16] Physical therapy significantly improves sensitivity, nerve conduction, and muscle strength in both BPI and ulnar neuropathy.[16]

Remedies for neuropathic pain range from noninvasive modalities like transcutaneous electrical nerve stimulation and medications to nerve blocks and surgery. Topical treatments include lidocaine and capsaicin.[17,18] Lidocaine is a local anesthetic that is available over the counter as 4% patches and by prescription as 5% patches. Capsaicin is derived from chili peppers. It attenuates nerve sensitivity to mechanical and chemical irritation.[17] It is available as a cream and as a patch. Gabapentin and pregabalin are calcium channel ligands shown to improve neuropathic pain and allodynia.[17] Allodynia refers the pain signals that neurons transmit in response to nonpainful stimuli.[17,18] Calcium channel ligands are used alone or in conjunction with either tricyclic antidepressants (eg, amitriptyline, nortriptyline) or serotonin norepinephrine reuptake inhibitors (eg, duloxetine).[17] Nerve blocks with lidocaine or other local anesthetics also decrease neuropathic pain and allodynia.[17]

Data regarding duration of neuropathic pain after sternotomy are not specific to peripheral nerve injuries.[19] Most of the literature regarding peripheral nerve injury in this population comes from dated case reports. Anecdotal evidence denotes resolution of symptoms within days to weeks up to a few months. Prospective randomized trials examining the average length of time to symptom resolution in patients with BPI and ulnar nerve injury are needed.

ACUTE POSTOPERATIVE PAIN

Acute postoperative pain is the most intense within the first 24 to 48 hours after surgery, and gradually improves during the postoperative period.[8] Pain severity is a subjective phenomenon. Some people have lower tolerance to nociceptive stimuli than others.[4] Personal factors associated with higher levels of periprocedural pain include the presence of anxiety or depression, age younger than 60 years, body mass index (BMI) $\geq$ 25, female gender, non-white ethnicity, and the presence of 1 or more comorbidities.[4,9] Use of the internal mammary artery for bypass grafting, opening of the pleural spaces, and operative time >3 hours are also related to more intense pain.[8,9]

Areas of discomfort may alternate during the healing process.[8] The sternotomy site, shoulders, back, and neck are commonly involved.[9] Minimally invasive surgery is associated with less pain than full sternotomy. Nociception is proportional to number and location of incisions, as well as the presence of chest tubes (**Table 1**).[9,20] Nerve trauma, bruising, and tenderness are more prevalent with open saphenous vein harvest compared with endoscopic vein harvest.[21] Endoscopic radial artery harvesting leads to significantly less pain at postoperative day 2 and at the time of discharge compared with open radial harvest.[22]

During rest periods, critical care patients experience moderate to severe pain.[4] Patients report worsening discomfort with routine activities such as incentive spirometry use, coughing, and movement.[9] Pain complicates recovery. It limits the depth of respiration and results in low-incentive spirometry volumes.[4,9] It inhibits ambulation and contributes to atelectasis and lower oxygen saturations.[4,8,9] In mechanically ventilated patients, pain may trigger ventilator dyssynchrony.[4] Common postoperative procedures, such as the insertion, manipulation, and/or removal of mechanical circulatory support, chest tubes, and other devices, such as arterial lines, central venous access devices, and bladder catheters, incite varying levels of pain.[4]

The American Pain Society (APS) recommends using validated pain scales along with objective data for measuring postoperative pain. A number of pain scales were reviewed during the creation of the Society of Critical Care Medicine's (SCCM) 2018 Management of Pain, Agitation, Delirium, Immobility, and Sleep (PADIS). The numeric rating visual (NRS-V) had significantly positive results in verbal patients compared with

Table 1 Indications for opioid use	
Pain	**Sedation**
Analgesia during times of impaired communication • Intubation • Neuromuscular blockade	Analgosedation • Opioids used for both pain control and sedative properties
Chest tubes, drains	
Moderate to severe pain due to the following: • Burn injury • Disease-related • Medical illness • Traumatic injury • Surgery	
Invasive monitoring lines	
Mechanical circulatory support	
Procedural pain	

Data from Refs.[4,7,9]

the visual analog scale (VAS) and the visual descriptor scale (VDS).[4] The 0 to 10 Faces Pain Thermometer (FPT) was initially validated on cardiac surgery patients. The review by SCCM demonstrated that the FPT is more reliable in adults than the Wong-Baker FACES scale, which was developed for pediatric pain assessment.[4] Behavioral pain scales are necessary for assessing pain in intubated patients. They are also useful in nonintubated patients with altered mentation and communication.[4] The Critical-Care Pain Observation Tool and the Behavioral Pain Scale in intubated (BPS) and non-intubated (BPS-NI) patients were deemed best for evaluating pain in this population.[4]

Postsurgical pain generally lasts several days to weeks, yet for some people it persists for months. The current literature estimates 17% to 56% of sternotomy patients have chronic pain 3 to 6 months after surgery.[8,9,19,23] Risk factors in the development of chronic postoperative cardiac surgery pain (CPOP) include the use of the internal thoracic (mammary) artery for bypass grafts and osteochondral avulsion and stainless steel sternal wire fixation in sternotomy patients and complex wound issues such as infection.[9,23] Intercostal nerve injury, rib fractures, and scar tissue formation are linked to CPOP in both cardiac and thoracic surgery patients.[9] Post-procedural pain that is intense, poorly controlled, and worse than anticipated along with protracted delays between a patient's request for and administration of "as-needed" analgesia increase the incidence of CPOP.[4,7,24] A large study examined the incidence of persistent pain in older adults after cardiac, thoracic, abdominal, or pelvic procedures. Those who underwent either minimally invasive (6.3%) or open (8.5%) thoracic surgery had the highest incidence of opioid use >90 days after surgery.[25] Overall, thoracic patients were 2.58 times more likely to have prolonged use than those who had nonthoracic procedures.[25]

PHYSIOLOGIC AND PSYCHOLOGICAL EFFECTS OF UNCONTROLLED PAIN

Physiologically, the body responses to uncontrolled pain and other stressors by triggering a neuroendocrine response.[26,27] This involves activation of the sympathetic nervous system (SNS), renin-angiotensin-aldosterone system (RAAS), and the hypothalamic pituitary adrenal axis (HPA).[26,27] SNS stimulation triggers catecholamine release from the adrenal medulla.[27] Epinephrine is a positive inotrope that stimulates cardiac β_1 receptors to increase heart rate and myocardial contractility.[27] Norepinephrine functions at α_1 receptors to induce vasoconstriction and β_1 receptors improve inotropy.[27] Activation of RAAS prompts release of angiotensin II from the kidneys.[27]

ATII has several physiologic properties. It raises blood pressure via vasoconstriction. It increases the risk of thrombus formation by stimulating plasminogen activator inhibitor protein (PAI-1 and PAI-2).[9,28] Moreover, ATII stimulates the HPA axis to augment mineralocorticoid and glucocorticoid production.[24,28] In addition, RAAS prompts secretion of the mineralocorticoid aldosterone from the zona glomerulosa region of the adrenal cortex.[28] Aldosterone promotes sodium reabsorption in the renal proximal tubules, which induces serum sodium and fluid retention, while lowering serum potassium levels.[28]

This pain-induced activation of the body's neurohormonal cascade generates elevations in heart rate, blood pressure, and fluid retention, while amplifying the likelihood of arrhythmias, such as atrial fibrillation.[4,24,27] All of these factors intensify myocardial oxygen demand (MVO$_2$). Higher MVO$_2$ combined with the potential for PAI-1/PAI-II–associated thrombin formation may induce myocardial ischemia.[28] Other consequences of this increased neurohormonal activation include worsening heart failure (HF). Aldosterone and vasopressin (antidiuretic hormone) secretion increase preload.[27] In patients with HF with reduced ejection fraction (HFrEF), the addition of this extra blood volume in the ventricle can negatively affect contractility (Starling's Law), reducing cardiac output. ATII and norepinephrine vasoconstrict, raising afterload and subsequently lowering cardiac output.[27] Chronic SNS activation is toxic to cardiac muscle cells, which contributes to worsening cardiac function over time.[27,29]

In addition to instigating adverse physiologic changes, untreated pain is related to a myriad of psychological phenomena including sleep deprivation, anxiety, depression, and delirium.[4,24] It may also contribute to the development of posttraumatic stress disorder (PTSD).[24]

STRATEGIES FOR PREVENTING POSTOPERATIVE PAIN

Current guidelines from SCCM and APS encourage anticipating and preemptively addressing periprocedural pain.[2,4] The APS recommends preoperative patient-centered and family-centered, culturally appropriate instruction that is tailored to both the patient's health literacy level and cognitive status.[2] Meetings like this should include provider questions aimed toward elucidating patient preferences (eg, "What pharmaceutical and nonpharmaceutical interventions have improved your pain in the past?").[2] Determining if the patient is reluctant to take opioids or other types of pain medications is essential in preventing uncontrolled pain after surgery.[9] If patient concerns exist, address them openly and honestly, while offering the patient options for pain management.[2,7]

Before surgery, patients may question whether or not they can continue taking their home medications while hospitalized.[2] Providers giving patients an idea of their expected medication regimen along with the rationale for these changes, may allay fears and decrease anxiety while fostering patient engagement, and promoting informed decision-making.[2] Last, good pain control and provider communication increase patient satisfaction.[9]

OPIOID PHARMACOLOGY AND DOSING

Morphine was derived from opium in the early nineteenth century. Since the mid-1800s, opioids have been the mainstay of postoperative patient management.[1] Opioids relieve pain by primarily binding to mu opioid receptors, which are located in the portions of the brain involved with nociception and to the outer laminae of the spinal cord's dorsal horn.[30,31] These receptors are also located in the gastrointestinal tract and in the bladder, which results in adverse effects such as constipation and urine retention.[24] Some opioid analgesics bind to delta opioid receptors located throughout the spinal cord's dorsal horn.[31] Some also bind to kappa opioid receptors, which are located in the outer lamina of the dorsal horn of the lumbosacral portion of the spinal cord.[31]

Prescribing opioid pain medication is an intricate process. Providers must assess the risk/benefit ratio of antinociceptive medications for each patient.[4] The APS cautions providers from ordering opioids based solely on patient-reported numeric or Behavioral Pain Scale ratings.[2] The APS guidelines recommend combining patient-reported pain scales with objective measures such as age, comorbidities such as renal or hepatic impairment, level of sedation, respiratory status, and the presence/level of opioid tolerance.[2] Frequent reassessment of pain allows for medication adjustments based on symptomatic relief, depth of sedation, and impact on functional ability, in addition to existence of any adverse effects.[2,32,33]

Hepatic and renal dysfunction alter metabolism and elimination of medications, respectively. Opioids are primarily metabolized by the liver and excreted by the kidneys.[33,34] The cytochrome P450 enzyme system metabolizes 80% of medications currently on the market. *CYP3A4* metabolizes more than 50% of opioids. Some opioids are processed through more than one isoenzyme (eg, oxycodone is metabolized by both *CYP2D6* and *CYP3A4*).[34] Drug interactions can occur if the substrate medications are processed through the same isoenzyme.[33] Induction or inhibition of an isoenzyme can lead to low or high levels of the substrate, respectively.[33] Patients with acute and/or chronic renal disease may not adequately clear opioids or their active metabolites.[33,35–37] For instance, morphine has 2 major metabolites that are eliminated by the kidneys: morphine-3-glucuronide (M3G) and morphine-6-glucuronide (M6G).[38] Both have high plasma concentrations and can cross the blood-brain barrier.[38] As creatinine clearance decreases during acute or chronic kidney injury, these metabolites accumulate.[36,38,39]

M6G is responsible for approximately 84.5% to 96.6% of morphine's analgesic effect depending on the route of administration.[38] It has more affinity for mu opioid receptor binding than its parent compound.[38] In a recent study of morphine pharmacokinetics, in patients with renal failure who received a one-time dose of intravenous morphine, morphine's analgesic effect was comparable to its effects in individuals with normal renal function.[38] However, with repeated doses, the analgesic effect in those with impaired kidney function increased to 100%.[38] M3G has the opposite affinity for the mu opioid receptor and may actually antagonize (prevent) morphine binding.[38] M3G is associated with morphine's adverse reactions, such as nausea and increased nociception.[38] Based on the available data, it is safer to prescribe morphine and other opioids at low doses and gradually titrate to effect.[34,36,38] Moreover, extreme caution should be used when calculating morphine doses in morbidly obese (BMI $\geq$ 40) patients with kidney dysfunction, as this magnitude of obesity alone significantly decreases M6G and M3G clearance.[40]

In addition to the risk of increased opioid or opioid metabolite levels in renal patients, clinicians should understand how hemodialysis (HD) alters drug levels. Some individuals may have increased nociception after HD treatments if their opioid medication is easily removed by dialysis. In general, drugs that have low molecular weights, low protein binding, low volume of distribution (V_d), and are hydrophilic are more dialyzable.[36] (There are several handbooks and smart phone applications regarding medications cleared by dialysis that are available for purchase.) In opioid-dependent patients, this may induce opioid withdrawal.[33] Consider adjusting medication dosages or administration times in this population.[33]

As previously mentioned, opioid response changes in response to patient characteristics that impact pharmacokinetics. Opioid potency also varies.[41,42] To determine the strengths of different agents, the efficacy of all opioids are compared with a standard criterion, morphine. This is based on the calculation of morphine milligram equivalents (MME). Having a standard morphine dosing equivalent (morphine equivalent daily dose [MEDD]) allows providers and pharmacists to evaluate the potency of a patient's daily opiate use, and allows for easier conversion from one opioid to another (**Box 1**).[6,43] Opioid conversion tables and online calculators are useful tools for clinicians[42,43] (https://opioidcalculator.practicalpainmanagement.com/).

- MEDD = strength per unit × (number of units/days of supply) × MME conversion factor[43]

OPIOID-INDUCED HYPERALGESIA

Opioid-induced hyperalgesia (OIH) is an exaggerated response to pain that is likely triggered by inflammation.[24,31] Chronic opioid exposure activates a process meant to prevent overstimulation of the central nervous system (CNS) by opioids.[24] During chronic exposure, the amount of G-protein coupled receptors decrease via downregulation.[24] Glutamate levels at the nerve synapses rise. N-methyl D-aspartate (NMDA) receptors are activated. Nociceptive signals are transmitted.[24] Opioids induce toll-like receptor activation of glial cells in the CNS resulting in inflammation.[24] This process alters the blood-brain barrier, facilitating peripheral macrophage entry into the CNS.[24] The overstimulated central and peripheral nerve cells are less sensitive to the effects of opioid analgesics leading to heightened pain perception.[24,31]

Risk factors for OIH include age, gender, and the presence of acute or chronic inflammation.[24] In critical care, inflammation occurs due to infection, physiologic stress, and/or high-dose or frequently administered opioids for analgesia or sedation, such as remifentanil.[24] OIH treatment strategies include daily interruption of opioid and sedative infusions, adding alternative analgesics (eg, ketamine, buprenorphine) as adjuncts to managing postoperative pain in this population, rotating opioid medications, or increasing the dose of the opioid.[24,31]

Ketamine is a noncompetitive NMDA antagonist that produces analgesia and anesthesia.[44] NMDA receptors are thought to intensify pain signal transmission.[45] Ketamine was developed in the 1960s from phencyclidine.[45] Because of its relationship to phencyclidine, ketamine produces dissociative effects, augmenting its anesthetic

---

Box 1
Risk factors for opioid-induced respiratory depression

- High doses of opioids during the postoperative period
- Patient-controlled analgesia
- Patient-controlled analgesia with a basal infusion rate
- Epidural opioids
- Sedatives
- Cardiac surgery
- Thoracic surgery

Data from Refs.[3,6,8,30]

properties.[45] It is thought to interfere with pain signal transmission by altering the activation of glial cells (astrocytes and microglia) in the CNS[45] (**Fig. 1**). When given preoperatively, it decreases the amount of opioids consumed after surgery.[2] Ketamine is sometimes used as a nonopioid adjunct to decrease postoperative opioid use.[31] It is thought that ketamine reduces OIH and opioid tolerance by antagonizing NMDA receptors in the CNS, leading to decreased sensitization.[45]

Despite anecdotal reports of its ability to reduce the need for opioids, varying reports in the literature contradict those claims. The Cochrane Database of Systematic Reviews evaluated several studies that demonstrated intraoperative intravenous ketamine administration reduced in postoperative opioid use in the first 24 to 48 hours after surgery.[46] Unfortunately many of the studies had low numbers of subjects in treatment groups. As a result, the Cochrane Review notes that ketamine "probably" decreases hyperalgesia and "likely" improves pain severity and decreases analgesic use.[46] Ketamine is generally well tolerated, but its adverse effects include anorexia, epigastric pain, and gastrointestinal bleeding.[45]

Buprenorphine is a partial opioid agonist with weak analgesic properties. It has a strong affinity for opioid receptors, preventing opioid binding at those sites.[24] Although it is typically used by itself to manage chronic pain or in conjunction with naloxone as medically directed treatment for substance abuse, it may attenuate OIH.[24] Avoid using buprenorphine in opioid-dependent patients because it can cause acute withdrawal.[34] Further research is needed to determine its efficacy in cardiothoracic surgery and critical care populations.

DEXMEDETOMIDINE AND OPIOID USE IN CARDIAC SURGICAL CRITICAL CARE

Although an in-depth discussion the sedation portion of SCCM's 2018 PADIS guidelines is beyond the scope of this article, a small control trial (DEXACET) examining the incidence of delirium in the first 48 hours after cardiac surgery demonstrated lower postoperative opioid usage in one of its experimental groups. DEXACET randomized patients (n = 140) to receive intravenous (IV) acetaminophen or placebo, along with an IV sedative infusion of either dexmedetomide or propofol within the first 48 hours after

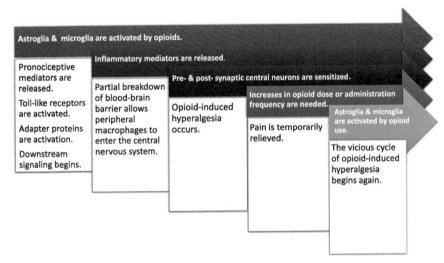

Fig. 1. The pathophysiology of opioid-induced hyperalgesia. (*Data from* Martyn JAJ, Mao J, Bittner EA. Opioid tolerance in critical illness. N Engl J Med 2019;380:365–78.)

surgery.[47] Dexmedetomidine is an alpha 2 (α_2) agonist that induces sedation by decreasing sympathetic outflow.[48] Propofol is a sedative-hypnotic with Food and Drug Administration (FDA) approval for both anesthesia and sedation.[49] Its mechanism of action is not fully understood, but its sedative effect may be related to regulation of gamma aminobutyric acid (GABA), an inhibitory neurotransmitter.[49] Interestingly, the use of IV acetaminophen combined with IV dexmedetomidine was associated with significantly decreased median opioid use compared with the combination of IV acetaminophen and IV propofol (328.8 vs 397.5 MME). Subjects who received the IV acetaminophen had significantly reduced delirium.[47] There were no major differences in the incidence of delirium in patients randomized to either sedative. However, the study may have been underpowered to determine if dexmedetomidine was superior to propofol in delirium reduction.[47] Further research with a larger number of subjects is needed to fully ascertain if one medication has more beneficial effects on delirium than the other.

DEVELOPMENT OF OPIOID TOLERANCE IN CRITICAL CARE

Patients with severe injuries and/or those requiring prolonged mechanical ventilation may have less pain relief from an opioid over time (tolerance).[24] Patients develop tolerance to the nausea, euphoria, sedation, and analgesia with repeated administration.[30,34] Abatement of the respiratory depressive effects takes longer.[30] Constipation is one adverse effect that does not improve over time. During periods of extended opioid exposure, extracellular molecules (first messengers) cause cells to release second messenger signals inside cells to downregulate opioid receptors.[50] In turn, escalating dosages or shorter time intervals between medication administration are required for adequate pain control.[24]

OPIOID-INDUCED IATROGENIC WITHDRAWAL SYNDROME

Critically ill patients who have prolonged exposure to opioids while in the intensive care unit (ICU) can experience withdrawal symptoms during rapid or gradual opioid weaning.[50] This is referred to as iatrogenic withdrawal syndrome (IWS).[50] Despite the widespread use of opioids in critically ill adult patients, there are more data on pediatric than adult IWS.[50,51] Given the paucity of data in adults, Wang and colleagues[50] evaluated the effect of opioid weaning on adult ICU patients receiving mechanical ventilation for >72 hours. They excluded those with a history of cognitive impairment, traumatic brain injury, and opioid or illicit drug (such as cocaine and heroin) use, and/or significant alcohol misuse. They used the criteria of the *Diagnostic and Statistical Manual of Mental Disorders, 5th edition* (DSM-V) criteria for opioid withdrawal, which may occur within minutes to days after stopping opioid use.[50] Incidence of IWS in this population was 16.7%.[50] Delirium was present in 44% of patients with IWS.[50] Based on the data, adults with IWS had higher cumulative opioid dosages and longer lengths of opioid exposure.[50] These findings are congruent with those of pediatric IWS.[50]

Opioid withdrawal is often likened to an influenza-type presentation that may include piloerection, muscle aches, diaphoresis, chills, fever, watery eyes and/or nose, nausea, or emesis.[30,50] Insomnia, agitation, and tremors are also common.[30,50] The Clinical Opioid Withdrawal Scale (COWS) is a valid, commonly used tool for assessing for opioid withdrawal in both inpatients and outpatients.[52] It helps clinicians assess the stage or severity of opioid withdrawal, in addition to determining the patient's degree of physical dependence on opioids.[53] Although COWS includes some objective data, its use of subjective measures limits its utility in intubated patients. Moreover, in their recent meta-analyses, Chiu and coworkers[51] were unable to find a valid tool that assesses IWS in adult critically ill patients, despite identifying 2 valid scales for use in the pediatric ICU.

Opioid withdrawal treatment is symptom-based. Alpha and beta-blockers decrease somatic symptoms.[54,55] Nausea and vomiting are treated with antiemetics, such as ondansetron or metoclopramide. If a patient is experiencing abdominal cramping, antispasmodic agents like dicyclomine or hyoscyamine may help.[55] If diarrhea occurs, loperamide and similar medications may decrease gastrointestinal motility.[55] Myalgias and arthralgias are usually responsive to acetaminophen or naproxen.[55] Anxiety and agitation may respond to nonbenzodiazepine medications with sedating effects such as hydroxyzine.[55]

OPIOID-INDUCED RESPIRATORY DEPRESSION

Opioid-induced respiratory depression (OIRD) is the most common cause of opioid-related deaths.[30] It is associated with increased hospital length of stay and higher costs.[6] Opioid binding to the mu opioid receptors in the brainstem leads to respiratory depression.[30] Without intervention, bradypnea (respiratory rate <12 breaths per minute) starts a chain reaction of carbon dioxide retention, hypoxia, and cardiac arrest.[34] Most cases of OIRD occur within the first 24 hours after surgery.[6] This is not surprising, as pain is typically the most severe in the first 24 hours after surgery and patients often require higher amounts of opioids for adequate pain relief.[3,8] Subjects in the OIRD group had 23% higher MEDD of postoperative opioids compared with those in the control group.[6] Patient-controlled analgesia, epidural opioid administration, and sedative use increase the risk of OIRD.[6] The incidence of OIRD is 19% in thoracic and vascular surgery patients.[6] This is not surprising, given its 3 main risk factors are coexisting cardiac disease, pulmonary disease, and obstructive sleep apnea.[6] Approximately 50% of patients who die from respiratory complications in the first 24 hours have OSA.[6] Vigilant monitoring and judicious use of opioids is imperative in preventing OIRD in all cardiothoracic surgery patients, especially those with OSA.

Naloxone is the medication of choice to reverse OIRD.[34] Naloxone is a pure opioid antagonist. Its mechanism of action is not completely understood. It competes with opioids at several opioid receptor sites in the CNS, but it has the most affinity for mu opioid receptors.[44] It is indicated for opioid reversal in patients with respiratory depression and/or impaired cardiovascular function (eg, tachycardia, hypotension).[34]

COMPARISON OF THORACIC EPIDURALS AND EXTENDED-RELEASE LIPOSOMAL BUPIVACAINE

Thoracic epidural analgesia (TEA) has been extensively used to manage perioperative thoracotomy pain.[56,57] In many institutions, these central nerve blocks are achieved using a continuous infusion of bupivacaine hydrochloride 0.125% in epidural space with or without opioid analgesics to reduce postoperative nociception in thoracotomy patients.[2,57] In a recent study, TEA with bupivacaine and fentanyl was compared with morphine PCA and oxycodone PCA.[56] Subjects randomized to TEA had lower postoperative pain both at rest and with movement, as well as improved patient satisfaction scores compared with those assigned to either PCA group.[56]

Despite the well-documented efficacy of epidural infusions in diminishing thoracotomy pain, these catheters are associated with several risks ranging from hypotension and urinary retention to more severe and potentially life-threatening complications such as spinal cord injury, cerebrospinal fluid leaks, epidural hematomas, and abscess development.[57] Successful catheter insertion relies on provider skill. Large body habitus and other physical characteristics of patients may make placement difficult or impossible.[57] Epidural or spinal anesthesia is not appropriate for all patients. Contraindications to neuraxial analgesia include history of spine surgery and conditions or medications that place a patient at risk for neurologic deterioration from neuraxial analgesia.[2]

Peripheral nerve blocks with paravertebral catheters and regional nerve blocks are effective alternatives to TEA.[2,7] Paravertebral catheters are placed between the parietal pleura and the chest wall during video-assisted thorascopic surgery (VATS) or open thoracotomy.[7] Because the catheters are not providing neuraxial analgesia, these paravertebral infusions use higher bupivacaine hydrochloride concentrations (0.25%) compared with TEA, and are associated with less hypotension and urinary retention.[58] Regional nerve blocks have typically used short-acting local anesthetics. Over the past few years, extended-release liposomal bupivacaine (LB) is becoming more popular among both thoracic and cardiac surgeons for minimally invasive surgeries.[7,59] LB is easy to administer under direct visualization.[7] Its formulation allows for a longer duration of pain relief.[7,57,60] Because it is long-acting, other non-bupivacaine local anesthetics such as lidocaine may cause immediate release of bupivacaine resulting in neurologic and/or cardiovascular toxicity.[60] The risk of methemoglobinemia increases with concurrent use of one or more drugs known to cause it (eg, nitroglycerin, nitroprusside, local anesthetics, phenytoin).[61]

Despite its higher price compared with traditional short-acting local anesthetics, many surgeons are now using it for nerve blocks with the goals of decreasing postoperative nociception and for its potential opioid-sparing effects.[57,60] Lee and colleagues[60] performed a small (n = 79) randomized controlled trial comparing the analgesic effects of parasternal nerve blocks with LB with saline placebo for 72 hours after coronary artery bypass graft (CABG) surgery. Patients who received the LB demonstrated significantly improved postoperative pain compared with those in the control group. However, there was no significant difference in opioid MMEs administered.

NONOPIOID ANALGESICS

Acetaminophen is widely used for pain relief in the outpatient setting. Because it is not a narcotic and is generally well-tolerated, its popularity for treating mild to moderate postoperative nociception is increasing.[7] The advent of IV acetaminophen has also renewed clinical interest in the drug. The parenteral route of administration eliminates concerns of poor absorption.[58] For most medications, the oral route is preferred over rectal administration because of erratic rectal absorption and patient discomfort.[7] After reviewing multiple studies, APS reports that there is no analgesia difference between IV or oral forms of the drug.[2]

Both gabapentin and pregabalin reduce opioid use after major surgery.[2] They are typically administered 1 to 2 hours before the procedure.[2] Although several dosing ranges for both drugs have been evaluated, the optimal dosing of each remains unclear.[2] Gabapentin is renally cleared and requires renal dosing.[33] Sedation occurs with higher doses and improves once the dose is lowered or the drug is stopped.[2] Gabapentin's more common adverse effects include ataxia, dizziness, nausea, peripheral edema, and tremor.[2] These also typically resolve once the drug is discontinued.

Over-the-counter and prescription nonsteroidal anti-inflammatory drugs (NSAIDs) are commonly used for pain relief. In 2010, an estimated 29 million Americans were either chronically or periodically taking NSAIDs.[62] They reduce pain by blocking the cyclooxygenase pathway preventing prostaglandin production. Although NSAIDs are a useful adjunct in decreasing nociception after thoracic surgery, they are often avoided in valvular or aortic surgery because of their risks of acute kidney injury, breakdown of the gastric mucosal barrier, and platelet inhibition.[2,9,47] In 2005, the FDA placed a black box warning on NSAIDs because of a higher incidence of stroke and myocardial infarction, and these drugs are contraindicated for perioperative pain management after CABG surgery.[2,63] This warning was strengthened in 2015.[63] Despite the black box warning, a retrospective pooled analysis from the PREVENT-IV and MEND-CABG II trials found that NSAIDs were used in 30.9% of CABG patients.[64] The 30-day outcomes were similar between the 2 groups and led the researchers to conclude there was no increased risk of using NSAIDs post-CABG.[64] Given the black box warning and the associated risks, more data are needed before prescribing NSAIDs post-CABG becomes a standard practice.

Tramadol is a synthetic centrally acting analgesic.[65] It is used to treat moderate pain. It is metabolized by *CYP2D6*. Its M1 metabolite has high affinity for binding to the mu opioid receptor.[65] Individuals with genetic polymorphisms of *CYP2D6* have varied responses to tramadol depending on their allele.[66] Those with little to no *CYP2D6* activity poorly metabolize tramadol, preventing the M1 metabolite formation Since the active metabolite is not formed, individuals with this allele have little to no pain relief from tramadol.[65] This mechanism of action increases the risks for drug misuse and respiratory depression. It weakly inhibits synaptic uptake of serotonin and dopamine. This increases the risk of developing seizures or serotonin syndrome if taken with any of the following antidepressant classes: selective serotonin reuptake inhibitors, selective serotonin-norepinephrine reuptake inhibitors, tricyclic antidepressants, or monoamine oxidase inhibitors.[65]

In addition to medications, there are multiple alternative therapies to alleviate nociception. For localized discomfort, applying heat or ice packs, or massage are often effective. Repositioning and increasing physical activity may provide relief. Some patients will benefit from biofeedback, image-guided therapy, and/or relaxation exercises.[33] Combining both modalities may synergistically decrease pain and improve patient outcomes.

ENHANCED RECOVERY AFTER SURGERY

Enhanced Recovery after Surgery (ERAS) for abdominal surgeries took hold in Europe in the 1990s.[67] It has been frequently used in thoracic surgery cases.[7,20] Cardiac surgeons, advanced practice providers, and other integral members of health care teams are increasingly interested in adopting a cardiac surgery–specific ERAS protocol. Several feasibility studies were completed, but protocols were not implemented in hospitals until recently. Williams and coworkers[3] developed the first ERAS Cardiac program in the United States. The ERAS Cardiac protocol incorporated several standard ERAS measures, including preoperative education, prehabilitation, optimization of nutrition, using multimodal opioid-sparing analgesia starting the morning of surgery and throughout the postoperative period, using short-acting anesthetics, prevention of nausea and vomiting, early ambulation, and priority discharge.[3,67] One-year results demonstrated 3 statistically significant outcomes, including a 30% reduction in intravenous opioid pain medication use in the first 24 hours postoperative. The other significant reductions were in hospital length of stay and ICU length of stay.[3] Ideally, future research on the ERAS Cardiac program will evaluate the overall effect multimodal therapies have on the quantity of MMEs administered during hospitalization and prescribed at discharge.

THE OPIOID EPIDEMIC AND PRESCRIBING LIMITS FOR ACUTE PAIN

Opioids are a mainstay for postoperative pain management, despite their addictive potential.[6] Several investigators list the overprescribing of opioid analgesics as a major factor in what is now called the "opioid epidemic."[30,68,69] The high incidence of chronic pain and the large numbers of opioid prescriptions filled each year, combined with pervasive drug diversion and misuse have become a public health crisis.[30,68,69] In 2016, 14,487 people died from overdoses of prescription opioids, including oxycodone, hydrocodone, and morphine.[43] In response, the Centers for Disease Control and Prevention developed a multifaceted approach aimed at ending the widespread misuse and abuse of these drugs. Monies awarded to states foster consumer education, cultivate prescription drug monitoring programs, and regulate the amount of opioids prescribed for acute pain.[43,70] As a whole, these interventions have reduced opioid prescriptions by 8.2% per year from 2014 to 2017. This is noteworthy compared with the 1.6% decline per year from 2010 to 2014.[43]

RESPONSIBLE PRESCRIBING AT DISCHARGE

A recent retrospective study evaluated opioid use in patients for 30 days before CABG surgery through 30 days after hospitalization. Those with a history of opioid exposure received a larger number of prescriptions for more than 150 mg of oxycodone and were significantly more likely to have chronic opioid dependence compared with their opioid-naïve counterparts (21.7% vs 3.2%).[71] These results highlight the necessity of maximizing multimodal pain control and minimizing opioid consumption.[71]

To stem the tide of opioid abuse, the Centers for Medicare and Medicaid Services established a 7-day maximum length of therapy for opioid prescriptions for acute pain.[72] To curb misuse, some third-party payers and pharmacies are now restricting the total daily dose of opioids in MME and/or the amount dispensed.[72] High-dose prescriptions are considered any prescription for ≥ 90 MME/d.[43] Before discharge, educate patients about tapering off medications to prevent withdrawal symptoms.[2] For example, oxycodone is safely tapered by decreasing the dosage 25% to 50% per day, while monitoring for withdrawal symptoms.[34] If symptoms occur, the dosage should be increased and tapering should occur more gradually.[34] Another strategy for reducing opioid use is prescribing a nonopioid analgesic such as acetaminophen for mild pain (pain scale rating 1–3) and limiting the use of the opioid for moderate to severe pain (pain scale rating 4–10).[2]

SUMMARY

Opioids remain the cornerstone for postoperative cardiothoracic surgery pain treatment.[1] Despite their efficacy, they are associated with a myriad of adverse effects, including respiratory depression, tolerance, dependence, and hyperalgesia.[2,6,24] Central nerve blocks remain the gold standard for managing thoracotomy pain. Peripheral nerve blocks with paravertebral catheters and long-acting local anesthetics are becoming more prevalent in preventing nociception in minimally invasive cardiac and thoracic procedures. Contemporary management is also moving toward multimodal analgesia to diminish opioid-associated risks and speed recovery times.[3] Good communication with patients and their families about expected postsurgery nociception and pain management options has been shown to improve patient satisfaction and decrease opioid consumption.[2] As part of the discharge planning process, clinicians should provide non-narcotic analgesics, such as acetaminophen, for mild pain.[2] Patient education should include information about opioid tapering to prevent opioid dependence. If patients reduce the opioid MMEs too rapidly, they may experience withdrawal symptoms. Teaching regarding the signs and symptoms of opioid withdrawal and to notify their provider if it occurs is another strategy for preventing dependence.[2,34]

ACKNOWLEDGEMENTS

Special thanks to Catherine Tierney, DNP, ACNP-BC for her thoughtful review of this article.

REFERENCES

1. Brook K, Bennett J, Desai SP. The chemical history of morphine: an 8000-year journey, from resin to de-novo synthesis. J Anesth Hist 2017;3:50–5.
2. Chou R, Gordon DB, de Leon-Casasola OA, et al. Management of postoperative pain: a clinical practice guideline from the American Pain Society, the American Society of Regional Anesthesia and Pain Medicine, and the American Society of Anesthesiologists' Committee on regional anesthesia, executive committee, and administrative council. J Pain 2016;17:131–57.
3. Williams JB, McConnell G, Allender JE, et al. One-year results from the first US-based enhanced recovery after cardiac surgery (ERAS Cardiac) program. J Thorac Cardiovasc Surg 2019;157(5):1881–8.
4. Devlin JW, Skrobik Y, Gelinas C, et al. Clinical practice guidelines for the prevention and management of pain, agitation/sedation, delirium, immobility, and sleep disruption in adult patients in the ICU. Crit Care Med 2018;46:e825–73.
5. Pedoto A, Amar D. Liposomal bupivacaine for intercostal nerve block: pricey or priceless? Semin Thorac Cardiovasc Surg 2017;29:538–9.
6. Gupta K, Nagappa M, Prasad A, et al. Risk factors for opioid-induced respiratory depression in surgical patients: a systematic review and meta-analyses. BMJ Open 2018;8:e024086.
7. Thompson C, French DG, Costache I. Pain management within an enhanced recovery program after thoracic surgery. J Thorac Dis 2018;10:S3773–80.
8. Zubrzycki M, Liebold A, Skrabal C, et al. Assessment and pathophysiology of pain in cardiac surgery. J Pain Res 2018;11:1599–611.
9. Huang AP, Sakata RK. Pain after sternotomy - review. Braz J Anesthesiol 2016;66: 395–401.
10. Ellison DL. Physiology of pain. Crit Care Nurs Clin North Am 2017;29:397–406.
11. Jellish WS, Oftadeh M. Peripheral nerve injury in cardiac surgery. J Cardiothorac Vasc Anesth 2018;32:495–511.
12. Healey S, O'Neill B, Bilal H, et al. Does retraction of the sternum during median sternotomy result in brachial plexus injuries? Interact Cardiovasc Thorac Surg 2013;17:151–7.
13. Arzillo S, Gishen K, Askari M. Brachial plexus injury: treatment options and outcomes. J Craniofac Surg 2014;25:1200–6.
14. Stoker GE, Kim HJ, Riew KD. Differentiating C8–T1 radiculopathy from ulnar neuropathy: a survey of 24 spine surgeons. Global Spine J 2014;4(1):1–6.
15. Gavazzi A, de Rino F, Boveri MC, et al. Prevalence of peripheral nervous system complications after major heart surgery. Neurol Sci 2016;37:205–9.
16. Milicin C, Sirbu E. A comparative study of rehabilitation therapy in traumatic upper limb peripheral nerve injuries. NeuroRehabilitation 2018;42:113–9.

17. Lovaglio AC, Socolovsky M, Di Masi G, et al. Treatment of neuropathic pain after peripheral nerve and brachial plexus traumatic injury. Neurol India 2019;67: S32–7.
18. Attal N, Bouhassira D. Pharmacotherapy of neuropathic pain: which drugs, which treatment algorithms? Pain 2015;156(Suppl 1):S104–14.
19. Guimaraes-Pereira L, Farinha F, Azevedo L, et al. Persistent postoperative pain after cardiac surgery: incidence, characterization, associated factors and its impact in quality of life. Eur J Pain 2016;20:1433–42.
20. Batchelor TJP, Rasburn NJ, Abdelnour-Berchtold E, et al. Guidelines for enhanced recovery after lung surgery: recommendations of the enhanced recovery after surgery (ERAS(R)) Society and the European Society of Thoracic Surgeons (ESTS). Eur J Cardiothorac Surg 2019;55:91–115.
21. Bisleri G, Muneretto C. Endoscopic saphenous vein and radial harvest: state-of-the-art. Curr Opin Cardiol 2015;30:624–8.
22. Kiaii BB, Swinamer SA, Fox SA, et al. A prospective randomized study of endoscopic versus conventional harvesting of the radial artery. Innovations (Phila) 2017;12:231–8.
23. Costa MA, Trentini CA, Schafranski MD, et al. Factors associated with the development of chronic post-sternotomy pain: a case-control study. Braz J Cardiovasc Surg 2015;30:552–6.
24. Martyn JAJ, Mao J, Bittner EA. Opioid tolerance in critical illness. N Engl J Med 2019;380:365–78.
25. Clarke H, Soneji N, Ko DT, et al. Rates and risk factors for prolonged opioid use after major surgery: population based cohort study. BMJ 2014;348:g1251.
26. Kinlein SA, Wilson CD, Karatsoreos IN. Dysregulated hypothalamic-pituitary-adrenal axis function contributes to altered endocrine and neurobehavioral responses to acute stress. Front Psychiatry 2015;6:31.
27. Xu B, Li H. Brain mechanisms of sympathetic activation in heart failure: roles of the renin-angiotensin system, nitric oxide and proinflammatory cytokines (Review). Mol Med Rep 2015;12:7823–9.
28. Patel S, Rauf A, Khan H, et al. Renin-angiotensin-aldosterone (RAAS): the ubiquitous system for homeostasis and pathologies. Biomed Pharmacother 2017; 94:317–25.
29. de Lucia C, Eguchi A, Koch WJ. New insights in cardiac beta-adrenergic signaling during heart failure and aging. Front Pharmacol 2018;9:904.
30. Volkow ND, McLellan AT. Opioid abuse in chronic pain–misconceptions and mitigation strategies. N Engl J Med 2016;374:1253–63.
31. Weinbroum AA. Postoperative hyperalgesia-a clinically applicable narrative review. Pharmacol Res 2017;120:188–205.
32. Balas MC, Pun BT, Pasero C, et al. Common challenges to effective ABCDEF bundle implementation: the ICU liberation campaign experience. Crit Care Nurse 2019;39:46–60.
33. Davison SN. Clinical pharmacology considerations in pain management in patients with advanced kidney failure. Clin J Am Soc Nephrol 2019. [Epub ahead of print].
34. Roxicodone (oxycodone hydrochloride) label - 021011s002lbl.pdf. Available at: https://www.accessdata.fda.gov/drugsatfda_docs/label/2009/021011s002lbl.pdf. Accessed March 2, 2019.
35. Parker K, Aasebo W, Haslemo T, et al. Relationship between cytochrome P450 polymorphisms and prescribed medication in elderly haemodialysis patients. SpringerPlus 2016;5:350.

36. Roberts DM, Sevastos J, Carland JE, et al. Clinical pharmacokinetics in kidney disease: application to rational design of dosing regimens. Clin J Am Soc Nephrol 2018;13:1254–63.

37. Lea-Henry TN, Carland JE, Stocker SL, et al. Clinical pharmacokinetics in kidney disease: fundamental principles. Clin J Am Soc Nephrol 2018;13:1085–95.

38. Klimas R, Mikus G. Morphine-6-glucuronide is responsible for the analgesic effect after morphine administration: a quantitative review of morphine, morphine-6-glucuronide, and morphine-3-glucuronide. Br J Anaesth 2014;113:935–44.

39. Liu T, Ivaturi V, Gobburu J. Integrated model to describe morphine pharmacokinetics in humans. J Clin Pharmacol 2019. [Epub ahead of print].

40. de Hoogd S, Valitalo PAJ, Dahan A, et al. Influence of morbid obesity on the pharmacokinetics of morphine, morphine-3-glucuronide, and morphine-6-glucuronide. Clin Pharmacokinet 2017;56:1577–87.

41. Data-Driven Prevention Initiative (DDPI) | Drug Overdose | CDC Injury Center. 2017. Available at: https://www.fda.gov/consumers/consumer-updates/fda-strengthens-warning-heart-attack-and-stroke-risk-non-steroidal-anti-inflammatory-drugs. Accessed May 30, 2019.

42. Chronic pain management toolkit - conversion table - conversion-table.pdf. 2019. Available at: https://www.aafp.org/dam/AAFP/documents/patient_care/pain_management/conversion-table.pdf. Accessed March 6, 2019.

43. 2018 Annual surveillance report of drug-related risks and outcomes: United States. Available at: https://www.cdc.gov/drugoverdose/pdf/pubs/2018-cdc-drug-surveillance-report.pdf. Accessed February 12, 2019.

44. Tucker C, Tucker L, Brown K. The intranasal route as an alternative method of medication administration. Crit Care Nurse 2018;38:26–31.

45. Bell RF, Kalso EA. Ketamine for pain management. Pain Rep 2018;3(5):e674.

46. Brinck EC, Tiippana E, Heesen M, et al. Perioperative intravenous ketamine for acute postoperative pain in adults. Cochrane Database Syst Rev 2018;(12):CD012033.

47. Subramaniam B, Shankar P, Shaefi S, et al. Effect of intravenous acetaminophen vs placebo combined with propofol or dexmedetomidine on postoperative delirium among older patients following cardiac surgery: the DEXACET randomized clinical trial. JAMA 2019;321:686–96.

48. Precedex (dexmedetomidine) safety info. Available at: https://www.pfizerpro.com/product/precedex/hcp. Accessed March 3, 2019.

49. Diprivan (propofol) prescribing information. Available at: http://diprivan-us.com/wp-content/themes/diprivan-us/docs/DIPRIVAN_PI.pdf. Accessed March 2, 2019.

50. Wang PP, Huang E, Feng X, et al. Opioid-associated iatrogenic withdrawal in critically ill adult patients: a multicenter prospective observational study. Ann Intensive Care 2017;7:88.

51. Chiu AW, Contreras S, Mehta S, et al. Iatrogenic opioid withdrawal in critically ill patients: a review of assessment tools and management. Ann Pharmacother 2017;51:1099–111.

52. Tompkins DA, Bigelow GE, Harrison JA, et al. Concurrent validation of the clinical opiate withdrawal scale (COWS) and single-item indices against the clinical institute narcotic assessment (CINA) opioid withdrawal instrument. Drug Alcohol Depend 2009;105:154–9.

53. Wesson DR, Ling W. The clinical opiate withdrawal scale (COWS). J Psychoactive Drugs 2003;35:253–9.

54. Burma NE, Kwok CH, Trang T. Therapies and mechanisms of opioid withdrawal. Pain Manag 2017;7:455–9.
55. Turner CC, Fogger SA, Frazier SL. Opioid use disorder: challenges during acute hospitalization. J Nurse Pract 2018;14:61–7.
56. Bialka S, Copik M, Daszkiewicz A, et al. Comparison of different methods of postoperative analgesia after thoracotomy-a randomized controlled trial. J Thorac Dis 2018;10:4874–82.
57. Medina M, Foiles SR, Francois M, et al. Comparison of cost and outcomes in patients receiving thoracic epidural versus liposomal bupivacaine for video-assisted thoracoscopic pulmonary resection. Am J Surg 2019;217(3):520–4.
58. Pun BT, Balas MC, Barnes-Daly MA, et al. Caring for critically ill patients with the ABCDEF bundle: results of the ICU Liberation collaborative in over 15,000 adults. Crit Care Med 2019;47:3–14.
59. Strike E, Arklina B, Stradins P, et al. Postoperative pain management strategies and delirium after transapical aortic valve replacement: a randomized controlled trial. J Cardiothorac Vasc Anesth 2019;33(6):1668–72.
60. Lee CY, Robinson DA, Johnson CA Jr, et al. A randomized controlled trial of liposomal bupivacaine parasternal intercostal block for sternotomy. Ann Thorac Surg 2019;107:128–34.
61. Exparel prescribing information highlights. Available at: https://www.exparel.com/hcp/prescriptioninformation.pdf. Accessed March 4, 2019.
62. Nelson DA, Marks ES, Deuster PA, et al. Association of nonsteroidal anti-inflammatory drug prescriptions with kidney disease among active young and middle-aged adults. JAMA Netw open 2019;2:e187896.
63. Commissioner Oot. Consumer updates - FDA strengthens warning of heart attack and stroke risk for non-steroidal anti-inflammatory drugs 2019. Available at: https://www.fda.gov/consumers/consumer-updates/fda-strengthens-warning-heart-attack-and-stroke-risk-non-steroidal-anti-inflammatory-drugs. Accessed May 30, 2019.
64. de Souza Brito F, Mehta RH, Lopes RD, et al. Nonsteroidal anti-inflammatory drugs and clinical outcomes in patients undergoing coronary artery bypass surgery. Am J Med 2017;130:462–8.
65. Ultram ER.pdf. Available at: https://www.janssen.com/us/sites/www_janssen_com_usa/files/products-documents/ultramer.pdf. Accessed March 7, 2019.
66. Vieira CMP, Fragoso RM, Pereira D, et al. Pain polymorphisms and opioids: an evidence based review. Mol Med Rep 2019;19(3):1423–34.
67. McConnell G, Woltz P, Bradford WT, et al. Enhanced recovery after cardiac surgery program to improve patient outcomes. Nursing 2018;48:24–31.
68. Volkow ND, Jones EB, Einstein EB, et al. Prevention and treatment of opioid misuse and addiction: a review. JAMA Psychiatry 2019;76:208–16.
69. Dever C. Treating acute pain in the opiate-dependent patient. J Trauma Nurs 2017;24:292–9.
70. State information | Drug overdose | CDC injury center. 2018. Available at: https://www.cdc.gov/drugoverdose/states/index.html. Accessed February 20, 2019.
71. Hirji SA, Landino S, Cote C, et al. Chronic opioid use after coronary bypass surgery. J Card Surg 2019;34:67–73.
72. Lowenstein M, Grande D, Delgado MK. Opioid prescribing limits for acute pain - striking the right balance. N Engl J Med 2018;379:504–6.

Acute Kidney Injury Following Cardiothoracic Surgery

Daniel L. Arellano, MSN, RN, ACNP-BC, CCRN, CEN[a,b,]*

KEYWORDS

- Acute kidney injury • Renal failure • Cardiothoracic surgery
- Cardiopulmonary bypass • KDIGO guidelines • Renal replacement therapy
- Biomarkers

KEY POINTS

- Inflammation and ischemia are 2 of the most common pathophysiologic factors for acute kidney injury in cardiothoracic surgery patients.
- Adherence to national guidelines for the prevention and treatment of acute kidney injury is recommended to improve outcomes.
- A multidisciplinary team in all areas of the perioperative environment should strategize to reduce elements associated with acute kidney injury.
- Biomarkers are an emerging tool for the management of acute kidney injury and are helpful in detection of acute kidney injury, evaluating the extent of renal injury, and monitoring response to therapy.

INTRODUCTION

Acute kidney injury (AKI) following cardiothoracic surgery (CTS) is a well-known phenomenon that has been described in the literature for many decades.[1–3] AKI occurs in approximately 30% of patients undergoing CTS and has been shown to increase mortality.[4] The etiology and treatment of AKI can be complex, and it is important to have a clear understanding of this condition to help reduce adverse outcomes. The process starts with identifying those patients at higher risk for AKI, treating patients across the operative spectrum, and using evidence-based strategies to reduce harmful events.

Disclosure: The author has nothing to disclose.
[a] Department of Undergraduate Studies, Cizik School of Nursing, University of Texas Health Science Center at Houston, Room # 775, 6901 Bertner Avenue, Houston, TX 77030, USA;
[b] Division of Anesthesiology, Critical Care, and Pain Medicine, Department of Critical Care, University of Texas MD Anderson Cancer Center, Houston, TX, USA
* Department of Undergraduate Studies, The University of Texas Health Science Center at Houston, Cizik School of Nursing, Room # 775, 6901 Bertner Avenue, Houston, TX 77030.
E-mail address: Daniel.L.Arellano@uth.tmc.edu

Crit Care Nurs Clin N Am 31 (2019) 407–417
https://doi.org/10.1016/j.cnc.2019.05.008
0899-5885/19/© 2019 Elsevier Inc. All rights reserved.

ccnursing.theclinics.com

The purposes of this paper are to discuss the pathophysiology of AKI, review risk prediction scoring models, detail diagnosis guidelines from the Kidney Disease Improving Global Outcomes (KDIGO) initiative, outline preventative strategies, discuss treatment modalities, and review new directions for research.

PATHOPHYSIOLOGY OF ACUTE KIDNEY INJURY WITH CARDIOTHORACIC SURGERY

It important to understand that there are many factors contributing to AKI in CTS, The 2 most common pathophysiologic factors are inflammation and ischemia. A clear understanding of these concepts will help to inform treatment decisions.

Inflammation

The process of cardiopulmonary bypass (CPB) has been shown to produce a systemic inflammatory response.[5,6] Contributors to this response include blood contact to CPB circuit surfaces, nonpulsatile blood flow, ischemia with reperfusion injury, and operative trauma.[7-9] Inflammatory mediators such as interleukin (IL)-6 and IL-8, as well as tumor necrosis factor α, are released and can remain peaked up to 4 hours after termination of CPB.[5] The humoral response associated with CPB-induced activation of the coagulation cascade causes neutrophil and monocyte activation that promotes the release of more proinflammatory cytokines. Diffuse organ ischemia secondary to CPB and operative techniques promotes the release of cytokines and free radicals, compounding the overall inflammatory response.[10-12] The CPB circuit pump can induce hemolysis and increase circulating plasma-free hemoglobin, deplete haptoglobin, and accelerate free radical production.[13-15] These inflammatory responses can produce deleterious effects to the kidneys by promoting cellular tissue death, edema, and toxin infiltration into the nephrons.

Ischemia

It has been well documented that CPB produces macroscopic and microscopic emboli.[16] These emboli can originate from activation of the coagulation cascade or from the introduction of gas into the CPB circuit. Surgical maneuvers can also generate emboli during aortic clamp placement, clamp manipulation, tissue manipulation, and during the process of CPB cannulation.[17] These emboli often travel to distal organs such as the kidneys and cause ischemia that contributes to AKI.[18] Hypoperfusion during the perioperative period causes oxidative stress, worsening the production of free radicals and limiting the production of antioxidants. Ischemia of the renal tissue can cause inflammation and initiate a vicious cycle whereby inflammation damages the endothelium, promoting vascular dysfunction and worsening the perfusion of tissues (**Fig. 1**).

RISK PREDICTION

There are multiple scoring systems helpful in predicting the risk of developing AKI in the CTS patient.[19-22] These scoring systems use a definition of AKI different from that defined by the KDIGO guidelines.[23] Most scores define AKI as the need for renal replacement therapy (RRT) in the postoperative course until discharge. The Cleveland Clinic Foundation Acute Renal Failure Scoring System is one of the most common well-validated tools used in practice today[19,24] (**Table 1**). This system was developed from a single-center trial representing approximately 30,000 patients undergoing CTS while excluding those who have had a renal transplant or were on preoperative hemodialysis.[19] The score uses 13 preoperative risk factors to provides a percentage risk for developing dialysis depending on acute renal failure (ARF). Interestingly, this was the

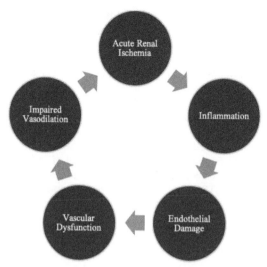

Fig. 1. The relationship between ischemia and inflammation in acute kidney injury.

only scoring system to incorporate gender and add a higher risk for female patients. Other risk factors include those with chronic disease such as chronic obstructive pulmonary disease, diabetes, and congestive heart failure (CHF).[19]

The Mehta Score is another validated tool to predict the need for RRT secondary to AKI. This scoring system used data from the Society of Thoracic Surgeons database

Table 1 Cleveland Clinic Foundation acute renal failure scoring system	
Risk Factor	**Points**
Female gender	1
Congestive heart failure	1
LVEF <35%	1
Preoperative use of IABP	2
COPD	1
Insulin-requiring diabetes	1
Previous cardiac surgery	1
Emergency surgery	2
Valve surgery only	1
CABG + valve surgery	2
Other cardiac surgeries	2
Preoperative creatinine 1.2–2.1 mg/dL	2
Preoperative creatinine >2.1 mg/dL	5
Risk for Dialysis-Dependent ARF	**Risk Percentage (%)**
0–2	0.4
3–5	1.8
6–8	9.5
9–13	21.3

Abbreviations: ARF, acute renal failure; CABG, coronary artery bypass graft; COPD, chronic obstructive pulmonary disease; IABP, intra-aortic balloon pump; LVEF, left ventricular ejection fraction.

and examined risk factors similar to those of the Cleveland Clinic system. New variables are included, such as the presence of cardiogenic shock, race, and age.[20] The complexity of these systems warranted the development of an easier tool for clinicians to use as a predictor of AKI. The Simplified Renal Index was validated using only 8 risk factors in patients who underwent CTS at 2 Canadian hospitals. It has also demonstrated adequate predictive value in this population.[22]

The Acute Kidney Injury after Cardiac Surgery (AKICS) score is a unique system developed in Brazil, and was validated on patients undergoing elective CTS. This score offers the advantage of predicting less severe forms of AKI (not requiring RRT) because it was validated using the KDIGO guideline definition of AKI as the outcome for validation.[21] Each score offers a unique set of variables that offers a variety of methodologies for clinicians to choose from to predict the risk of a patient developing AKI following CTS. The KDIGO guidelines generally recommend the use of scoring systems to help stratify the risk of developing AKI in all applicable procedures.[23]

DIAGNOSIS OF ACUTE KIDNEY INJURY

The timely diagnosis of AKI using consensus guidelines is paramount in patients undergoing CTS. Marginal increases in serum creatinine have been noted to be a poor prognostic indicator.[25] KDIGO Guidelines define AKI as a 0.3 mg/dL increase in the serum creatinine from baseline within 48 hours of surgery, a 50% increase in serum creatinine from baseline within 7 days of surgery, or a decrease in urine output of less than 0.5 mL/kg/h for 6 hours.[23] It is important to evaluate each patient based on both serum creatinine and urinary output. Individualized assessment of the patient's volume status will be required. Therefore, promoting accurate nursing measurement and documentation of hourly output is recommended. Recall that oliguria is common after CTS and is often secondary to hypovolemia. Formal differentiation between prerenal, intrarenal, and postrenal causes of AKI should be performed. This may include diagnostics such as serum and urine electrolytes and/or a renal ultrasonography. Clinicians should also be trending creatinine measurements, observing volume status, and monitoring for serious electrolyte and acid-base disorders. Nephrology consultation is warranted for patients with progressive AKI. Advanced diagnostics such as microscopic urine examination may be indicated.

KDIGO guidelines offer 3-tiered staging criteria for AKI.[23] Baseline creatinine measurements in addition to hourly urinary output are important components of this process. Further research is indicated to assess whether the poor outcomes in CTS patients experiencing stage 1 AKI are associated with actual renal dysfunction or the systemic process that contributed to the AKI. Establishing universal consensus of these stages will help to measure incidence and outcomes, and to monitor intervention effectiveness in AKI.

PREVENTION OF ACUTE KIDNEY INJURY
General Strategies

There is a multitude of strategies to prevent AKI in the CTS patient. However, clinicians should start with identification of patients at higher risk using scoring systems previously discussed. Those patients at higher risk of developing AKI should be optimized before surgery as much as possible.[26] This includes management of hydration status, blood pressure, and CHF. Discontinue nephrotoxic medications as appropriate including nonsteroidal anti-inflammatory drugs and unnecessary antibiotics. Withholding angiotensin-converting enzyme inhibitors (ACEi) or angiotensin receptor blockers (ARBs) before surgery is still a point of debate.[27] However, appropriate management of blood pressure will be paramount before surgery. Patients with contrast-induced ARF may require delayed CTS to prevent adverse outcomes.

Pharmacologic Strategies

Managing fluid balance in the perioperative period is likely the best strategy to prevent AKI in CTS patients. Cardiac surgery can be associated with edema and microvascular tissue injury.[28] Therefore, it is important to maintain targeted management of fluids and avoid fluid overload.[29] Optimize stroke volume to improve renal perfusion with the use of balanced crystalloids and albumin. Normal saline has been associated with hyperchloremic metabolic acidosis and renal injury, whereas balanced solutions are less likely to cause acidosis and have been shown to reduce the need for RRT.[30,31] Colloids been shown to be no more effective than some crystalloids for fluid resuscitation; however, they remain common practice in the clinical setting.[32] The use of albumin is recommended over starch solutions because compared with saline, albumin decreased the odds of AKI by 76% whereas starch solutions increased the odds of AKI by 92%.[33] Starch solutions have also been shown to increase mortality in many populations.[33] Again, targeted fluid management with use of invasive or noninvasive cardiac output monitoring may be helpful in preventing fluid overload.

The use of vasoactive agents to improve renal perfusion is generally not recommended. Examples of these vasoactive medications include fenoldopam and low-dose dopamine. Fenoldopam is a dopamine agonist that is thought to dilate renal vasculature and therefore increase perfusion to the kidneys. The evidence supporting the use of this medication is mixed. KDIGO guidelines do not support the use of fenoldopam, and therefore it is typically not used in practice.[23] Low-dose dopamine is also thought to cause vasodilation by increasing cyclic AMP. However, it has been well established that this medication does not reduce AKI in patients undergoing CTS.[34]

Other pharmacologic agents thought to prevent AKI in CTS include steroids, N-acetylcysteine, and sodium bicarbonate. As discussed earlier, one of the major causes of AKI in CTS is inflammation. However, routine use of corticosteroids to reduce inflammation has shown no benefit in this population.[35] N-Acetylcysteine is thought to minimize vasoconstriction, block inflammation, and reduce oxidative stress. However, this medication has not been extensively examined in a prospective methodology in this population and is therefore not recommended to reduce the risk of AKI.[23] Lastly, sodium bicarbonate has been shown to decrease renal oxygen consumption and is commonly used in the treatment of AKI. However, it has also not been demonstrated to prevent AKI in patients with CTS.[23]

Maintaining fluid balance, avoiding nephrotoxins, and selection of appropriate pharmacologic therapy are the best ways to prevent AKI in CTS patients.

PERIOPERATIVE CONSIDERATIONS

There are multiple factors that may affect AKI in the perioperative setting (**Table 2**). Early identification, rapid treatment, and use of evidence-based practice may improve outcomes.

Preoperative

Patients who have CTS often experience conditions in the preoperative period that may increase their chances for the development of AKI. For example, a new-onset myocardial infarction may cause the patient to experience impaired left ventricular function, which decreases perfusion to the kidney. Global tissue ischemia may cause

Table 2
Perioperative considerations for AKI

Preoperative	Intraoperative	Postoperative
Prerenal ARF	Cardiopulmonary bypass	Hypoperfusion
Dehydration	Embolic events	Vasoactive agents
Impaired LV function	Aortic clamp time	Hypovolemia
Medications	Hypoperfusion	Shock
IV Contrast	Vasoactive agents	Anemia
ACEi/ARB	Hypovolemia	Nephrotoxins
Age		Inflammation
Comorbid conditions		Sepsis
HTN		
CKD		
PVD		

Abbreviations: ACEi, angiotensin-converting enzyme inhibitor; ARB, angiotensin receptor blocker; ARF, acute renal failure; CKD, chronic kidney disease; HTN, hypertension; IV, intravenous; LV, left ventricular; PVD, peripheral vascular disease.

nausea and vomiting and limit oral intake, precipitating dehydration and prerenal azotemia. Diagnostic interventions for myocardial infarction, such as coronary angiography, introduces toxic intravenous contrast medium the nephron and causes acute tubular necrosis. This may be exacerbated by existent medications such as ACEi or ARBs. Age and other comorbid conditions such as hypertension, chronic kidney disease, and peripheral vascular disease may also increase the chance of developing AKI in this period.

Intraoperative

The intraoperative period is a critical time to consider events that may contribute to AKI. Patients are exposed to anesthesia and CPB, which may induce hemodynamic instability, inflammation, and ischemia. As previously noted, CPB has many effects on the body that can contribute to renal dysfunction. In addition, surgical techniques such as cardiac manipulation, vessel repair, and aortic clamping can increase the chances of embolic formations. These emboli can travel to the kidney and become a cause of prerenal ARF. Hypoperfusion may also be present because of hypovolemia and the use of vasoactive agents for hemodynamic instability. It is essential that the multidisciplinary operative team strategize to reduce these harmful intraoperative events.

The off-pump coronary artery bypass (OpCAB) was developed to eliminate the potential harmful effects of CPB for CTS. However, this surgical technique can cause hemodynamic instability secondary to cardiac manipulation required to access the coronary arteries. OpCAB is associated with a lower incidence of postoperative AKI.[36] However, despite multiple large-scale trials and meta-analyses, the research remains unclear as to whether this surgical technique will affect the need for RRT or will improve outcomes.[36] Many studies cite the lack of a clear definition for AKI in the CTS population. The KDIGO guidelines stop short of recommending OpCAB to reduce AKI or the need for RRT.[23] Results were similar in transcatheter aortic valve replacement versus on-pump aortic valve replacement. A large randomized trial found no significant difference in AKI or initiation of RRT between CPB groups.[37]

Postoperative

Events in the postoperative period are complementary to those that normally occur in any intensive care unit (ICU) environment. Hypoperfusion is common secondary to the use of vasoactive agents, hypovolemia, anemia, and shock. Protocol-based management may be helpful in maintaining adequate hemodynamics and oxygenation to prevent evolving AKI.[23] Massive systemic inflammation after cardiac surgery is common and multifactorial. Nephrotoxins should be avoided at this critical stage, and patients should be monitored closely for sepsis, which may hasten AKI.

TREATMENT OF ACUTE KIDNEY INJURY

Treating AKI in CTS patients starts with attenuating ischemia and inflammation. This approach should be used in all areas of the perioperative environment. If these interventions prove unsuccessful, the patient may require further supportive care. Discontinue nephrotoxic medications when possible. Manage acid-base disturbances and electrolyte abnormalities carefully. Ensure electrolyte levels remain on target to prevent postoperative atrial fibrillation. Monitor serial laboratory tests and urinary output. Consult nephrology, if indicated, to assist with the need for RRT or assist in the evaluation of AKI. Indications for RRT include oliguria, profound fluid overload, refractory acidemia (pH < 7.2), hyperkalemia (potassium >6 mEq/L), and severe azotemia, among others.[23] Trending these laboratory tests rather than treating an isolated value is an important factor when considering RRT. Some trials have indicated that starting RRT earlier may improve mortality rates and decrease the length of stay in the ICU.[38] In fact, one study indicated that early RRT decreased mortality by more than 26% and decreased ventilator days by almost a week.[39] Further research regarding early versus late RRT is indicated.

There is no evidence to suggest that the selection of continuous versus intermittent dialysis will improve outcomes.[40] The modality is often chosen based on experience, preference, and the clinical situation. Selection bias may exist for patients in the ICU to receive continuous RRT because they are already in a highly monitored environment with intensive nursing care. This would reduce intermittent hemodialysis schedules and increase the availability of these resources to the other parts of the hospital. One must recognize that the selection of continuous hemodialysis in the CTS population may decrease mobility initiatives that would normally reduce the length of stay in the ICU.

Nutrition is an extremely important factor for healing and should not be neglected in CTS patients who develop AKI. Malnourished patients have been shown to have an increased risk of mortality.[41] Therefore, enteral nutrition should be started as early as possible. Goals should include the administration 20 to 30 kcal/kg/d and approximately 1.0 g/kg/d of protein. Patients may require higher energy and protein goals if they are transitioned to RRT.[23] Maintaining glycemic control is also recommended for those patients developing AKI. Hyperglycemia has been associated with increased mortality rates and, therefore, insulin therapy should be used to maintain a target glucose level between 110 and 149 mg/dL.[23] It is unclear whether hyperglycemia itself causes worse outcomes or is simply a marker of the critically ill patient. Regardless, CTS and KDIGO guidelines both recommend maintaining euglycemia.[23]

Mesenchymal stem cells are an evolving therapy for the treatment of AKI. These stem cells possess anti-inflammatory and tissue-repair properties that have demonstrated efficacy in animal models.[42] They are typically collected from the bone marrow and administered via intravenous infusion. The stem cells target the injured kidney, and can repair damaged nephrons and reverse AKI. There are ongoing studies using these cells in a variety of different organs to evaluate their strong reparative properties.[43] Mesenchymal stem cells may provide a novel therapy for AKI in the CTS population and deserve further investigation.

AREAS FOR FUTURE RESEARCH

Biomarkers are an emerging tool for the management of AKI and proved to be helpful in detecting AKI earlier, monitoring response to therapy, and evaluating the extent of renal injury. Research has yielded the discovery of many biomarkers, but few are commercially available and approved by the Food and Drug Administration (FDA). The biomarkers discussed in this review are displayed in **Fig. 2**, reflecting the site of expression within the nephron.

Urinary insulin-like growth factor binding protein 7 and tissue inhibitor of metalloproteinases 2 are common biomarkers used in practice today and approved by the FDA. These urinary markers are measured to help assess the risk of developing stage-2 to 3 AKI within the first 12 hours of cardiac surgery.[44] Once identified, clinicians can rapidly treat and reduce moderate to severe AKI by more than 33%.[44] Further testing is needed to validate the use of these markers across the spectrum of care.

Serum and urine cystatin C can also be helpful in predicting AKI in CTS patients.[45] Serum cystatin C has proved to be more sensitive and specific for renal injury, although other factors such as inflammation, race, and age can affect the use of this biomarker.[46,47] Neutrophil gelatinase-associated lipocalin (NGAL) has been used in conjunction with kidney injury molecule 1 and urine IL-18 to indicate renal damage. NGAL has been compared with creatinine and has demonstrated positive predictive value for length of stay in ICU and hospital as well as use of RRT.[48,49] Despite the abundance of these biomarkers, few are used in practice for reasons of availability and cost. Additional research is needed to improve the technology and practicality for their use.

Another area for future research is the impact of AKI staging. The KDIGO guidelines outline specific staging criteria that include urinary output, but few studies have examined the impact of fluid balance, diuretic use, and different weights (actual, ideal, and lean body weights). The impact of various urinary catheter devices that help monitor urinary flow and consistency should also be explored.[23] Research targeting the use

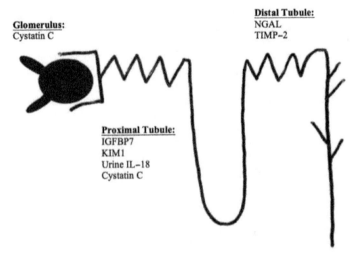

Glomerulus:
Cystatin C

Distal Tubule:
NGAL
TIMP-2

Proximal Tubule:
IGFBP7
KIM1
Urine IL-18
Cystatin C

Fig. 2. Biomarkers of acute kidney injury. IGFBP, insulin-like growth factor binding protein; IL, interleukin; KIM, kidney injury molecule; NGAL, neutrophil gelatinase-associated lipocalin; TIMP, tissue inhibitor of metalloproteinases.

of estimated glomerular filtration rate may also prove to be helpful. Many clinicians ignore this laboratory value and instead focus on daily serum measurements of blood urea nitrogen and creatinine.

Perioperative use of ACEi and ARBs should also be examined more closely. Recall that these medications are commonly used according to guideline recommendations for patients with CHF and heart disease. Ongoing debate remains as to whether these medications should be stopped before surgery. Closer examination of AKI rates in patients taking these agents will be helpful. Finally, determination of outcomes associated with early versus late RRT should also be explored. Current practice guidelines do not offer solid recommendations for this population.[23] Comparing these data with those that require long-term hemodialysis will be beneficial.

SUMMARY

AKI in the CTS patient is a known contributor to mortality. Mitigating the inflammation and ischemia associated with CTS will minimize the risk of disease development. This article provides a foundation for the pathophysiology and treatment across the operative spectrum. Additional prevention, diagnosis, and treatment strategies are in development and may work toward improving the length of stay in ICU, length of stay in hospital, and mortality rates. Until novel therapies are introduced, closely following established CTS surgery guidelines and the KDIGO guidelines offers the best chance for AKI resolution and prevention of adverse outcomes.

REFERENCES

1. Bhat JG, Gluck MC, Lowenstein J, et al. Renal failure after open heart surgery. Ann Intern Med 1976;84(6):677–82.
2. Andersson L, Ekroth R, Bratteby L, et al. Acute renal failure after coronary surgery-a study of incidence and risk factors in 2009 consecutive patients. J Thorac Cardiovasc Surg 1993;41(04):237–41.
3. Ostermann M, Taube D, Morgan C, et al. Acute renal failure following cardiopulmonary bypass: a changing picture. Intensive Care Med 2000;26(5):565–71.
4. Lagny M-G, Jouret F, Koch J-N, et al. Incidence and outcomes of acute kidney injury after cardiac surgery using either criteria of the RIFLE classification. BMC Nephrol 2015;16(1):76.
5. Cremer J, Martin M, Redl H, et al. Systemic inflammatory response syndrome after cardiac operations. Ann Thorac Surg 1996;61(6):1714–20.
6. Taylor KM. SIRS—the systemic inflammatory response syndrome after cardiac operations. Ann Thorac Surg 1996;61(6):1607–8.
7. Hornick P, Taylor K. Pulsatile and nonpulsatile perfusion: the continuing controversy. J Cardiothorac Vasc Anesth 1997;11(3):310–5.
8. Kirklin JK, Blackstone EH, Kirklin JW. Cardiopulmonary bypass: studies on its damaging effects. Blood Purif 1987;5(2–3):168–78.
9. Czerny M, Baumer H, Kilo J, et al. Inflammatory response and myocardial injury following coronary artery bypass grafting with or without cardiopulmonary bypass. Eur J Cardiothorac Surg 2000;17(6):737–42.
10. Paparella D, Yau T, Young E. Cardiopulmonary bypass induced inflammation: pathophysiology and treatment. An update. Eur J Cardiothorac Surg 2002;21(2):232–44.
11. Kirklin JK, Westaby S, Blackstone E, et al. Complement and the damaging effects of cardiopulmonary bypass. J Thorac Cardiovasc Surg 1983;86(6):845–57.

12. Sheridan AM, Bonventre JV. Cell biology and molecular mechanisms of injury in ischemic acute renal failure. Curr Opin Nephrol Hypertens 2000;9(4):427–34.

13. Billings FT, Yu C, Byrne JG, et al. Heme oxygenase-1 and acute kidney injury following cardiac surgery. Cardiorenal Med 2014;4(1):12–21.

14. Loebl EC, Baxter CR, Curreri PW. The mechanism of erythrocyte destruction in the early post-burn period. Ann Surg 1973;178(6):681.

15. Haase M, Bellomo R, Haase-Fielitz A. Novel biomarkers, oxidative stress, and the role of labile iron toxicity in cardiopulmonary bypass-associated acute kidney injury. J Am Coll Cardiol 2010;55(19):2024–33.

16. Blauth CI. Macroemboli and microemboli during cardiopulmonary bypass. Ann Thorac Surg 1995;59(5):1300–3.

17. Barbut D, Hinton R, Szatrowski T, et al. Cerebral emboli detected during bypass surgery are associated with clamp removal. Stroke 1994;25(12):2398–402.

18. Sreeram GM, Grocott HP, White WD, et al. Transcranial Doppler emboli count predicts rise in creatinine after coronary artery bypass graft surgery. J Cardiothorac Vasc Anesth 2004;18(5):548–51.

19. Thakar CV, Arrigain S, Worley S, et al. A clinical score to predict acute renal failure after cardiac surgery. J Am Soc Nephrol 2005;16(1):162–8.

20. Mehta RH, Grab JD, O'brien SM, et al. Bedside tool for predicting the risk of postoperative dialysis in patients undergoing cardiac surgery. Clin J Am Soc Nephrol 2006;114(21):2208–16.

21. Palomba H, De Castro I, Neto A, et al. Acute kidney injury prediction following elective cardiac surgery: AKICS Score. Kidney Int 2007;72(5):624–31.

22. Wijeysundera DN, Karkouti K, Dupuis J-Y, et al. Derivation and validation of a simplified predictive index for renal replacement therapy after cardiac surgery. JAMA 2007;297(16):1801–9.

23. Kidney Disease: Improving Global Outcomes (KDIGO) Acute Kidney Injury Work Group. KDIGO clinical practice guideline for acute kidney injury. Kidney Int Suppl 2012;2:1–138.

24. Englberger L, Suri RM, Li Z, et al. Validation of clinical scores predicting severe acute kidney injury after cardiac surgery. Am J Kidney Dis 2010;56(4):623–31.

25. Lassnigg A, Schmidlin D, Mouhieddine M, et al. Minimal changes of serum creatinine predict prognosis in patients after cardiothoracic surgery: a prospective cohort study. J Am Soc Nephrol 2004;15(6):1597–605.

26. Rosner MH, Okusa MD. Acute kidney injury associated with cardiac surgery. Clin J Am Soc Nephrol 2006;1(1):19–32.

27. Devbhandari MP, Balasubramanian SK, Codispoti M, et al. Preoperative angiotensin-converting enzyme inhibition can cause severe post CPB vasodilation—current UK opinion. Asian Cardiovasc Thorac Ann 2004;12(4):346–9.

28. Rehm M, Bruegger D, Christ F, et al. Shedding of the endothelial glycocalyx in patients undergoing major vascular surgery with global and regional ischemia. Circulation 2007;116(17):1896–906.

29. Giglio M, Dalfino L, Puntillo F, et al. Haemodynamic goal-directed therapy in cardiac and vascular surgery. A systematic review and meta-analysis. Interact Cardiovasc Thorac Surg 2012;15(5):878–87.

30. Semler MW, Self WH, Wanderer JP, et al. Balanced crystalloids versus saline in critically ill adults. N Engl J Med 2018;378(9):829–39.

31. Krajewski M, Raghunathan K, Paluszkiewicz S, et al. Meta-analysis of high-versus low-chloride content in perioperative and critical care fluid resuscitation. Br J Surg 2015;102(1):24–36.

32. Finfer S, Bellomo R, Boyce N, et al. A comparison of albumin and saline for fluid resuscitation in the intensive care unit. N Engl J Med 2004;350(22):2247–56.

33. Wiedermann CJ, Dunzendorfer S, Gaioni LU, et al. Hyperoncotic colloids and acute kidney injury: a meta-analysis of randomized trials. Crit Care 2010;14(5): R191.

34. Lassnigg A, Donner E, Grubhofer G, et al. Lack of renoprotective effects of dopamine and furosemide during cardiac surgery. J Am Soc Nephrol 2000;11(1): 97–104.

35. Loef B, Henning R, Epema A, et al. Effect of dexamethasone on perioperative renal function impairment during cardiac surgery with cardiopulmonary bypass. Br J Anaesth 2004;93(6):793–8.

36. Seabra VF, Alobaidi S, Balk EM, et al. Off-pump coronary artery bypass surgery and acute kidney injury: a meta-analysis of randomized controlled trials. Clin J Am Soc Nephrol 2010;5:1734–44.

37. Smith CR, Leon MB, Mack MJ, et al. Transcatheter versus surgical aortic-valve replacement in high-risk patients. N Engl J Med 2011;364(23):2187–98.

38. Liu Y, Davari-Farid S, Arora P, et al. Early versus late initiation of renal replacement therapy in critically ill patients with acute kidney injury after cardiac surgery: a systematic review and meta-analysis. J Cardiothorac Vasc Anesth 2014;28(3): 557–63.

39. Leite TT, Macedo E, Pereira SM, et al. Timing of renal replacement therapy initiation by AKIN classification system. Crit Care 2013;17(2):R62.

40. Davenport A, Bouman C, Kirpalani A, et al. Delivery of renal replacement therapy in acute kidney injury: what are the key issues? Clin J Am Soc Nephrol 2008;3(3): 869–75.

41. Fiaccadori E, Lombardi M, Leonardi S, et al. Prevalence and clinical outcome associated with preexisting malnutrition in acute renal failure a prospective cohort study. J Am Soc Nephrol 1999;10(3):581–93.

42. Bianchi F, Sala E, Donadei C, et al. Potential advantages of acute kidney injury management by mesenchymal stem cells. World J Stem Cells 2014;6(5):644.

43. Humphreys BD, Bonventre JV. Mesenchymal stem cells in acute kidney injury. Annu Rev Med 2008;59:311–25.

44. Meersch M, Schmidt C, Hoffmeier A, et al. Prevention of cardiac surgery-associated AKI by implementing the KDIGO guidelines in high risk patients identified by biomarkers: the PrevAKI randomized controlled trial. Intensive Care Med 2017;43(11):1551–61.

45. Zhang Z, Lu B, Sheng X, et al. Cystatin C in prediction of acute kidney injury: a systemic review and meta-analysis. Am J Kidney Dis 2011;58(3):356–65.

46. Stevens LA, Schmid CH, Greene T, et al. Factors other than glomerular filtration rate affect serum cystatin C levels. Kidney Int 2009;75(6):652–60.

47. Parikh CR, Coca SG, Thiessen-Philbrook H, et al. Postoperative biomarkers predict acute kidney injury and poor outcomes after adult cardiac surgery. J Am Soc Nephrol 2011;9:1737–47.

48. Bennett M, Dent CL, Ma Q, et al. Urine NGAL predicts severity of acute kidney injury after cardiac surgery: a prospective study. Clin J Am Soc Nephrol 2008; 3(3):665–73.

49. McIlroy DR, Wagener G, Lee HT. Neutrophil gelatinase-associated lipocalin and acute kidney injury after cardiac surgery: the effect of baseline renal function on diagnostic performance. Clin J Am Soc Nephrol 2010;5:211–9.

The Role of Venoarterial Extracorporeal Membrane Oxygenation in Postcardiotomy Cardiogenic Shock

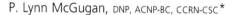

P. Lynn McGugan, DNP, ACNP-BC, CCRN-CSC*

KEYWORDS

- VA ECMO • Postcardiotomy cardiogenic shock • Ventricular assist device
- Oxygenators

KEY POINTS

- Postcardiotomy cardiogenic shock has a high mortality rate. Venoarterial (VA) extracorporeal membrane oxygenation (ECMO) may be used to provide systemic perfusion while myocardial recovery occurs or other treatment options are investigated.
- VA ECMO can be cannulated either peripherally or centrally, each strategy has benefits and drawbacks.
- Management of patients on VA ECMO includes the need for patient and circuit assessment, anticoagulation, nutrition, sedation, and ventilator management.
- Complications, including limb ischemia, bleeding, upper body hypoxia, thrombi, altered kidney function, left ventricular distension, infection, and stroke, may occur, in addition to pump complications.
- Quality of life may be affected after initiation of VA ECMO, but in initial studies, it seems to not differ from patients who have chronic health-related issues.

Postcardiotomy cardiogenic shock (PCCS) occurs at a rate of 0.5% to 6% and has a poor prognosis, with a mortality rate of 60%.[1,2] Cardiogenic shock results in tissue hypoperfusion, and multiple interventions may be needed to restore perfusion and prevent end-organ damage. Venoarterial (VA) extracorporeal membrane oxygenation (ECMO) is the most intense, invasive therapy to date used for PCCS.

DEFINITION

PCCS has variable definitions in the literature; therefore, the incidence is difficult to predict.[1,3] From the available definitions, PCCS occurs with an incidence of

Disclosure Statement: The author has nothing to disclose.
CTICU, Duke University Hospital, ACNP, Durham, NC, USA
* Box 3677 Duke University Medical Centre, Durham, NC 27705.
E-mail address: Lynn.mcgugan@duke.edu

approximately 0.5% to 6%.[1] The time frame ranges between 0 and 48 hours after cardiac surgery.[4] Classic cardiogenic shock requirements of systolic blood pressure (SBP) less than 90 mm Hg, left atrial pressure greater than 18 mm Hg, cardiac index less than 1.8 L/min/m[2], and pulmonary capillary wedge pressure greater than 16 mm Hg (or pulmonary edema of a nonrespiratory cause) without inotropes or mechanical devices are typically used in addition to the postoperative timeframe; however, some definitions include the need for mechanical circulatory support (MCS) at any time during the index hospital stay.[1,3]

PATHOPHYSIOLOGY

PCCS can occur from right ventricular (RV), left ventricular (LV), or biventricular failure and has many potential causes (**Box 1**).[5] If untreated, poor cardiac function results in a reduced supply of oxygenated blood being delivered to tissues. RV failure manifests as an elevated central venous pressure and RV dilation, and leads to systemic hypoperfusion due to underfilling of the LV. LV failure manifests as an elevated pulmonary capillary wedge pressure and leads to pulmonary edema as blood backs up into the pulmonary circulation. Systemic hypoperfusion results because the heart is either unable to fill adequately or, if able to fill, contract adequately. Poor tissue perfusion leads to anaerobic metabolism, leading to lactate production and acidosis. Acidosis results in cell membrane dysfunction and failure of the sodium pump; digestive enzymes are released by intracellular lysosomes and toxic substances enter the circulation and damage the capillary endothelium, which causes cell destruction, dysfunction, and death.[6]

TREATMENTS

Initial treatments for PCCS from LV failure are inotropes and placement of an intra-aortic balloon pump (IABP), if not already present. RV failure is initially treated by optimizing preload, vasodilation of the pulmonary vasculature, and the use of inotropes.[7] MCS is not considered until these strategies have been used or considered.[8] Preoperative IABPs may be prophylactically placed for certain patients (**Box 2**).[9] The use of an IABP alone for cardiogenic shock is associated with a mortality rate of 27% to 54%, escalating therapies include short-term or long-term ventricular assist devices (VADs), and VA ECMO.[10] Two types of ECMO exist. Venovenous (VV) ECMO drains and returns blood to the venous system after oxygenation and is effective for pulmonary failure. VA ECMO drains blood from the venous system and returns it to the arterial system after oxygenation, and is effective for both cardiac and pulmonary failure.

Box 1
Potential causes of postcardiotomy cardiogenic shock

Bradycardia	RV dysfunction
Arrhythmias	Vasoplegia
Coronary artery graft/native coronary artery thrombus	Surgical or technical problems
Incomplete revascularization	LV outflow tract obstruction
Myocardial stunning	Kinking of a graft after coronary artery bypass
Coronary artery spasm	Air embolus to a native coronary artery/graft

Data from Fitzsimmons MG. Management of intraoperative problems after cardiopulmonary bypass. In: Mark JB, Nussmeier NA, editors. UpToDate. Waltham, MA: UpToDate, 2018, www. uptodatecom. Accessed January 9, 2019.

Box 2
Conditions for prophylactic intraaortic balloon pump insertion

Myocardial ischemia	Pulmonary edema or hemodynamic instability from mitral regurgitation
Low ejection fractions (<25%)	

Data from Beca J, Wilcox T, Hall RMO. Mechanical cardiac support. In: Sidebotham D, McKee A, Gillham M, Levy JH, editors. Cardiothoracic critical care. Philadelphia, PA: Elsevier; 2007.

Durable VADs are not commonly placed for PCCS; less permanent devices are used until functional recovery status is verified. In biventricular failure with intact respiratory function, the choice of a short-term VAD versus ECMO may be determined by the surgeon's preference and experience.[10] Many centers may have algorithms for device choice in MCS. One has been published in the literature that considers family and patient wishes, neurologic status, coagulation status, and hemodynamic stability.[11]

Intraaortic Balloon Pump

An IABP is often the first-line or second-line therapy for PCCS, and the IABP may remain, even if VA ECMO is inserted. Many centers place an IABP concurrently with VA ECMO for cardiogenic shock.[12,13] Potential benefits include reducing the blood volume of the LV by decreasing afterload and encouraging forward flow, improved diastolic and pulmonary capillary wedge pressures, improved coronary flow, and increased organ perfusion.[12] The presence of an IABP may allow for easier weaning from VA ECMO, although it does not affect survival to discharge.[14]

Short-Term Ventricular Assist Device

Short-term VADs placed for PCCS may be inserted either centrally or peripherally. RV failure is common after left VAD (LVAD) placement and/or orthotopic heart transplantation (OHT). A right VAD (RVAD) may be placed in this situation. Cannulation with short-term VADs for biventricular failure results in more cannulation sites than are required for VA ECMO; however, this strategy allows for 1 ventricle to be supported for a longer time in cases of unequivocal ventricular recovery and avoids the complications of ECMO.[10]

Oxygenators Added to Ventricular Assist Devices

VAD patients frequently develop pulmonary complications in the early postoperative period. Short-term VAD patients have an advantage in this situation because an oxygenator can be added into the cannulas and support the oxygen requirements of the patient. This option is not available to patients who have intracorporeal VADs implanted.[15,16]

An RVAD, with or without an oxygenator, instead of VA ECMO, may be the best choice for an LVAD patient in cardiogenic shock. An RVAD can be kept in place for a period of time, and weaned slowly when the patient appears ready.[17–19] If an oxygenator is in place, it may be removed even before the RV has fully recovered.[18,19]

Venoarterial Extracorporeal Membrane Oxygenation

Depending on the site of cannulation, blood flows from either a large vein or the right atrium through the VA ECMO drainage cannula, through the oxygenator, which removes carbon dioxide and adds oxygen, and delivered back to the body through a cannula to either a large peripheral artery or the aorta (**Fig. 1**). A centrifugal pump

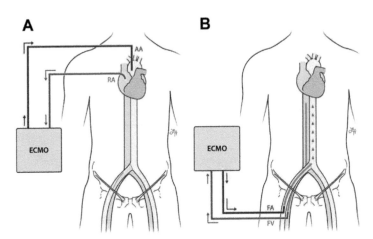

Fig. 1. Central (*A*) versus peripheral (*B*) VA ECMO. AA, ascending aorta; FA, femoral artery; FV, femoral vein; RA, right atrium. (*Illustrated by* Lauren Halligan, MSMI; copyright Duke University; with permission under a CC BY-ND 4.0 license.)

propels blood into the arterial circulation, and a heat exchanger either warms or cools the returned blood. Advantages of VA ECMO compared with short-term VAD support are the ability to support both ventricles, immediate insertion at the bedside, and the ability to oxygenate the blood.[20]

A recent analysis compared short-term VAD support with the CentriMag LVAD (Abbott, Chicago, Illinois, USA), with either peripheral or central ECMO cannulation.[10] Patients on ECMO received more blood and platelet transfusions; had more limb ischemia, systemic inflammatory response syndrome (SIRS), and septic shock; and required reexploration almost twice as often as the VAD group.[10] VAD patients had higher discharge rates and survival rates than the ECMO patients at 30 days, 6 months, 1 year, and 4 years.[10]

VENOARTERIAL EXTRACORPOREAL MEMBRANE OXYGENATION CANNULATION STRATEGIES
Central

Central cannulation is most commonly obtained with the venous cannula in the right atrium (or both superior and inferior venae cavae) and the arterial cannula in the aorta. This method allows for the most complete drainage of the heart while also supplying oxygenated blood to all branches of the aorta via antegrade flow.[21] It requires access to the right atrium and aorta, most commonly a median sternotomy, although aortic cannulation can also be accomplished via anterior thoracotomy.[22–24] This type of cannulation may be used to liberate the patient from the cardiopulmonary bypass pump in the operating room. Central cannulation is not usually seen outside of the PCCS population.[20]

Peripheral

Peripheral cannulation is often preferred owing to the ease of cannula insertion and the less invasive nature of peripheral cannulas. Peripheral cannulation requires access to a large vein and large artery, commonly the femoral vein and artery, although the internal jugular vein and axillary artery can also be used.[25] Cannulas can be placed directly in the vessels or through side grafts attached to the vessels.[26] The most recent guidelines from the Extracorporeal Life Support Organization (ELSO) recommend ultrasound guidance before peripheral cannulation to assess anatomy and estimate vessel size before and during cannula insertion to prevent complications.[27] Although axillary artery cannulations are not commonly used for PCCS patients, the subclavian artery may be used for peripheral VA ECMO access.[22]

Advantages and Disadvantages of Both

Central cannulation is usually performed in the operating room. Larger cannulas can be used when the patient is centrally cannulated and may provide the ability for higher flows.[20,22] Femoral cannulation is commonly used for patients undergoing cardiopulmonary resuscitation (CPR) or those who are too unstable to take to the operating room. Peripheral cannulation allows for chest closure but may cause poor oxygenation to the head vessels and limb ischemia, although the latter risk is lessened with the insertion of a distal perfusion catheter (DPC) (**Fig. 2**).[22,23] Vascular complications occur more often in peripherally cannulated patients.[25] Centrally cannulated patients have more bleeding, require reoperations, and require renal replacement therapy more often than peripherally cannulated patients, but there is no increase in mortality, sepsis, limb ischemia, or stroke.[25,28,29]

INITIATION OF VENOARTERIAL EXTRACORPOREAL MEMBRANE OXYGENATION

Successful deployment of VA ECMO restores hemodynamic stability. One study found mean arterial pressure (MAP) was noted to increase approximately 15 mm Hg, and mean pulmonary artery pressure decreased 11 mm Hg after cannulation.[3] Lactate measurements have long been used to assess tissue perfusion; serial

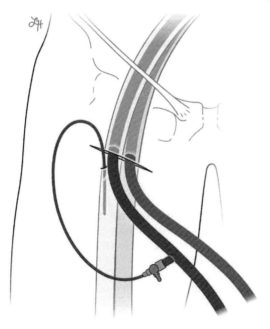

Fig. 2. Distal Perfusion Catheter. (*Illustrated by* Lauren Halligan, MSMI; copyright Duke University; with permission under a CC BY-ND 4.0 license.)

measurements are useful in determining the extent of tissue hypoxia and are used to predict outcomes. Many researchers have found lower initial lactate levels and faster lactate clearance were associated with improved survival.[3,13,30]

VENOARTERIAL EXTRACORPOREAL MEMBRANE OXYGENATION MANAGEMENT
Anticoagulation

As the blood flows through the artificial surfaces of the ECMO tubing, inflammatory and coagulation cascades are activated, increasing thrombotic risk for both the patient and ECMO circuit. Thrombosis can cause circuit failure, oxygenator failure, hemolysis, and thrombotic events such as stroke and limb ischemia.[31] ELSO recommends a heparin bolus when initiating ECMO, even if the patient is coagulopathic and bleeding.[32]

The anticoagulation goal is preventing circuit or patient thrombus, while not causing bleeding. Anticoagulation for PCCS patients is started when bleeding has subsided, usually less than 50 mL/h. Anticoagulation may be delayed but is especially important in the patient who has little to no native contractility because thrombi will form in the aortic root or LV if blood is not ejected from the LV to the aorta.[23] The ELSO Anticoagulation Guidelines recommend an activated clotting time (ACT) of 180 to 220 seconds and supports the use of both unfractionated heparin and a direct thrombin inhibitor (DTI).[32] Thromboelastograms, activated partial thromboplastin times, and anti-Xa levels may be helpful in addition to looking at the ACT.[32] The level of antithrombin should be checked to ensure it is adequate.[32]

Running a VA ECMO circuit without anticoagulation is occasionally done and, according to Sy and colleagues,[31] may be safe in short VA ECMO runs. A small cohort of nonanticoagulated VA ECMO subjects found only 12 thromboembolic events over 2 days.[33] Most anticoagulation on ECMO has been accomplished by using heparin, but DTI are increasingly used. Bivalirudin is the most commonly used DTI; studies have not found a difference in time to therapeutic anticoagulation, neurologic complications, thrombosis, or bleeding.[34,35]

Sedation Vacation

Pharmacokinetics are altered when patients are on ECMO, and patients may require higher doses of sedatives to allow optimal hemodynamics and ventilation. Sedatives should be titrated to effect. If the patient requires sedation, then daily sedation vacations are important to elicit changes in neurologic functioning that may change patient management and indicate prognosis.

Ventilator Management

With peripheral cannulation, positive end-expiratory pressure (PEEP) and the fraction of expired oxygen (Fio$_2$) are used to oxygenate blood flowing through the lungs and out into the aorta where it perfuses the coronary and cerebral vasculature. For the patient on VA ECMO, tissue oxygenation is a result of the blood delivered from the ECMO return cannula mixed with the blood ejected from the native heart, with most of the oxygenation delivered by the ECMO circuit.[34] The mixing of the blood occurs in the aortic root if the patient is centrally cannulated but occurs at somewhere in the mid-aorta if the patient is femorally cannulated.[34] If the patient is stable, they may be extubated.

Flow or Mean Arterial Pressure Goal

A MAP greater than 90 mm Hg has been associated with greater survival and less risk of renal injury. A recent study found subjects on VA ECMO did not survive if their average MAP was less than 70 mm Hg.[35] Extracorporeal flow depends on cannula size, the size of the vena cava, volume status, thoracic and abdominal pressures, oxygenator flow capacity, and the minimal positive and negative pressures that can be tolerated without causing hemolysis.[36] After initiation, blood flow is increased to determine the maximal pump flow, then decreased to the lowest level that will provide support; ideally, to a level that allows a 10 mm Hg pulse pressure difference so that blood is ejected.[7,21,34] Monitoring central venous saturations may be the best way to determine adequate perfusion, with a goal greater than 75%.[34]

ASSESSMENT
Pulsatility

The presence of retrograde flow into the aorta causes increased afterload on the LV. Blood return to the LV includes native pulmonary blood flow, as well as bronchial return and any leakage from an incompetent aortic valve. LV distention may occur if the contractility of the LV is not enough to overcome the afterload and may cause pulmonary edema, hemorrhage, and acute lung injury.[36] Pulsatility on the arterial line, in the absence of counterpulsation (IABP) and aortic regurgitation, indicates that the LV is ejecting, making LV distention, pulmonary edema, and thrombi less likely.[36] Ten to 20 mm Hg of pulsatility on the arterial waveform is usually considered adequate.[21]

Circuit

The circuit should be inspected frequently for thrombi and leaks, despite new materials for manufacturing device components making both less prevalent. Loss of circuit integrity on the venous side of the circuit will entrain air, whereas on the arterial side of the circuit it will result in blood loss.[34] Fibrin or clot formation should be monitored but only intervened on when presenting a risk to pump function or patient emboli.[34]

Extremities

Cannulated extremities must be assessed frequently for adequate perfusion. The presence of a DPC makes malperfusion less likely, but the catheter itself can also develop clots. Inserting arterial cannulas through side grafts may eliminate the need for a DPC,[8] although Cakici and colleagues[26] found cannulas inserted through the side graft insertion strategy had a higher incidence of surgical site bleeding and hypoperfusion.

PHARMACOKINETICS

Sequestration of drugs in the circuit, increased volume of distribution, and changes in drug clearance modify drug pharmacokinetics in VA ECMO patients.[37,38] The pharmacokinetics of lipophilic agents (fentanyl, morphine, midazolam) are thought to change markedly when ECMO is initiated because they are more likely to be sequestered in the circuit.[37] As organ function improves, more of a drug may be required.[37]

NUTRITION

Studies show that 55% to 79% of patients receive goal nutrition while on ECMO.[39,40] Ferrie and colleagues[40] found tube feeding intolerance occurred frequently in both VV and VA ECMO patients, but most intolerances could be managed by adding promotility agents. Early enteral nutrition (within 2 days of initiation) was found to be associated with lower mortality in VA ECMO patients than nutrition started after day 3.[41]

WEANING

Improved systolic and diastolic blood pressure without increasing inotropes or vasopressors and increased pulsatility on the arterial line may indicate myocardial recovery.[36,42,43] Echocardiographic findings associated with successful decannulation from VA ECMO were aortic time velocity integral greater than 10 cm and LV ejection fraction greater than 20% to 25%, whereas preoperative SBP less than 90 mm HG, pre-ECMO pH of less than 7.2, a lactate level greater than 8 after 24 hours on ECMO, and mixed venous oxygen saturation of less than 65% sampled from the venous ECMO cannula predicted poor weaning outcomes.[13,42] Before weaning, inotropes and pulmonary vasodilators can be started to enhance myocardial performance. Anticoagulation is optimized because less flow increases risk for thrombus and then flow is decreased.[43] Weaning occurs by decreasing flow, but the sweep gas is never turned off. Although the lungs may appear to be functioning, if they are not and sweep gas is turned off, then deoxygenated blood will be supplied to the coronary and cerebral vessels. Flow may be decreased rapidly, but may also be decreased by 0.5 L/min increments over time to evaluate changes in hemodynamics and end organ function.[34] Flow is generally kept above 1 to 2 L/min during wean trials.[8,21,42,44,45]

VENOARTERIAL EXTRACORPOREAL MEMBRANE OXYGENATION COMPLICATIONS

Many complications are a result of ECMO components and therapies, others occur as a result of hypoperfusion in the period before ECMO cannulation, and still others occur due to the effects ECMO has on the body. Complications are not infrequent or minor, and this should be considered during the risks and benefits discussion.[46]

Bleeding

Bleeding is much more common than clotting: 27% versus 8%.[31] Patients may have multiple preexisting conditions predisposing them to bleeding.[3] The anticoagulation required to prevent thrombi also puts the patient at risk. The most common sites of bleeding are cannula sites, followed by surgical sites, although intracranial bleeding is the most serious.[34] Even minor procedures may cause uncontrollable bleeding.[34] Kallikrein inhibitors may be given to enhance platelet function and prevent breakdown of clots.[34] When bleeding occurs, anticoagulation should be decreased or paused, and blood components given to restore normal coagulation values.

Hemolysis

Hemolysis is noted by increased levels of plasma-free hemoglobin (PFHgb) and lactate dehydrogenase (LDH), and decreased levels of haptoglobin. Some centers restrict total blood flow, so as not to cause red blood cell destruction, but the pump itself should not cause hemolysis unless inlet pressures are excessive or there are circuit clots.[13,34] PFHgb should be checked and should be less than 10 mg/dL; any value greater than 50 mg/dL should be investigated.[34]

Emboli or Thrombi

Polymethylpentene oxygenators, heparin-coated tubing, and centrifugal pumps have reduced the amount of circuit thrombosis.[34] Thrombi form in the oxygenator and at sites of stasis or turbulent flow. When a thrombus forms in the oxygenator, it increases the resistance of the system, and reduces blood flow and the amount of oxygenated hemoglobin delivered.[34] Eventually, the oxygenator or system components may have to be replaced. Thrombi can occur anywhere in the body or ECMO circuit. If femorally cannulated, retrograde flow may not be adequate to reach the aortic root and thrombi may develop, which may be seen on echocardiography. Intracardiac thrombi may form in conditions of low or stagnant flow, inadequate anticoagulation and proinflammatory conditions, and may embolize to anywhere in the arterial tree.

Acute Kidney Injury

Acute kidney injury (AKI) during ECMO is common and usually multifactorial, resulting from hypoperfusion, infection, or inflammation.[47] Oliguria is among of the earliest indicators and is used as a reflection of additional end organ damage. Urine output (UOP) in the first 24 hours is a good predictor of mortality for PCCS patients on VA ECMO; the more UOP, the better chance of survival the patient has.[48] Yan and colleagues,[49] and Lin and colleagues,[50] found AKI predictive of poor outcomes on ECMO.

Left Ventricular Distention

Distention of the LV occurs in 10% to 60% of patients on VA ECMO.[51] If left untreated, cardiac and pulmonary damage can occur due to pressure within the cardiac chambers and retrograde flow into the pulmonary circulation, and thrombi may form. LV decompression may be done surgically, or an Impella (Abiomed, Danvers, MA, USA) catheter can be placed as an LV vent, which has the benefit of being peripheral so that no further chest surgery is required.[12,52] Patients in cardiogenic shock who had a left-sided Impella placed had a reduced mortality and need for inotropes by day 2 after ECMO initiation compared with patients who did not receive an Impella.[53]

Upper Body Hypoxia

Also referred to as Harlequin syndrome, or north-south syndrome, upper body hypoxia may occur in peripheral cannulation.[21] As the heart starts to recover function, blood that may not be well-oxygenated is ejected into the aorta and delivered to the coronary and cerebral circulation. Mixing of deoxygenated blood from the heart and oxygenated blood from the ECMO return cannula may result in the upper body being more poorly oxygenated than the lower body. With the return cannula in the aorta, central cannulation ensures well-oxygenated blood is mixed with whatever blood is ejected from the heart.[22] Upper body hypoxia can be detected by measuring the partial pressure of oxygen in the right upper extremity as the arteries of the right arm branch off the right subclavian artery from the proximal aortic arch.[36] Upper body hypoxia may require the placement of an additional return cannula in the internal jugular or subclavian vein if increasing the Fio_2 is not effective. The additional cannula returns oxygenated blood, ensuring that the blood flowing through the heart and lungs is oxygenated.[54]

Stroke

Stroke can both embolic and hemorrhagic.[36] Cerebral ischemia can occur due to upper body hypoxia, as previously mentioned. Ischemic stroke is the most common type, whereas hemorrhagic stroke has been linked to risk factors, including rapid carbon dioxide change at the time of ECMO initiation, female sex, central cannulation, and thrombocytopenia.[55] Ischemic stroke has not been associated with increased mortality but hemorrhagic stroke has.[55]

Limb Complications

The large arterial cannulas used for VA ECMO and the hemodynamic instability of most patients before cannulation are 2 main reasons for limb ischemia in peripherally cannulated patients.[20,22] Cannulas greater than 20 French, female sex, younger age, difficulties with cannulation, and the presence of peripheral vascular disease are associated with greater risk of vascular injury.[22] Yen and colleagues[56] also found that greater numbers of vasoactive infusions, smaller femoral artery size, presence of peripheral vascular disease, and the absence of a pulse immediately before or immediately after cannula insertion are risk factors for limb ischemia. The common femoral artery increases in size as patients age, so younger patient are at higher risk for limb ischemia. Near-infrared spectrometry can be used to evaluate for limb ischemia, a SpO2 of 40 and a pressure of 50 mm Hg is required to perfuse the limbs and prevent ischemia.[57,58] Mortality greatly increases when limb ischemia occurs.[22,56,59] Compression of the femoral vein and the venous cannula may compromise venous flow, leading to venous congestion and ischemia.[3,36] Pseudoaneurysm, hematomas, arterial dissection, or retroperitoneal bleeding can also occur.[22]

Distal perfusion catheter
A DPC, also called a reperfusion catheter or a superior femoral artery (SFA) catheter, placed at time of ECMO decreases the risk of limb ischemia by providing perfusion via antegrade flow to the distal extremity. This catheter is attached to the ECMO circuit and provides oxygenated blood into the SFA. Anticoagulation also lessens the risk of limb ischemia.[22]

Pump Complications

Higher perfusion pressures increase the risk for circuit leaks or blowouts, pressures below 400 mm Hg are considered safe.[34] High postpump pressures (>300 mm Hg) indicate resistance to flow somewhere, either due to high patient MAP or resistance (possibly due to clots) in the return cannula, the oxygenator, or the tubing from the oxygenator to the cannula.[34] If high pressure occurs suddenly, a tubing kink or embolus may be the cause.[34]

Air in the circuit
Air in the circuit is detected by the bubble detector. False alarms can occur when fluid boluses are administered rapidly to the patient, diluting the regional blood flow in the vicinity of the bubble detector and making it appear as though there is an air bubble. A true air bubble occurs from air in intravenous medications or fluids, or through the drainage cannula either at the site of cannulation or through a stopcock.[34] Air on the drainage side of the ECMO circuit is usually absorbed by the oxygenator and is less of a problem than on the return side. Air entering the return side can occur if the oxygenator is higher than the patient and if the blood side pressure is lower than the gas side pressure.[34]

Circuit clots
Clots are detected by using a light to inspect the tubing and circuit.[34] They are most commonly found in areas of turbulence or of low flow. Circuit changes, or changing a portion of the circuit should be discussed if clots are enlarging or are on the infusion side of the circuit.[34] Thrombin strands occur at areas of high flow, and are clots that have not yet accumulated red blood cells due to the high flow areas they form in.[34] Not only can thrombi embolize into the arterial tree and cause ischemia, they also cause hemolysis due to turbulent flow.

Mechanical complications
The circuit is designed to switch to battery backup if electrical power failure occurs. The water bath for the heat exchanger drains the most energy, turning this off during the power failure will provide more time on battery backup while the cause is

investigated or the pump switched out for the emergency backup pump.[34] If the battery backup fails or is drained, a low-flow alarm will occur and the backup hand crank should be used.

Decannulation

If the drainage cannula is lost, air enters the circuit and will stop the pump, requiring insertion of another cannula and a circuit change.[34] If the return cannula is lost, volume and perfusion for the patient are lost.[34] In a decannulation situation, clamp both the return and the drainage cannulas to the ECMO circuit, increase ventilator and inotropic support, and institute advanced cardiac life support and CPR, if needed, while reinserting the cannula and changing out the pump or circuit if needed. Preventing decannulation can be accomplished by securing the cannulas to at least 2 sites, inspecting these sutures frequently, and by keeping the patient calm.[34]

Infection or Sepsis

Large cannulas in the vasculature put patients at risk for cannula-related infections and bacteremia. Most patients are intubated and have indwelling bladder catheters, putting them at risk for pneumonia and urinary tract infections. Ventilator-associated pneumonia (VAP) has been shown to be the primary infection for ECMO patients; patients with VAP were also the ones who were most likely to become septic.[60] Cannula site infections may also occur, especially if the patient is obese or malnourished,[22] and mediastinitis is also a possibility for PCCS patients.[21] Patients on VA ECMO have higher infection rates than those patients on VV ECMO.[34] The probability of infection increases with time spent on ECMO and how acutely ill patients were before being placed on ECMO.[60,61] Patients who acquire infections while on ECMO have longer days of ECMO support, longer duration of mechanical ventilation, and spend longer in the intensive care unit (ICU).[59–63] Gram-negative infections seem to be most common.[64] Infection and sepsis put the ECMO patient at risk for circuit dysfunction because the coagulation cascade is activated, leading to thrombotic complications.[63] ELSO does not have a policy for standard antibiotics, although many centers choose to provide some antibacterial coverage.[34]

OUTCOMES FOR VENOARTERIAL EXTRACORPOREAL MEMBRANE OXYGENATION PATIENTS

Postcardiotomy shock as a cause for VA ECMO initiation has among the highest mortality and morbidity rates of all indications for VA ECMO initiation; however, these have decreased in the last 10 years despite increased numbers of ECMO patients and the amount of comorbidities they have.[64]

Myocardial Recovery

Recovery of myocardial function is the desired outcome for all PCCS patients. Device weaning occurs when there is evidence of myocardial recovery; then ECMO is decannulated with the assistance of inotropes or an IABP.[21]

Transition to Ventricular Assist Device or Heart Transplant

The mortality rate of patients who undergo VA ECMO before OHT has decreased over time and, in recent years, has been found to be no different than those who did not require temporary MCS before transplant; however, strokes, renal and liver failure, bleeding complications, and sepsis were all increased in patients on VA ECMO before transplant.[65]

Futility

Some patients will not recover enough cardiac function to be weaned from ECMO, nor will they be transplant or VAD candidates. ELSO recommends this discussion take place with the family (and patient, if possible) before ECMO is initiated and, if there is no cardiac recovery within 3 days and the patient does not have options for durable devices or transplant, that a discussion of ECMO removal occur.[34] PCCS is rarely anticipated, making discussions with the patient or family before ECMO initiation for PCCS unrealistic in this situation.

Mortality

The mortality rate for PCCS patients placed on VA ECMO, excluding OHT, is among the highest causes for VA ECMO placement, potentially due to PCCS patients being older and having higher comorbidity scores.[4,65] In their meta-analysis of PCCS patients, Khorsandi and colleagues[66] found a survival to discharge rate of 30.8%, whereas Biancari and colleagues[67] reported this rate at 36.1%. An analysis of the National Inpatient Sample showed mortality for PCCS patients on ECMO decreased almost 50% in the last several years, from 60.3% to 31.2%.[64] Survival at 30 days is key; those who survive until 30 days are likely to survive long-term.[68]

Heart transplant patients who develop PCCS have a consistently higher survival rate than patients who have had other cardiac surgeries. Studies have shown 50% to 74% survival for OHT patients placed on ECMO for primary graft dysfunction, potentially due to the short-term nature of post-OHT cardiogenic shock.[22,69,70]

Prognostic indicators

Although survival after VA ECMO has increased in recent years, mortality remains high. The Survival after VA ECMO (SAVE) score, available at www.save-score.com, used data from more than 3800 patients in cardiogenic shock to elicit factors associated with survival (**Box 3**).[36,71] The retrospective nature of the study meant only patients who were already on ECMO had variables evaluated.[71]

Khorsandi and colleagues[66] found advanced age, renal failure, and extended duration of ECMO support to be negative prognostic indicators. Biancari and colleagues[67] found younger age and lower lactate levels at the time of ECMO initiation were positive prognostic indicators. Few studies have looked at longer term outcomes; survival at one year has been found to be anywhere from 24-30%, and midrange survival at 3-5 years has been found to be 18%.[4,67,72] In addition to finding that oliguria was associated with decreased survival on ECMO for the PCCS patient, Distelmaier and colleagues[48] found that adding oliguria to SAPS-3 (Simplified Acute Physiology Score) and SOFA (Sequential Organ Failure Assessment) scores enhanced their risk stratification capacity. Liver injury also seems to have a prognostic component; bilirubin levels greater than 30 g/dL were associated with 100% mortality, 90% of patients died with a bilirubin greater than 11 g/dL.[73]

End of Life

Organ failure, family request, hemorrhage, or a diagnosis incompatible with life are the common reasons for discontinuing ECMO support.[74] Do not attempt resuscitation (DNAR) orders are contradictory in VA ECMO patients because resuscitation is provided that is more intense and effective than traditional resuscitation. Experts recommend that when patients are placed on VA ECMO discussions of DNAR status should likely not occur, owing to the confusion that may be created.[75] Patients are placed on ECMO as a bridge-to-destination VAD, recovery or transplantation, although some patients will not recover or be VAD or transplant candidates; then then issue of the

---

Box 3
Precannulation variables included in survival after VA-ECMO (SAVE) score

Acute cardiogenic shock diagnosis
Age
Weight

Acute pre-ECMO organ failures

Chronic renal failure

Duration of intubation in hours
  pre-ECMO cannulation

Peak inspiratory pressure <20 mm Hg
Pre-ECMO cardiac arrest
Diastolic blood pressure before ECMO
  cannulation >40 mm Hg
Pulse pressure before ECMO
  cannulation <20 mm Hg
Bicarbonate value before ECMO
  cannulation ≤15 mmol/L

Data from Schmidt M, Burrell A, Roberts L, et al. Predicting survival after ECMO for refractory cardiogenic shock: the survival after veno-arterial-ECMO (SAVE)-score. Eur Heart J. 2015;36(33):2246–56.

---

so-called bridge to nowhere arises.[76] Patients are kept alive on ECMO but have no viable destination that allows continued survival. According to ethicists, withdrawing a life-sustaining technology is the same as withholding one, although withdrawing requires an action and may appear different to clinicians.[77] End-of-life care for patients on ECMO can be traumatic and cause distress. An ethics, stress management, and/or palliative care consult should be considered if distress is suspected in families or staff.

QUALITY OF LIFE AFTER VENOARTERIAL EXTRACORPOREAL MEMBRANE OXYGENATION

Recovering from ECMO is a long and unpredictable process, with many potential complications, which may be unexpected and stressful, having long-term effects on mental and physical health, which affect quality of life (QoL).[78]

Norkiene and colleagues[78] looked at the presence of posttraumatic stress disorder (PTSD) and QoL in PCCS patients, comparing them with patients who had cardiac surgery but did not require ECMO and patients with coronary artery disease (CAD) who did not have surgery. Health-related QoL measured by the Short Form 36 (SF-36) Health Survey tool was no different in patients who received ECMO and the CAD patients who did not have surgery, although it was higher in those who had elective cardiac surgery who did not require ECMO. PTSD was present in 28.5% of patients, although the investigators point out that the prevalence of PTSD in ICU patients has been reported to be up to 52%.[78]

Combes and colleagues[79] studied QoL in VA ECMO patients, including those with PCCS, and found self-reported results for physical and mental functioning using the SF-36 were lower than age-matched or sex-matched controls in physical and social functioning but equal in vitality and mental health. When compared with patients with endstage renal disease on dialysis, congestive heart failure, and those who had adult respiratory distress syndrome, the results were very comparable. It seems that, even though QoL may be affected after VA ECMO, it may not be different than patients who have serious medical problems or who have required intensive care.

Financial

Financial constraints due to extended hospitalizations and aftercare can cause anxiety and problems for patients and their families.[78] More than 1 in 4 families report financial burdens as a result of medical bills.[80] Chiu and colleagues[81] reported hospital charges for VA ECMO patients averaged more than 1.2 million (USD). Case managers and financial care counsellors should be engaged early in the care of ECMO patients to discuss and provide education around financial issues.

SUMMARY

Venoarterial ECMO is currently the most intense therapy available for patients in PCCS. Not only is it resource intensive but mortality remains high for VA ECMO patients after PCCS, and further research is needed to determine prognostic indicators and which patients will benefit the most from VA ECMO.

REFERENCES

1. Fukahara S, Takeda K, Garan AR, et al. Contemporary mechanical circulatory support therapy for postcardiotomy shock. Gen Thorac Cardiovasc Surg 2016; 64(4):183–91.
2. Pappalardo F, Montisci A. Veno-arterial extracorporeal membrane oxygenation (VA ECMO) in postcardiotomy cardiogenic shock: how much pump flow is enough? J Thorac Dis 2016;8(10):E1444–8.
3. Truby L, Mundy L, Kalesan B, et al. Contemporary outcomes of venoarterial extracorporeal membrane oxygenation for refractory cardiogenic shock at a large tertiary care center. ASAIO J 2015;61(4):403–9.
4. Chen M, Evans A, Gutsche J. Post-cardiotomy shock extracorporeal membrane oxygenation. J Cardiothorac Vasc Anesth 2018. https://doi.org/10.1053/j.jvca. 2018.05.029 [pii:S1053-0770(18)30362-30368].
5. Fitzsimmons MG. Management of intraoperative problems after cardiopulmonary bypass. In: Mark JB, Nussmeier NA, editors. UpToDate. Waltham (MA): UpToDate; 2018. Available at: www.uptodatecom. Accessed January 9, 2019.
6. Gaieski DF, Mikkelson ME. Definition, classification, etiology, and pathophysiology of shock in adults. In: Parsons PE, Finlay G, editors. UpToDate. Waltham (MA): UpToDate; 2018. Available at: www.uptodate.com. Accessed January 7, 2019.
7. Kapur NK, Esposito ML, Bader Y, et al. Mechanical circulatory support devices for acute right ventricular failure. Circulation 2017;136(3):314–26.
8. Ariyaratnam P, McLean LA, Cale AR, et al. Extra-corporeal membrane oxygenation for the post-cardiotomy patient. Heart Fail Rev 2014;19(6):717–25.
9. Beca J, Wilcox T, Hall RMO. Mechanical cardiac support. In: Sidebotham D, McKee A, Gillham M, et al, editors. Cardiothoracic critical care. Philadelphia: Elsevier; 2007. p. 342–64.
10. Mohite PN, Sabashnikov A, Koch A, et al. Comparison of temporary ventricular assist devices and extracorporeal life support in post-cardiotomy cardiogenic shock. Interact Cardiovasc Thorac Surg 2018. https://doi.org/10.1093/icvts/ivy185.
11. Takayama H, Truby L, Koekort M, et al. Clinical outcome of mechanical circulatory support for refractory cardiogenic shock in the current era. J Heart Lung Transplant 2013;32(1):106–11.
12. Cheng R, Hachamovitch R, Makkar R, et al. Lack of survival benefit found with use of intraaortic balloon pump in extracorporeal membrane oxygenation: a pooled experience of 1517 patients. J Invasive Cardiol 2015;27(10):453–8.
13. Hsu PS, Chen JL, Hong GJ, et al. Extracorporeal membrane oxygenation for refractory cardiogenic shock after cardiac surgery: predictors of early mortality and outcome from 51 adult patients. Eur J Cardiothorac Surg 2010;37(2):328–33.
14. Wang L, Xing Z. Short-term outcomes of intra-aortic balloon pump combined with venoarterial extracorporeal membrane oxygenation: a systematic review and meta-analysis. Artif Organs 2018. https://doi.org/10.1111/aor.13397.

15. Sertic F, Ali A. Acute-right-ventricular-failure post-cardiotomy: RVAD as a bridge to a successful recovery. J Surg Case Rep 2018;(6):rjy140.

16. Mohite PN, Patil NP, Popov AF, et al. Oxygenator in short-term LVAD circuit: a rescue in post-LVAD pulmonary complications. Perfusion 2016;31(7):608–10.

17. Shekar K, Mullany DV, Thomson B, et al. Extracorporeal life support devices and strategies for management of acute cardiorespiratory failure in adult patients: a comprehensive review. Crit Care 2014;18(3):219.

18. Mohite PN, Sabashnikov A, De Robertis F, et al. Oxy-RVAD: rescue in pulmonary complications after LVAD implantation. Perfusion 2015;30:596–9.

19. Khorsandi M, Schroder J, Daneshmand M, et al. Outcomes of extra-corporeal right ventricular assist with durable left ventricular assist device. Ann Thorac Surg 2018. https://doi.org/10.1016/j.athoracsur.2018.11.051 [pii:S0003-4975(18) 31851-31854].

20. Extracorporeal Life Support Organization. ELSO adult cardiac failure supplement to the ELSO general guidelines. Available at: https://www.elso.org/Portals/0/IGD/Archive/FileManager/e76ef78eabcusersshyerdocumentselsoguidelinesforadultc ardiacfailure1.3.pdf. Accessed January 2, 2019.

21. Jayaraman AL, Cormican D, Shah P, et al. Cannulation strategies in adult veno-arterial and veno-venous extracorporeal membrane oxygenation: techniques, limitations, and special considerations. Ann Card Anaesth 2017;20(Suppl):S11–8.

22. Pillai AK, Bhatti Z, Bosserman AJ, et al. Management of vascular complications of extra-corporeal membrane oxygenation. Cardiovasc Diagn Ther 2018;8(3):372–7.

23. Rabin J, Kaczorowski DJ. Perioperative management of the cardiac transplant recipient. Crit Care Clin 2019;35(1):45–60.

24. Rubino A, Costanzo D, Stanszus D, et al. Central veno-arterial extracorporeal membrane oxygenation (C-VA-ECMO) after cardiothoracic surgery: a single center experience. J Cardiothorac Vasc Anesth 2018;32(3):1169–74.

25. Ranney DN, Benrashi E, Meza JM, et al. Central cannulation as a viable alternative to peripheral cannulation in extracorporeal membrane oxygenation. Semin Thorac Cardiovasc Surg 2017;29(2):188–95.

26. Cakici M, Ozcinar E, Baran C, et al. A retrospective cohort analysis of percutaneous versus side-graft perfusion techniques for veno-arterial extracorporeal membrane oxygenation in patients with refractory cardiogenic shock. Perfusion 2017;32(5):363–71.

27. Nanjayya VB, Murphy D. Ultrasound guidance for extra-corporeal membrane oxygenation general guidelines 2015. Available at: https://www.elso.org/Portals/0/Files/elso_Ultrasoundguideance_ecmogeneral_guidelines_May2015.pdf. Accessed December 7, 2018.

28. Kanji HD, Schulze CH, Oreopoulos A, et al. Peripheral versus central cannulation for extracorporeal membrane oxygenation: a comparison of limb ischemia and transfusion requirements. Thorac Cardiovasc Surg 2010;58(8):459–62.

29. Raffa GM, Kowalewski M, Brodie D, et al. Meta-analysis of peripheral or central ECMO in postcardiotomy and non-postcardiotomy shock. Ann Thorac Surg 2019;107(1):311–22.

30. Li CL, Wang H, Jia M, et al. The early dynamic behavior of lactate is linked to mortality in postcardiotomy patients with extracorporeal membrane oxygenation support: a retrospective observational study. J Thorac Cardiovasc Surg 2015;149(5): 1445–50.

31. Sy E, Sklar MC, Lequier L, et al. Anticoagulation practices and the prevalence of major bleeding, thromboembolic events, and mortality in venoarterial

extracorporeal membrane oxygenation: a systematic review and meta-analysis. J Crit Care 2017;39:87–96.

32. Extracorporeal Life Support Organization. ELSO anticoagulation guidelines. Available at: https://www.elso.org/Portals/0/Files/elsoanticoagulationguideline8-2014-table-contents.pdf. Accessed December 7, 2018.

33. Lamarche Y, Chow B, Bédard A, et al. Thromboembolic events in patients on extracorporeal membrane oxygenation without anticoagulation. Innovations (Phila) 2010;5(6):424–9.

34. Extracorporeal Life Support Organization. ELSO guidelines for cardiopulmonary extracorporeal life support. Available at: https://www.elso.org/Portals/0/IGD/Archive/FileManager/929122ae88cusersshyerdocumentselsoguidelinesgeneralalleclsversion1.3.pdf. Accessed January 4, 2019.

35. Tanaka D, Shimada S, Mullin M, et al. What is the optimal blood pressure on veno-arterial extracorporeal membrane oxygenation? Impact of mean arterial pressure on survival. ASAIO J 2018. https://doi.org/10.1097/MAT.0000000000000824.

36. Meuwese CL, Ramjankhan FZ, Braithwaite SA, et al. Extracorporeal life support in cardiogenic shock: indications and management in current practice. Neth Heart J 2018;26(2):58–66.

37. Touchard C, Aubry A, Eloy P, et al. Predictors of insufficient peak amikacin concentration in critically ill patients on extracorporeal membrane oxygenation. Crit Care 2018;22(1):199.

38. Sanfilippo F, Asmussen S, Maybauer DM, et al. Bivalirudin for alternative anticoagulation in extracorporeal membrane oxygenation: a systematic review. J Intensive Care Med 2017;32(5):312–9.

39. Bear DE, Smith C, Barrett NA. Nutrition support in adult patients receiving extracorporeal membrane oxygenation. Nutr Clin Pract 2018;33(6):738–46.

40. Ferrie S, Herkes R, Forrest P. Nutrition support during extracorporeal membrane oxygenation (ECMO) in adults: a retrospective audit of 86 patients. Intensive Care Med 2013;39(11):1989–94.

41. Ohbe H, Jo T, Yamana H, et al. Early enteral nutrition for cardiogenic or obstructive shock requiring venoarterial extracorporeal membrane oxygenation: a nationwide inpatient database study. Intensive Care Med 2018;44(8):1258–65.

42. Aissaoui N, Luyt CE, Leprince P, et al. Predictors of successful extracorporeal membrane oxygenation (ECMO) weaning after assistance for refractory cardiogenic shock. Intensive Care Med 2011;37(11):1738–45.

43. Williams B, Bernstein W. Review of venoarterial extracorporeal membrane oxygenation and development of intracardiac thrombosis in adult cardiothoracic patients. J Extra Corpor Technol 2016;48(4):162–7.

44. Pappalardo F, Pieri M, Arnaez Corada B, et al. Timing and strategy for weaning from veno-arterial ECMO are complex issues. J Cardiothorac Vasc Anesth 2015;29(4):906–11.

45. Cavarocchi NC, Pitcher HT, Yang Q, et al. Weaning of extracorporeal membrane oxygenation using continuous hemodynamic transesophageal echocardiography. J Thorac Cardiovasc Surg 2013;146(6):1474–9.

46. Xie A, Phan K, Tsai YC, et al. Venoarterial extracorporeal membrane oxygenation for cardiogenic shock and cardiac arrest: a meta-analysis. J Cardiothorac Vasc Anesth 2015;29(3):637–45.

47. Tsai T, Chien H, Tsai F, et al. Comparison of RIFLE, AKIN, and KDIGO classifications for assessing prognosis of patients on extracorporeal membrane oxygenation. J Formos Med Assoc 2017;116(11):844–51.

48. Distelmaier K, Roth C, Binder C, et al. Urinary output predicts survival in patients undergoing extracorporeal membrane oxygenation following cardiovascular surgery. Crit Care Med 2016;44(3):531–8.
49. Yan X, Jia S, Meng X, et al. Acute kidney injury in adult postcardiotomy patients with extracorporeal membrane oxygenation: evaluation of the RIFLE classification and the Acute Kidney Injury Network criteria. Eur J Cardiothorac Surg 2010;37:334–8.
50. Lin CY, Chen YC, Tsai FC, et al. RIFLE classification is predictive of short-term prognosis in critically ill patients with acute renal failure supported by extracorporeal membrane oxygenation. Nephrol Dial Transplant 2006;21:2867–73.
51. Rupprecht L, Florchinger B, Schopka S, et al. Cardiac decompression on extracorporeal life support: a review and discussion of the literature. ASAIO J 2013;59: 547–53.
52. Cheng A, Swartz MF, Massey HT. Impella to unload the left ventricle during peripheral extracorporeal membrane oxygenation. ASAIO J 2013;59(5):533–6.
53. Patel SM, Lipinski J, Al-Kindi SG, et al. Simultaneous Venoarterial Extracorporeal membrane oxygenation and percutaneous left ventricular decompression therapy with Impella is associated with improved outcomes in refractory cardiogenic shock. ASAIO J 2019;65(1):21–8.
54. Brasseur A, Scolletta S, Lorusso R, et al. Hybrid extracorporeal membrane oxygenation. J Thorac Dis 2018;10(Suppl 5):S07–715.
55. Le Guennec L, Cholet C, Huang F, et al. Ischemic and hemorrhagic brain injury during venoarterial-extracorporeal membrane oxygenation. Ann Intensive Care 2018;8(1):129.
56. Yen CC, Kao CH, Tsai CS, et al. Identifying the risk factor and prevention of limb ischemia in extracorporeal membrane oxygenation with femoral artery cannulation. Heart Surg Forum 2018;21(1):E018–22.
57. Steffen RJ, Sale S, Anandamurthy B, et al. Using near-infrared spectroscopy to monitor lower extremities in patients on venoarterial extracorporeal membrane oxygenation. Ann Thorac Surg 2014;98(5):1853–4.
58. Huang SC, Yu HY, Ko WJ, et al. Pressure criterion for placement of distal perfusion catheter to prevent limb ischemia during adult extracorporeal life support. J Thorac Cardiovasc Surg 2004;128(5):776–7.
59. Yang F, Hou D, Wang J, et al. Vascular complications in adult postcardiotomy cardiogenic shock patients receiving venoarterial extracorporeal membrane oxygentation. Ann Intensive Care 2018;8(1):72.
60. Schmidt M, Bréchot N, Hariri S, et al. Nosocomial infections in adult cardiogenic shock patients supported by venoarterial extracorporeal membrane oxygenation. Clin Infect Dis 2012;55(12):1633–41.
61. Aubron C, Cheng AC, Pilcher D, et al. Infections acquired by adults who receive extracorporeal membrane oxygenation: risk factors and outcome. Infect Control Hosp Epidemiol 2013;34(1):24–30.
62. Grasselli G, Scaravilli V, Di Bella S, et al. Nosocomial infections during extracorporeal membrane oxygenation: incident, etiology, and impact on patients' outcome. Crit Care Med 2017;45(10):1726–33.
63. Biffi S, Di Bella S, Scaravilli V, et al. Infections during extracorporeal membrane oxygenation: epidemiology, risk factors, pathogenesis and prevention. Int J Antimicrob Agents 2017;50(1):9–16.
64. Li B, Sun G, Cheng Z, et al. Analysis of nosocomial infections in post-cardiac surgery extracorporeal membrane oxygenation support therapy. Heart Surg Forum 2018;21(5):E387–91.

65. Sanaiha Y, Bailey K, Downey P, et al. Trends in mortality and resource utilization for extracorporeal membrane oxygenation in the United States: 2008-2014. Surgery 2018. https://doi.org/10.1016/j.surg.2018.08.012 [pii:S0039-6060(18)30522-1].

66. Khorsandi M, Dougherty S, Bouamra O, et al. Extra-corporeal membrane oxygenation for refractory cardiogenic shock after adult cardiac surgery: a systematic review and meta-analysis. J Cardiothorac Surg 2017;12(1):55.

67. Biancari F, Perrotti A, Dalén M, et al. Meta-analysis of the outcome after postcardiotomy venoarterial extracorporeal membrane oxygenation in adult patients. J Cardiothorac Vasc Anesth 2018;32(3):1175–82.

68. Flécher E, Anselmi A, Corbineau H, et al. Current aspects of extracorporeal membrane oxygenation in a tertiary referral centre: determinants of survival at follow-up. Eur J Cardiothorac Surg 2014;46(4):665–71.

69. Marasco SF, Vale M, Pellegrino V, et al. Extracorporeal membrane oxygenation in primary graft failure after heart transplantation. Ann Thorac Surg 2010;90:1541–6.

70. D'Alessandro C, Aubert S, Golmard JL, et al. Extra-corporeal membrane oxygenation temporary support for early graft failure after cardiac transplantation. Eur J Cardiothorac Surg 2010;37:343–9.

71. Schmidt M, Burrell A, Roberts L, et al. Predicting survival after ECMO for refractory cardiogenic shock: the survival after veno-arterial-ECMO (SAVE)-score. Eur Heart J 2015;36(33):2246–56.

72. Wang L, Wang H, Hou X. Clinical outcomes of adult patients receiving extracorporeal membrane oxygenation for postcardiotomy cardiogenic shock: a systematic review and meta-analysis. J Cardiothorac Vasc Anesth 2018;32(5):2087–93.

73. Masha L, Peerbhai S, Boone D, et al. Yellow means caution: correlations between liver injury and mortality with the use of VA-ECMO. ASAIO J 2018. https://doi.org/10.1097/MAT.0000000000000895.

74. Smith M, Vukomanovic A, Brodie D, et al. Duration of veno-arterial extracorporeal life support (VA ECMO) and outcome: an analysis of the Extracorporeal Life Support Organization (ELSO) registry. Crit Care 2017;21(1):45.

75. Meltzer EC, Ivascu NS, Fins JJ. DNR and ECMO: a paradox worth exploring. J Clin Ethics 2014;25(1):13–9.

76. Makdisi T, Makdisi G. Ethical challenges in extra corporeal membrane oxygenation use. Ann Palliat Med 2017;6(Suppl 2):S128–31.

77. Williams SB, Dahnke MD. Clarification and mitigation of ethical problems surrounding withdrawal of extracorporeal membrane oxygenation. Crit Care Nurse 2016;36(5):56–65.

78. Norkiene I, Jovaisa T, Scupakova N, et al. Long-term quality of life in patients treated with extracorporeal membrane oxygenation for postcardiotomy cardiogenic shock. Perfusion 2018. https://doi.org/10.1177/0267659118815291. 267659118815291.

79. Combes A, Leprince P, Luyt CE, et al. Outcomes and long-term quality-of-life of patients supported by extracorporeal membrane oxygenation for refractory cardiogenic shock. Crit Care Med 2008;36(5):1404–11.

80. Cohen RA, Kirzinger WK. Financial burden of medical care: a family perspective. NCHS Data Brief 2014;(142):1–8. Available at: http://citeseerx.ist.psu.edu/viewdoc/download?doi=10.1.1.650.4193&rep=rep1&type=pdf. Accessed January 5, 2019.

81. Chiu R, Pillado BS, Sareh S, et al. Financial and clinical outcomes of extracorporeal mechanical support. J Card Surg 2017;32(3):215–21.

Cardiac Surgical Resuscitation
State of the Science

S. Jill Ley, MS, RN, CNS*

KEYWORDS

- Cardiac surgery • Cardiac arrest • Resuscitation • Resternotomy

KEY POINTS

- Patients who arrest after cardiac surgery should be treated using algorithms tailored specifically for this population in an intensive care unit environment, in preference to advanced cardiac life support, for optimal survival.
- If initial interventions to correct arrhythmias with shocking or pacing and airway troubleshooting are unsuccessful, the team should prepare for immediate resternotomy.
- Epinephrine should not be administered following cardiac surgical arrest due to potentially life-threatening rebound hypertension, proarrhythmic properties, and lack of efficacy.
- Experiential training of first responders to acute cardiac arrest provides an opportunity for skill acquisition, review of infrequently used equipment, and teambuilding that optimally prepares for these low-volume, high-risk events.

INTRODUCTION

An endless barrage of new literature creates challenges for clinicians trying to keep abreast of evidence-based practices when only a subset may be actionable, particularly with respect to resuscitation science. Professional societies have weighed in with specific grading recommendations to prioritize findings, highlighting the importance of randomized trials compared with observational studies, with the coveted guideline status awarded to a relatively few noteworthy contributions that warrant immediate consideration for implementation. The International Liaison Committee on Resuscitation (ILCOR) was created in 1992 to evaluate the scientific literature and strive for international consensus regarding resuscitation science, with provision of

Disclosure: The author acknowledges being a member of the Cardiac Surgical Unit Advanced Life Support (CSU-ALS) North America Advisory Board and is an instructor in CSU-ALS programs.
Surgical & Interval Services, California Pacific Medical Center, 1101 Van Ness Avenue #4403, San Francisco, CA 94109, USA
* 62 Paseo Way, Greenbrae, CA 94904.
E-mail address: leyj@sutterhealth.org

Crit Care Nurs Clin N Am 31 (2019) 437–452
https://doi.org/10.1016/j.cnc.2019.05.010
0899-5885/19/© 2019 Elsevier Inc. All rights reserved.

ccnursing.theclinics.com

scheduled updates in the form of Consensus on Cardiopulmonary Resuscitation [CPR] and Emergency Cardiovascular Care Science With Treatment Recommendations (CoSTR) publications.[1] Questions formulated in the population, intervention, comparator, outcome (PICO) format undergo detailed evidence reviews and are graded as high, moderate, low, or very low. Unless new evidence is graded as overwhelmingly conclusive, the status quo is maintained. This lofty standard leads to the continuation of historical practices that are themselves often based on weak or conflicting evidence, if more recent data are underpowered to change course. Through ILCOR participation, the European Resuscitation Council (ERC) and the American Heart Association (AHA) have become standard-bearers for the determination and dissemination of resuscitation standards throughout Europe and the United States, respectively.

To date, these efforts have yielded universal algorithms largely based on out-of-hospital cardiac arrest (OHCA) data that anticipate an unwitnessed event in a deoxygenated patient, attended by layperson rescuers without advanced cardiac life support (ACLS) resources. Given the obvious disparity in this scenario versus an in-hospital cardiac arrest (IHCA) occurring hours after heart surgery in an intensive care unit (ICU), it is not surprising that the Society of Thoracic Surgeons (STS) and the European Association of Cardiothoracic Surgery (EACTS) sought a more evidence-based approach for their unique patient population. In addition, the widespread adoption of circulatory support technologies using ventricular assist devices or extracorporeal membrane oxygenation (ECMO) has created a highly specialized subset within cardiac surgery that requires device-specific variations in resuscitation protocols. This article addresses the most current, evidence-based treatment standards specific to surgical IHCAs that are endorsed by the STS, EACTS, and ERC; identifies important modifications from AHA guidelines; and review pertinent literature addressing these recommendations.

UNIQUE FEATURES OF CARDIAC SURGICAL ARRESTS

The rationale for modifying ACLS after cardiac surgery is based on the interaction between arrest pathophysiology and the environment in which it occurs: "... external massage is ineffective for an arrest due to tamponade or hypovolemia (bleeding), and therefore these subsets of patients will receive inadequate cerebral perfusion during cardiac arrest in the absence of resternotomy."[2] Cardiac surgical arrests are somewhat predictable in their frequency, cause, timing, and relatively high potential for success. Up to 8% of these patients experience a perioperative arrest, and a high percentage (30%–50%) present with a shockable rhythm (ie, ventricular fibrillation [VF] or pulseless ventricular tachycardia [VT]). An additional 28% of arrests after cardiac surgery are due to mechanical events such as tamponade or graft failure.[2] Anthi and colleagues[3] confirmed the early timing of these events; more than half occurred within 3 hours of ICU arrival and 80% were within 8 hours. They implemented a successful strategy of prompt ICU resternotomy that yielded a laudable survival-to-discharge rate of 79%. In one of the few recent papers reporting this outcome, LaPar and colleagues,[4] identified survival rates of 17% to 50% in 17 Virginia hospitals that presumably followed conventional ACLS protocols. This review indicates the most common postoperative cardiac surgical arrest scenario occurs as a monitored event in a patient either intubated or well-oxygenated, with readily available defibrillators, pacemakers, blood products, and the potential for resuming cardiopulmonary bypass if needed. Recommendations for these resuscitations are far outside the scope of current ACLS algorithms. Given the clear limitations of CPR and vasopressors in these scenarios, an STS task force was formed to conduct a detailed literature review that followed The American College of Cardiology and AHA clinical practice guideline methodology. This author was part of a multidisciplinary group that developed the STS Expert Consensus Statement position paper to provide the best evidence on this topic.[2]

CARDIOPULMONARY RESUSCITATION VERSUS DEFIBRILLATION: EVIDENCE SUMMARY

The AHA emphasizes that both the initiation of high-quality CPR and early defibrillation "...are key interventions associated with improved outcome from adult cardiac arrest."[1] The importance of timely defibrillation was demonstrated by Chan and colleagues,[5] who studied IHCA from shockable rhythms and showed that survival decreased from 39% to 22% when defibrillation took longer than 2 minutes. In weighing the importance of an initial therapy, a shockable rhythm is present in up to half of cardiac surgical arrests, and the ready availability of defibrillators and personnel trained in their use presents an important opportunity to prioritize this treatment modality versus CPR. Additionally, harm from CPR has been demonstrated in 32% to 45% of the general population (eg, rib fracture, pulmonary embolism).[6] Shortly after cardiac surgery, external cardiac massage can expose the right ventricle to sharp sternal edges and/or protruding wires, contributing to laceration and hemorrhage.[7,8] Numerous studies have concluded there is no benefit to a brief period of CPR (less than 4 minutes) before defibrillation for a witnessed arrest, and the AHA now advises that the defibrillator be used as soon as possible.[9] In weighing the relative risks and benefits of immediate CPR or defibrillation for cardiac surgical arrest the STS recommends throughout

---

> If the electrocardiogram shows ventricular fibrillation/pulseless ventricular tachycardia, you may delay external cardiac massage for up to one minute to administer shocks (Class IIA, Level B).

NUMBER OF SHOCKS: EVIDENCE SUMMARY

Historical changes to the AHA algorithms led Davis and colleagues[10] to examine the success of defibrillating with 3 sequential stacked shocks (2005–2008), a single shock then 2 minutes of CPR before each defibrillation (2008–2011), or a protocol of 3 escalating shocks (2011–2013) in a single-center, longitudinal study. They found that survival was lowest with a single shock followed by 2 minutes of CPR, whereas the highest survival was seen after using the shock escalation protocol (14%–25% vs 65%–68%, $P<.01$). In a separate study, Bradley and colleagues[11] reviewed the AHA "Get with the Guidelines Registry" data between 2004 and 2012 in 172 US Department of Veterans Affairs hospitals to evaluate the impact of rapid sequence shocks versus a deferred second shock in 2733 adults with VF or VT. They found that for patients whose shockable rhythm persisted following a first defibrillation attempt, outcomes were superior with delivery of subsequent shocks within 1 minute versus more delayed. The unadjusted risk ratio (RR) for return of spontaneous circulation (ROSC) was 62.5 versus 57.4% (RR 0.92, $P<.01$), 24-hour survival was 43.6% versus 38.4% (RR 0.88, $P<.01$), and survival to discharge was 30.8% versus 24.7% (RR 0.80, $P<.01$). These investigators emphasize that contemporary, 1-shock protocols were developed for OHCA patients and should be abandoned in favor of stacked shocks in witnessed IHCA or procedural settings, which is the current ERC recommendation. In weighing the relative risks versus benefits of sequential defibrillation attempts for shockable rhythms, the STS recommends throughout

> For patients with VF or pulseless VT, three sequential shocks should be given without intervening external cardiac massage (Class I, Level B).

MEDICATIONS: EVIDENCE SUMMARY
Epinephrine

Epinephrine (EPI) remains on the ACLS algorithm for VF/VT despite any studies documenting improved neurologically intact survival after its use. The long-awaited PARA-MEDIC2 trial is a randomized, double-blind, placebo-controlled study from the United Kingdom that compared outcomes of EPI administered for OHCA.[12] They examined data from 8014 subjects, which included 19% with a shockable rhythm. Both the EPI and placebo groups demonstrated disappointing overall survival rates, but the administration of EPI, for the first time, was shown to result in improved 30-day survival (3.2% vs 2.4%, $P = .02$). However, EPI was associated with worse neurologic outcomes; a higher percentage of severe neurologic dysfunction occurred in survivors receiving EPI versus placebo (31% vs 17.8%), with one-third of all survivors ultimately experiencing withdrawal of treatment. Few patients or surgeons would argue that survival with a severe neurologic impairment is a successful outcome; the evidence reveals no advantage and potential harm from use of EPI after OHCA.

For IHCA, there is not only a lack of evidence in support of its use, there are important adverse effects, including increased myocardial oxygen demand and precipitation of arrhythmias, which are particularly dangerous in this population. Andersen and colleagues[13] determined that premature use of EPI, which can occur in the treatment of witnessed, in-hospital events, can lead to increased risk of harm. They reported that IHCA subjects with shockable rhythms who received EPI within the first 2 minutes of a failed first shock had significantly lower rates of ROSC, survival, and neurologically intact survival (odds ratio 0.71, 0.70, 0.69, respectively; $P<.001$) versus later administration. Premature use of EPI is a deviation from ACLS protocols that they found in 60% of arrests in 2016 (n = 1510). An additional concern described in multiple case reports is the risk for rebound hypertension with EPI administration.[14,15] Prompt restoration of the cardiac output in combination with EPI stimulation can result in profound hypertension, potentially causing iatrogenic bleeding and surgical reexploration. There are instances of hypotension in which the use of EPI may be beneficial before arrest, but small doses of 50 to 100 mcg are recommended.[2] The STS provides this level C recommendation regarding EPI administration:

> We recommend that neither epinephrine nor vasopressin be given during the cardiac arrest unless directed by a clinician experienced in their use (Class III [harm], Level C).

ADDITIONAL MEDICATIONS: EVIDENCE SUMMARY
Antiarrhythmics

Current recommendations for antiarrhythmic drug therapy in the treatment of refractory VF/VT are extrapolated from OHCA data, such as the Amiodarone, Lidocaine, or

Placebo Study (ALPS), which showed no survival benefit with either drug.[16] On further analysis restricted to bystander-witnessed events, they identified that amiodarone and lidocaine both modestly improved survival-to-discharge rates by approximately 4%. However, for arrests witnessed by emergency personnel (ie, those most closely resembling witnessed IHCA events), discharge survival was significantly higher with amiodarone than placebo (38.6% vs 16.7%, $P = .01$) but not lidocaine (23.3%). Current adult ACLS algorithms now advocate a single agent, amiodarone, for treatment of refractory VF/VT, whereas pediatric advanced life support algorithms include use of either amiodarone or lidocaine. Pediatric recommendations are based on a recent multicenter review from Valdes and colleagues,[17] which showed that lidocaine improved ROSC and 24-hour survival but provided no benefit in discharge outcomes for patients 18 years of age or younger. Given the modest survival benefit with antiarrhythmic drug therapy versus the effectiveness of electrical defibrillation when applied early, initial efforts should focus on immediate defibrillation rather than preparing medications. The STS endorses the following interventions for refractory VF/VT:

After three failed attempts at defibrillation for VF/pulseless VT, a bolus of 300 mg intravenous amiodarone should be given through the central line (Class IIA, Level A).

Continuous Infusions

Administration of various fluid and medication infusions is a routine part of any cardiac operation, and creates the possibility of mistakenly bolusing a vasoactive drug or causing a significant medication error, leading to arrest. For this reason, in an ongoing resuscitation not readily reversed, the STS recommends throughout

---

In an established cardiac arrest, all infusions before arrest should be stopped (Class IIA, Level C). If there is concern about awareness, it is acceptable to continue the sedative infusions. Other infusions can be restarted as indicated by the clinical situation by an experienced clinician (Class IIA, Level C).

USE OF PACING STRATEGIES: EVIDENCE SUMMARY

Intraoperative placement of epicardial pacing wires provides a unique strategy for emergency management of asystole or profound bradycardia beyond the administration of vasopressors recommended in ACLS algorithms.[9] Approximately 25% of valve patients require pacing during the perioperative period, which can occur days after the operation.[18] Temporary pacing strategies using epicardial or transcutaneous systems are widely available with virtually no risk of harm (other than the potential for rhythm competition) and offer great benefit in cases of impaired impulse formation. The STS recommendation regarding asystole management states

---

If the ECG [electrocardiogram] shows asystole, you may delay external massage for as long as a minute to maximize the temporary pacemaker output (Class IIA, Level C).

Maximal outputs from both atrial and ventricular settings should be used in an asynchronous mode (ie, DOO), which is achieved via the emergency button of standard temporary pacing generators. Failure to capture that is not immediately remedied by troubleshooting epicardial connections (ie, patient-to-cable, cable-to-device) or battery replacement warrants the immediate institution of CPR as a bridge to resternotomy, with consideration of a chronotrope or transcutaneous pacing if deemed timely and appropriate. In the event of a pulseless arrest with a paced rhythm (ie, PEA), the pacemaker should be paused briefly to better evaluate the underlying rhythm without pacing artifacts. This may unmask fine VF and provide a strategy of immediate defibrillation that might otherwise be missed.

AIRWAY MANAGEMENT: EVIDENCE SUMMARY

Cardiac surgical patients are most likely intubated at the time of arrest and may suffer from issues such as right mainstem intubation, hemothorax, or pneumothorax. Standard principles of advanced airway management apply; a monitored cardiac arrest should prompt an immediate bedside review of airway, breathing, and circulation (ABC), beginning with airway patency. Promptly performing bag-valve ventilation on 100% oxygen enables assessment of airway patency and lung compliance while optimizing oxygen delivery and venous return through removal of positive end-expiratory pressure (PEEP). Malpositioning or obstruction of the endotracheal tube (ETT) should be excluded or corrected, and a tension pneumothorax should be ruled out or treated with large-bore cannula insertion in the second intercostal space. Continuous monitoring of end tidal carbon dioxide ($ETCO_2$) is useful in identifying respiratory abnormalities, as well as monitoring progress during a resuscitation event; persistent $ETCO_2$ below 10 mm Hg is associated with nonsurvival.[9] Once airway and breathing are established and the respiratory status is stable, ventilation on 100% oxygen without PEEP should continue. The STS recommendations for emergency management of airway and breathing include

- Immediately increase the inspired oxygen to 100% (Class I, Level C); positive end-expiratory pressure should be removed (Class IIA, Level C).
- For ventilated patients, the ventilator should be disconnected and a bag-valve used. Look and listen for breath sounds on both sides with equal chest movement, specifically examining for a pneumothorax or a hemothorax. Confirm the presence of end-tidal carbon dioxide (Class I, Level C).
- If you suspect a tension pneumothorax, place a large-bore needle into the second intercostal space, anterior midclavicular line, followed either by a chest drain or opening of the pleura at resternotomy (Class I, Level C).

ARREST PROTOCOL AFTER CARDIAC SURGERY: EVIDENCE SUMMARY

As current AHA/ACLS recommendations for arrest management are primarily based on OHCA data, it is not surprising that the STS, EACTS, and ERC would pursue evidence for the optimal approach to the unique circumstance of arrest after cardiac surgery. The final resuscitation protocol mirrors current AHA goals in being evidence-based, simple to follow, and easily duplicated for training purposes (**Fig. 1**).[2] All cardiac surgical societies worldwide now recommend this approach for postoperative cardiac surgical arrests in preference to AHA/ACLS algorithms.[19,20] The protocol

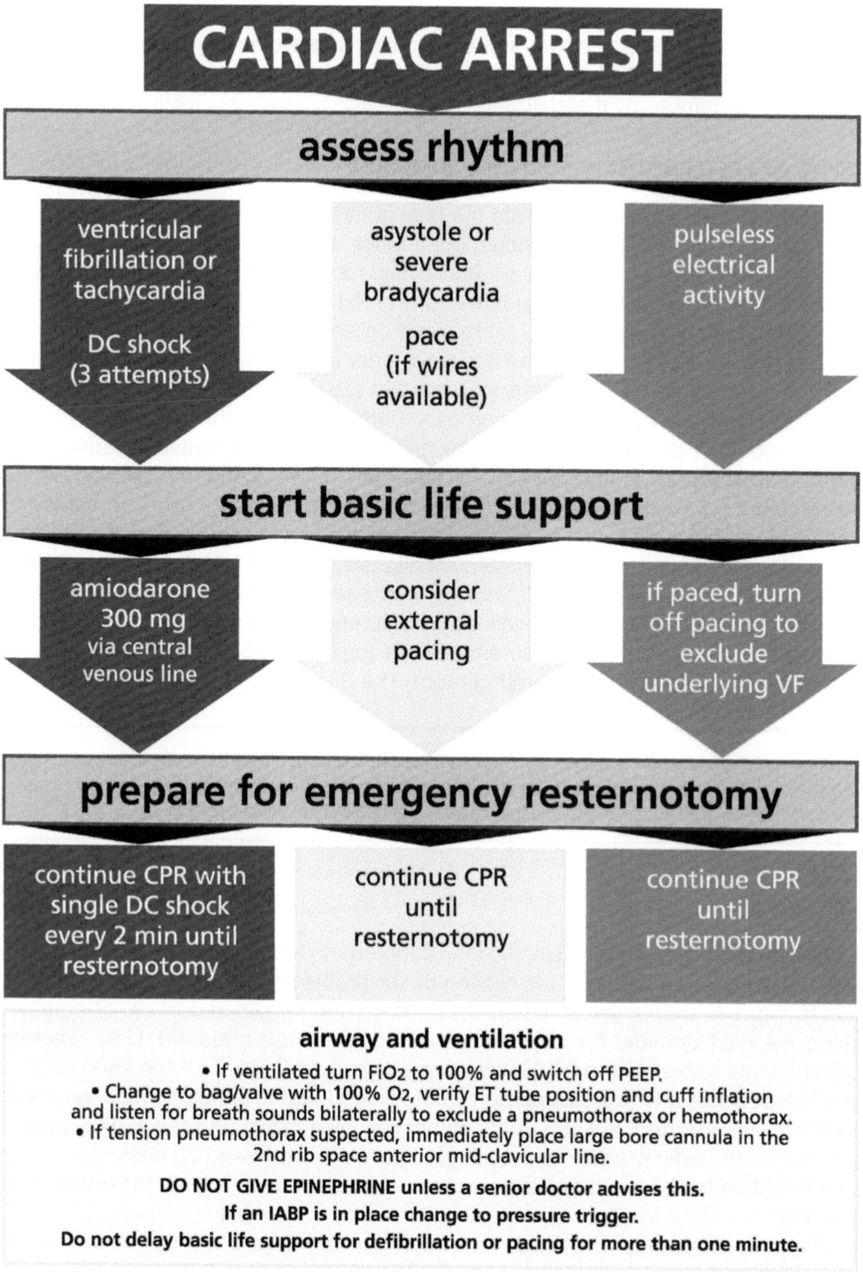

CARDIAC ARREST

assess rhythm

ventricular fibrillation or tachycardia	asystole or severe bradycardia	pulseless electrical activity
DC shock (3 attempts)	pace (if wires available)	

start basic life support

amiodarone 300 mg via central venous line	consider external pacing	if paced, turn off pacing to exclude underlying VF

prepare for emergency resternotomy

continue CPR with single DC shock every 2 min until resternotomy	continue CPR until resternotomy	continue CPR until resternotomy

airway and ventilation

• If ventilated turn FiO_2 to 100% and switch off PEEP.
• Change to bag/valve with 100% O_2, verify ET tube position and cuff inflation and listen for breath sounds bilaterally to exclude a pneumothorax or hemothorax.
• If tension pneumothorax suspected, immediately place large bore cannula in the 2nd rib space anterior mid-clavicular line.

DO NOT GIVE EPINEPHRINE unless a senior doctor advises this.

If an IABP is in place change to pressure trigger.

Do not delay basic life support for defibrillation or pacing for more than one minute.

Fig. 1. Protocol for management of arrest after cardiac surgery endorsed by STS and EACTS. ET, endotracheal; Fio_2, fraction of inspired oxygen; O_2, oxygen. (*From* Dunning J, Levine A, Ley SJ, et al. Used with permission from: The Society of Thoracic Surgeons expert consensus statement for the resuscitation of patients who arrest after cardiac surgery. Ann Thorac Surg. 2017;103:1007; with permission.)

encompasses initial strategies for arrhythmia management that prioritize defibrillation or pacing before CPR, and airway troubleshooting specific to this in-hospital population (ie, malpositioned ETT, tension pneumothorax), followed by rapid progression to emergency resternotomy if stabilization efforts fail.

TIMING OF RESTERNOTOMY: EVIDENCE SUMMARY

Emergency resternotomy represents the final common pathway for the cardiac surgery resuscitation protocol and should commence within 5 minutes of arrest to optimize neurologically intact survival. Pottle and colleagues[21] saw an increase in cardiac surgery postarrest survival rates from 17% to 48% when reopening occurred within 5 minutes of arrest onset. Mackay and colleagues[22] saw similar results when reopening took place no later than 10 minutes after the onset of arrest. Timely reentry is driven by the proven superiority of internal versus external cardiac massage in achieving adequate cerebral and coronary perfusion pressure (CPP).[23,24] Paradis and colleagues[25] demonstrated that maximal CPP was an essential determinant of ROSC in adult arrest victims, with a CPP less than 15 predicting nonsurvival. Arterial line monitoring provides immediate feedback about perfusion. Failure to achieve a systolic blood pressure target of 60 mm Hg heralds the need for immediate intervention; during CPR this degree of hypotension signals the need to proceed immediately with chest reopening and internal massage. In cases of tamponade, reopening even a portion of the sternum relieves physiologic compression and often restores perfusion immediately, whereas full resternotomy allows for direct visualization and potential stabilization for return to the operating room. The STS recommends throughout

---

Internal cardiac massage is superior to external cardiac massage. In patients with a recent sternotomy in whom resuscitative efforts are likely to last more than 5 minutes, emergency resternotomy is indicated to perform internal cardiac massage (Class IIA, Level C).

OUTCOME DATA

Survival after cardiac arrest is significantly affected by delays in recognition and treatment, particularly immediate defibrillation of shockable rhythms. Despite ongoing efforts to improve outcomes of arrest, these data have remained somewhat stagnant during the past decade. For OHCA, survival-to-discharge rates are 12%, whereas IHCA patients experience a 24.8% discharge-to-survival rate.[26] Of the 2500 to 5000 arrests that occur after cardiac surgery in the United States annually, wide variations in survival are reported. In 1998, Anthi and colleagues[3] demonstrated a 79% survival rate when reportedly practicing a strategy of initial CPR followed by chest opening in the ICU within 3 to 5 minutes, but no other details about arrest management were provided.

LaPar and colleagues[4] provided more contemporary results in a report on a 17-facility collaborative in Virginia where cardiac arrest occurred in 3.7% to 8.5% of patients, with survival rates of 31% to 51%, presumably using a standard ACLS approach. Karhunen and colleagues[27] demonstrated an 82% discharge survival rate with early resternotomy in coronary bypass subjects who arrested postoperatively and found long-term (15-year) survival was equivalent to matched controls. Maccaroni and colleagues[28] reported an improvement in survival outcomes after they stopped the practice of scoop-and-run arrest management, in which patients were moved to an operating room for resuscitation, after determining it required a 9-minute transit time. On training their team to use the European version of the STS protocol in 2009, the need for urgent resternotomy decreased by 19% in 2 years ($P = .06$) and survival to discharge increased from 36.3% to 63.8% ($P = .08$). Ley and colleagues[29] also reported a significant improvement in survival outcomes after implementing the European resuscitation protocol in their ICU. Although the overall arrest rate declined modestly from 3.4% to 2.9% ($P = .50$), the incidence of failure to rescue following cardiac arrest decreased significantly from 64.5% to 34.6% in the 4 years after implementation ($P = .034$).

EVIDENCE-BASED TRAINING TO PREPARE FOR CARDIAC SURGICAL ARRESTS

Educating clinical staff to respond to a cardiac arrest in a manner that deviates from ACLS is a critical yet challenging aspect of improving arrest outcomes for these low-volume, high-risk events. The STS Expert Consensus Statement includes additional recommendations regarding the conduct of cardiac surgical arrests, which has been standardized to support this training. Six essential roles have been delineated for optimal arrest management and timely resternotomy (**Fig. 2**). Key responsibilities for these providers, as well as the reopening team, are outlined in **Table 1**. Training is organized to foster hands-on, simulated role performance at a rapid pace, with focused debriefing. With an understanding of essential duties, providers can take action without waiting for physician orders, preparing for an emergency resternotomy like a coordinated racing team pit crew with a goal of reopening within 5 minutes. Key differences from traditional ACLS include prioritization of defibrillation or pacing before CPR by first responders, attention to internal defibrillation and pacing needs by the third responder, and preparations by the reentry team. The ICU nursing lead and team leader work closely together to notify surgeons and others who may be needed for the response, and allocate appropriate resources and personnel to proceed quickly to resternotomy, if indicated.

Equipment needed to assist the ICU reopening team includes a small resternotomy set containing only the items needed for urgent reentry, including a scalpel (and possibly scissors) for incising the skin and sutures, a wire cutter or puller for removal of sternal wires, a sternal retractor for visualization and access, and a sterile suction handle and tubing to evacuate bleeding (**Figs. 3 and 4**). The ready availability of this set is critical to the efficient conduct of these events and is recommended by the STS:

> A small emergency resternotomy set should be available in every ICU, containing only the instruments necessary to perform the resternotomy. This small set should be in addition to a full cardiac surgery sternotomy set, which need not be opened until after the emergency resternotomy has been performed. These sets should be clearly marked and checked regularly (Class I, Level C).

Rapid resternotomy using aseptic technique is the highest priority; efficiencies are created by avoiding prolonged searches by ICU providers unfamiliar with surgical instruments, as well as the application of a sterile drape encompassing the patient and bed, thus creating a large sterile field for safely depositing needed equipment (eg, suction, internal defibrillator paddles, instrument set). Handwashing and application of sterile attire by all team members is not essential and creates delay; in the interest of time, only the reentry team is required to don standard surgical attire. No significant increase in deep sternal wound infections has been identified for emergent resternotomy, largely due to prior skin prep and antibiotic administration that inevitably precedes sternal reentry,

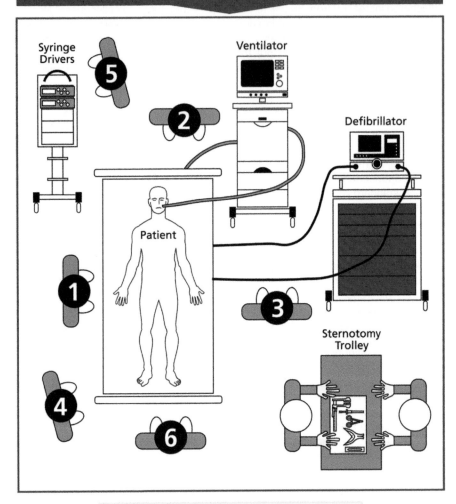

Six key roles in the cardiac arrest

Syringe Drivers

Ventilator

Defibrillator

Patient

Sternotomy Trolley

Six key roles in the cardiac arrest:

1. External cardiac massage
2. Airway and breathing
3. Defibrillation
4. Team leader
5. Drugs and syringe drivers
6. ICU co-ordinator

Fig. 2. Provider roles during initial management of arrest after cardiac surgery. At least 2 additional sterile providers are needed for sternal reopening. (*From* Dunning J, Levine A, Ley SJ, et al. Used with permission from: The Society of Thoracic Surgeons expert consensus statement for the resuscitation of patients who arrest after cardiac surgery. Ann Thorac Surg. 2017;103:1012; with permission.)

Table 1
Key role functions during management of postoperative cardiac surgical arrest

Role	Key Role Functions
1. First responder	• Identify arrest • Call for help • Manage rhythm with defibrillation or pacing • After failing 3 shocks or pacing, initiate external massage
2. Airway	• Increase fraction of inspired oxygen (Fio$_2$) to 100% • Remove PEEP • Implement bag-valve ventilation • Assess airway and breathing • Rule out malpositioned ETT or tension pneumothorax
3. Defibrillation and pacing	• Place defibrillator pads on patient and connect to defibrillator • Administer 3 sequential shocks at 150–200 J and administer subsequent defibrillations • Sequester temporary pacemaker generator nearby in case of use before drape placement; initiate or manage pacing as appropriate • On placement of sterile drape, initiate defibrillator cable change to, halt external compressions and remove chest dressings • Change defibrillator cable to convert from external to internal paddles; decrease energy output to 20 J
4. Team leader	• Direct code responses by team members • Ascertain cause of arrest and order treatments or diagnostic tests • Initiate appropriate therapies and consultations • Initiate timely preparations for resternotomy
5. Medication administration	• VT/VF: administer amiodarone after 3 failed shocks • Stop all infusions • Question use of epinephrine unless directed by senior clinician
6. Critical care nursing leader	• Oversee personnel resources: assemble appropriate emergency responders and notify surgeon and others • Oversee equipment resources: direct team to obtain needed resternotomy cart or sterile items for reentry • Oversee diagnostic testing resources: deploy point-of-care testing resources to code team
7. Resternotomy provider #1 (sterile) 8. Resternotomy provider #2 (sterile)	• Don sterile gown and gloves using aseptic technique • Apply large sterile drape to cover patient and bed • Cut skin along prior incision using scalpel • Remove wires by first cutting, then pulling, until all removed • Place retractor completely under sternum and open widely • Apply suction to clear bleeding using sterile Yankauer • Initiate 2-handed internal massage • Insert internal paddles carefully for internal defibrillation

the common practice to continue antibiotics, and surgical irrigation and wash-out.[30] Boeken and colleagues[31] determined the most important risk factor associated with infection after emergency resternotomy for bleeding was time; patients who developed subsequent infections were reoperated an average of 11.1 hours postoperatively versus 5.3 in those without infection ($P<.05$). The STS recommends throughout

Two to three staff members should put on gown and gloves as soon as a cardiac arrest is called, and prepare the emergency resternotomy set (Class IIA, Level C).

Handwashing is not necessary before closed-sleeve donning of gloves (Class IIA, Level C).

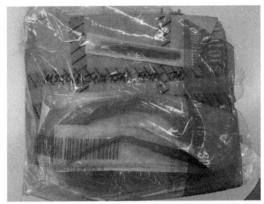

Fig. 3. Exterior packaging of mini-resternotomy set used for reopening during ICU emergencies.

Further guidance for providers who perform the resternotomy is delineated in the STS document and should be rehearsed during team training exercises. Identification of these personnel carries significant implications for training and competency verification, as well as medical-legal implications of providing 24-7 coverage for such emergencies. In acknowledging that this provider may be a nonsurgeon, the STS states, "Physician assistants and advanced practice nurses, or senior intensive care nurses, may be the ideal clinicians to undergo this training and provide the necessary coverage on site, although it is up to local units to allocate these roles and ensure adequate training to ensure competency."[2] Nurse practice acts vary by state and should be consulted to determine if they view participating in emergency resternotomy as within scope of practice. The preparation and training needed by an organization seeking to implement this change includes surgeon champions, infrastructure assessment, delineation of responder roles for events in or outside the ICU, committee approvals, equipment updates, and additional steps, as outlined by Ley.[32]

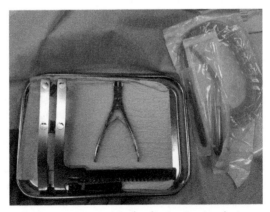

Fig. 4. Mini-resternotomy set contents: sterile chest retractor, instrument to cut and pull sternal wires.

SPECIAL CIRCUMSTANCES: NONTRADITIONAL INCISIONS AND MECHANICAL SUPPORT DEVICES

The traditional median sternotomy incision is no longer standard and many cardiac surgery patients undergo alternative approaches, such as port access, thoracotomy, or hemisternotomy. In these patients, as well as those receiving alternative chest closure techniques (eg, bone cement, Talon®), these special circumstances will require altering the previously described approaches to resternotomy. Comprehensive guidance for performing a resternotomy with these techniques is lacking; therefore, the STS advises surgeons to discuss with the ICU team, on arrival, any such alteration in closure and their recommendations for emergency management.

Patients who have been placed on circulatory support devices, such as ECMO or a left ventricular assist device (LVAD), pose special resuscitation challenges, including the timely recognition of arrest in those with a nonpalpable blood pressure. Device-specific algorithms incorporating available monitoring data should be available to providers to enable accurate recognition and appropriate emergency responses, which

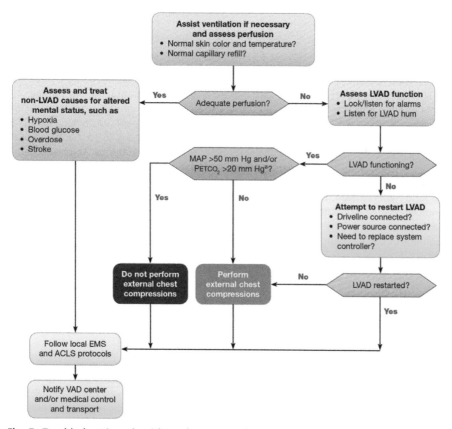

Fig. 5. Troubleshooting algorithm when responding to an unresponsive patient with an LVAD. [a] The PETCO$_2$ cutoff >20 mm Hg should be used only when an ET tube or tracheostomy is used to ventilate the patient. Use of supraglottic (eg, King) airway results in a falsely elevated PETCO$_2$ value. (*From* Peberdy AM, Gluck JA, Ornato JP, et al. Cardiopulmonary resuscitation in adults and children with mechanical circulatory support. A scientific statement from the American Heart Association. Circulation 2017;135:e1124; with permission.)

typically begin with device troubleshooting to optimize flow.[33] Knowledge of device-specific troubleshooting, as well as the surgical approach during insertion or implant, is critical to rescuers; for example, if the aortic valve is incompetent and has been oversewn, responders should anticipate that flow patterns will be restricted to going through the device. When device maneuvers fail, the need for restoration of perfusion takes priority versus concerns about accidental decannulation, and external cardiac massage should be initiated in a timely manner. An excellent AHA algorithm has been developed to illustrate the decision-making process in the resuscitation of LVAD patients (**Fig. 5**). With increasing numbers of device patients in and outside the ICU, resuscitation approaches must be well-delineated and disseminated to likely first responders. The STS recommends following the same universal algorithm for LVAD patients as those without a device, although IABP patients require altering the trigger mode:

In cardiac arrest with an IABP in place, the IABP should be set to pressure trigger mode (Class IIA, Level C).

SUMMARY

Arrest after cardiac surgery is a predictable event that carries a high potential for survival when using appropriate strategies. The unique characteristics of these patients and the environment where arrests are likely to occur mandate important modifications to standard ACLS methods to achieve optimal patient outcomes. The STS recently developed a unique, evidence-based protocol aligned with an identical European guideline that should replace ACLS for patients who arrest after cardiac surgery.[2,19] These strategies reduce patient harm by prioritizing management of life-threatening arrhythmias before CPR, avoid use of vasopressors that can trigger rebound hypertension, and efficiently proceed toward standardized emergency resternotomy within 5 minutes if initial interventions prove ineffective. With release of this guidance comes a new opportunity to provide standardized, evidence-based management of cardiac surgical emergencies for universal use after cardiac surgery, as well as training strategies that promote optimal learning. Implementation of this consensus document, similar to reopening a chest, requires skilled collaboration and teamwork among surgeons and their teams to be effective. With the potential to save hundreds of lives annually, this challenge is long overdue and one that the cardiac surgical community is ready to undertake.

REFERENCES

1. Kleinman MD, Perkins GD, Bhanji F, et al. ILCOR scientific knowledge gaps and clinical research priorities for cardiopulmonary resuscitation and emergency cardiovascular care: a consensus statement. Resuscitation 2018;127: 132–46.
2. Dunning J, Levine A, Ley SJ, et al. The Society of Thoracic Surgeons expert consensus statement for the resuscitation of patients who arrest after cardiac surgery. Ann Thorac Surg 2017;103:1005.
3. Anthi A, Tzelepis GE, Alivizatos P, et al. Unexpected cardiac arrest after cardiac surgery: incidence, predisposing causes, and outcome of open chest cardiopulmonary resuscitation. Chest 1998;113:15–9.

4. LaPar DJ, Ghanta RK, Kern JA, et al. Hospital variation in mortality from cardiac arrest after cardiac surgery: an opportunity for improvement? Ann Thorac Surg 2014;98:534–9 [discussion: 539–40].

5. Chan PS, Krumholz HM, Nichol G, et al. Delayed time to defibrillation after in-hospital cardiac arrest. N Engl J Med 2008;358:9–17.

6. Miller AC, Rosati SF, Suffredini AF, et al. A systematic review and pooled analysis of CPR-associated cardiovascular and thoracic injuries. Resuscitation 2014;85: 724–31.

7. Bohrer H, Gust R, Bottiger BW. Cardiopulmonary resuscitation after cardiac surgery. J Cardiothorac Vasc Anesth 1995;9:352.

8. Kempen PM, Allgood R. Right ventricular rupture during closed-chest cardiopulmonary resuscitation after pneumonectomy with pericardiotomy: a case report. Crit Care Med 1999;27:1378–9.

9. American Heart Association. Highlights of the 2015 American Heart Association guidelines update for CPR and ECC. Available at: www.heart.org/cpr. Accessed April 22, 2016.

10. Davis D, Aguila SA, Sell R, et al. A focused investigation of expedited, stack of three shocks versus chest compressions first followed by single shocks for monitored ventricular fibrillation/ventricular tachycardia cardiopulmonary arrest in an in-hospital setting. J Hosp Med 2016;11(4):264–8.

11. Bradley SM, Liu W, Chan PS, et al. Defibrillation time intervals and outcomes of cardiac arrest in hospital: retrospective cohort study from Get with the Guidelines-Resuscitation registry. BMJ 2016;353:i1653.

12. Perkins GD, Ji C, Deakin CD, et al. A randomized trial of epinephrine in out-of-hospital cardiac arrest. N Engl J Med 2018;379(8):711–21.

13. Andersen LW, Kurth T, Chase M, et al. Early administration of epinephrine (adrenaline) in patients with cardiac arrest with initial shockable rhythm in hospital: propensity score matched analysis. BMJ 2016;353:i1577.

14. Lin S, Callaway CW, Shah PS, et al. Adrenaline for out-of-hospital cardiac arrest resuscitation: a systematic review and meta-analysis of randomized controlled trials. Resuscitation 2014;85:732–40.

15. Webb ST. Caution in the administration of adrenaline in cardiac arrest following cardiac surgery. Resuscitation 2008;78:101 [author reply: 101–2].

16. Kudenchuk PJ, Brown SP, Daya M, et al. Amiodarone, lidocaine, or placebo in out-of-hospital cardiac arrest. N Engl J Med 2016;374(18):1711–22.

17. Valdes SO, Donoghue AJ, Hoyme DB, et al. Outcomes associated with amiodarone and lidocaine in the treatment of in-hospital pediatric cardiac arrest with pulseless ventricular tachycardia or ventricular fibrillation. Resuscitation 2014; 85(3):381–6.

18. AlWaqfi NR, Ibrahim KS, Khader YS, et al. Predictors of temporary epicardial pacing wires use after valve surgery. J Cardiothorac Surg 2014;9(33):1–7.

19. Dunning J, Fabbri A, Kolh PH, et al. Guideline for resuscitation in cardiac arrest after cardiac surgery. Eur J Cardiothorac Surg 2009;36:3–28.

20. Truhlar A, Deakin CD, Soar J, et al. European Resuscitation Council guidelines for resuscitation 2015 section 4. Cardiac arrest in special circumstances. Resuscitation 2015;95:148–201.

21. Pottle A, Bullock I, Thomas J, et al. Survival to discharge following open chest cardiac compression (OCCC). A 4-year retrospective audit in a cardiothoracic specialist centre–Royal Brompton and Harefield NHS Trust, United Kingdom. Resuscitation 2002;52(3):269–72.

22. Mackay JH, Powell SJ, Osgathorp J, et al. Six-year prospective audit of chest re-opening after cardiac arrest. Eur J Cardiothorac Surg 2002;22(3):421–5.
23. Sanders AB, Kern KB, Atlas M, et al. Importance of the duration of inadequate coronary perfusion pressure on resuscitation from cardiac arrest. J Am Coll Cardiol 1985;6:113–8.
24. Twomey D, Das M, Subramanian H, et al. Is internal massage superior to external massage for patients suffering a cardiac arrest after cardiac surgery? Interact Cardiovasc Thorac Surg 2008;7:151–6.
25. Paradis NA, Martin GB, Rivers EP, et al. Coronary perfusion pressure and the return of spontaneous circulation in human cardiopulmonary resuscitation. JAMA 1990;263(8):1106–13.
26. American Heart Association. Statistical update. CPR & first aid emergency cardiovascular care 2015. Available at: https://cpr.heart.org/AHAECC/CPRAndECC/ResuscitationScience/UCM_477263_AHA-Cardiac-Arrest-Statistics.jsp%5BR=301,L,NC%5D. Accessed January 23, 2019.
27. Karhunen JP, Jokinen JJ, Raivio PM, et al. Long-term survival and quality of life after cardiac resuscitation following coronary artery bypass grafting. Eur J Cardiothorac Surg 2011;40(1):249–54.
28. Maccaroni MF, Watson ND, NGaage DL. Managing cardiac arrest after cardiac surgery: the impact of a five year evolving re-sternotomy policy and a review of the literature. Analg Resusc: Curr Res 2013;S1. https://doi.org/10.4172/2324-903X. S1-008.
29. Ley SJ, Gaudiani VG, Egrie GE, et al. Cardiac arrest after open heart surgery; improved processes save lives. Society of Thoracic Surgeons, 51st annual meeting, poster presentation. San Diego, CA, 2015.
30. Yap E, Levine A, Strang T, et al. Should additional antibiotics or an iodine washout be given to all patients who suffer an emergency resternotomy on the cardiothoracic intensive care unit? Interact Cardiovasc Thorac Surg 2008;7(3):464–9.
31. Boeken U, Eisner J, Feindt P, et al. Does the time of resternotomy for bleeding have any influence on the incidence of sternal infections, septic courses or further complications? Thorac Cardiovasc Surg 2001;49(1):45–8.
32. Ley SJ. Standards for resuscitation after cardiac surgery. Crit Care Nurse 2015; 35:30–8.
33. Peberdy AM, Gluck JA, Ornato JP, et al. Cardiopulmonary resuscitation in adults and children with mechanical circulatory support. A scientific statement from the American Heart Association. Circulation 2017;135:e1115–34.

End-of-Life Care in Cardiothoracic Surgery

Barbara Birriel, PhD, ACNP-BC[a],*, Katrina D'Angelo, MSN, AGACNP-BC[b]

KEYWORDS

- End of life • Cardiac surgery • Thoracic surgery • Critical care
- Potentially inappropriate treatment • Futility

KEY POINTS

- Prolonged intensive care unit stays and complications are unexpected after cardiothoracic surgery, resulting in stress for patients, families, and clinicians.
- Patient, families, and clinicians can all have difficulty changing expectations when complications occur.
- Clinicians have a moral imperative to provide optimal end-of-life care for patients and families.
- End-of-life care following cardiothoracic surgery involves 3 phases: acknowledgment that end of life is near, comfort care, and withdrawal of treatment.
- Support for clinicians providing end-of-life care is vital to ensuring appropriate patient and family care.

INTRODUCTION

Cardiothoracic surgical procedures are a common cause of intensive care unit (ICU) admissions as part of routine postoperative care. Although these procedures are most often planned, rather than emergent, they do carry a risk of mortality. Coronary artery bypass grafting (CABG) is the most frequently performed cardiac operation, followed by aortic valve replacement (AVR), combined CABG and AVR, and mitral valve replacement.[1] Operative mortality for cardiac surgeries in 2016 ranged from 1.1% to 9.5%, depending on the specific procedure.[1] Major thoracic surgeries requiring ICU admission include pulmonary lobectomy, pneumonectomy, and esophagectomy. The Society of Thoracic Surgeons General Thoracic Surgery Database relates a mortality of 1% for lobectomy,[2] 5% for pneumonectomy, and 3.4% for esophagectomy.[3]

Disclosure: The authors have nothing to disclose.
[a] The Pennsylvania State University College of Nursing, 90 Hope Drive, 1300 ASB/A110, Hershey, PA 17033, USA; [b] Heart and Vascular Intensivist Service, Penn State Health Milton S. Hershey Medical Center, 500 University Drive, Hershey, PA 17033, USA
* Corresponding author.
E-mail address: bbirriel@psu.edu

Crit Care Nurs Clin N Am 31 (2019) 453–460
https://doi.org/10.1016/j.cnc.2019.05.011
0899-5885/19/© 2019 Elsevier Inc. All rights reserved.

ccnursing.theclinics.com

Although some newer cardiothoracic surgery texts[4] have begun to include content on palliative care and end-of-life care, most common texts do not discuss it.[5,6] Almost all education-focused articles and guidelines in cardiothoracic surgery address routine care and life-sustaining treatment.[7-10] For clinicians seeking information on best practices in end-of-life care following cardiothoracic surgery, little is to be found. This article explores the current literature related to end-of life care following cardiothoracic surgery and develops evidence-based guidelines for provision of care.

LITERATURE ON END-OF-LIFE CARE: CARDIAC SURGERY

The postoperative course for cardiac surgery patients generally consists of a brief stay in intensive care followed by a short inpatient stay before discharge.[11] Thirty-day mortalities are currently reported as being low.[1,11] In combination with the surgical culture of never giving up, this has led to the perception that there is reluctance for providers to alter postoperative goals of care and carry end-of-life discussions.[11,12] With cardiac surgery being performed on an increasing number of high-risk individuals because of advanced age and multiple comorbidities, there is an increasing societal push for transparency and end-of-life discussions for the cardiac surgery patient population.

In the United States, more than 400,000 patients per year undergo cardiac surgery and are at risk of potential complications such as cardiac arrest, cardiac tamponade, postcardiotomy cardiogenic shock requiring mechanical circulatory support, and major bleeding postoperatively.[10,13] Evaluating and characterizing risks of inpatient mortality may provide the multidisciplinary team with more encompassing information to aid family members in making difficult decisions about end-of-life care.[11] Risks such as cardiac arrest, deep sternal wound infection, stroke, and pneumonia have been associated with mortality timing postoperatively.[11]

There are several barriers that health care professionals may encounter that detour or delay end-of-life discussions. One is the notion that it is the provider's duty to cure the patient, as well as the sense of responsibility that may be felt for patient outcomes.[14] In addition, cardiac surgery in several states requires 30-day mortality reporting, and it has been suggested that this metric may lead to delays in decision making and withdrawal of life-sustaining therapies.[12] However, Hua and colleagues[12] found that this metric was unlikely to have a major impact on the delivery of appropriate end-of-life care, but that a surgeon's personal sense of responsibility for patient outcomes may contribute to the hesitancy of end-of-life discussions. Nurses in this specialty area are aware of these barriers. Most (59.3%) surgery nurses at 2 Florida academic medical centers reported rarely or never having end-of-life discussions with patients and their families.[15] Because of the extensive amount of time spent with patients and families at the bedside, nurses can be critical in identifying when end-of-life discussions are necessary and appropriate.

Presenting potential surgical risks and complications should not only be explained to the patient but to the patient's surrogate and family members. Many family members express that they have the expectation of a successful operation and do not expect that the patient will die during or shortly after surgery.[16] The integration of patient-centered advance care planning (PC-ACP) was investigated to evaluate whether preoperative discussions can help patients and families understand the complexity and potential risks associated with cardiac surgery.[14] PC-ACP was thought to aid in facilitating conversations about advance care planning, patient-surrogate congruence, and alleviating decision conflict.[14] In one study, PC-ACP was conducted by a nurse facilitator in a preoperative setting and dyads in this treatment group thought that they were better informed and had a better understanding of the benefits and burdens of surgery.[14] Interventions such as PC-ACP may aid in decreasing feelings of anger, despair, and shock that family members have when they are informed about a patient's irreversible critical condition or death after cardiac surgery.[16]

LITERATURE ON END-OF-LIFE CARE: THORACIC SURGERY

With many surgical referrals for procedures of palliation, thoracic surgery is a specialty that is experienced with discussing the end of life.[17] Facilitating conversations about goals of care and setting clear surgical expectations for patients and families is an integral part of this particular surgical specialty. Thoracic surgery patients often have malignant diseases of the chest, and surgeries are often meant to alleviate symptoms rather than be curative.[18]

Many of the procedures completed by thoracic surgeons involve complex illnesses that are incurable and only symptom relief can be offered. Potential diagnoses requiring thoracic surgery for palliation include dysphagia, tracheobronchial obstruction, pleural effusions, and tracheoesophageal fistula.[17] Individuals who received palliative interventions for these conditions were investigated; Freeman and colleagues[17] found that of their patients receiving a palliative procedure, 11% died before leaving the hospital and 21% were discharged to hospice. Families of patients with low projected survival and advanced disease may be able to prepare and experience less anxiety if discussions about end of life and postoperative expectations are communicated early in care.[17]

Because of the nature of these ailments and that the interventions provided are not curative, thoracic surgery providers and nursing may be more at ease with initiating end-of-life discussions, patient goals of care, and preparing patient families in the event that the patient dies in the hospital. By clearly communicating that interventions are palliative and not designed to prolong life, families may be able to plan for any complication accordingly rather than experiencing shock and despair associated with an unexpected death.

WHY SO LITTLE ATTENTION TO END-OF-LIFE CARE?

The need for palliative care and goals-of-care discussions in patients with advanced cardiovascular disease is accepted.[19,20] It is less clear why this changes following cardiothoracic surgery. It is known that major cardiac and thoracic operations involve a risk of significant complications and mortality, but end-of-life discussions are delayed or may not occur at all. In the case of most cardiac surgeries, the goals of the operation are to improve function, eliminate symptoms, and prolong life. It can be difficult to transition to the acknowledgment that the goals cannot be met and that life will end.

It has been noted that, for many thoracic surgeries, the goal of the operation is at least partially palliation. The patients often have a primary oncology diagnosis. It seems that the transition to end-of-life care when appropriate would be easier in those cases. However, those discussions may not occur within the surgical care team but be left to oncology.

The cardiothoracic surgery literature shows that clinicians are reluctant to move to end-of-life discussions and care. What are clinicians to do when it becomes clear that a patient will not survive following surgery? There is a paucity of studies specific to the cardiothoracic surgery population to guide provision of end-of-life care. The critical care literature provides some guidance.

END-OF-LIFE CARE IN THE INTENSIVE CARE UNIT

Critical care nurses, at the bedside 24 hours a day, are most involved in the care of critically ill patients at the end of life. Berlin[21] identified setting realistic expectations, compassionate communication, shared decision making, and management of both physical and nonphysical symptoms as imperatives in the delivery of quality end-of-life care. Dyspnea and respiratory distress are the among the worst symptoms patients can experience at the end of life. Assessment and intervention by the nurse is a vital part of optimal care.[22] The American College of Critical Care Medicine recommends palliative care consultation for all patients with a prolonged ICU stay.[23]

The most common obstacles in providing end-of-life care, as described in a survey of 2000 members of the American Association of Critical-Care Nurses, were families in denial, families going against patient wishes and advance directives, and families directing care that negatively affected patients.[24] Recommendations to improve end-of-life care in that same study included ensuring characteristics of a good death, improving physician communication with patients and families, adjusting nurse/patient ratios to 1:1, recognizing and avoiding futile care, increasing end-of-life education, having physicians who are present and "on the same page," not allowing families to override patients' wishes, and the need for more support staff. These findings have not changed over the past 17 years.[25]

When conflict is identified in end-of-life decision-making, it is most often a situation in which a patient or family wants to continue aggressive care that the health care team believes will be ineffective. Physician approach to this type of conflict ranges from deference to family wishes to a variety of persuasive strategies designed to change families' minds.[26] A policy statement from multiple critical care societies described a model for responding to requests for these potentially inappropriate treatments.[27] Recommendations include:[27]

- Implement strategies to prevent intractable treatment conflicts. These strategies include proactive communication and expert consultation (eg, ethics, palliative care).
- Use of the term potentially inappropriate rather than futile to describe treatments that have some chance of achieving an effect, although clinicians think there are competing ethical considerations (eg, use of a pressor can improve blood pressure but the primary diagnosis of end-stage heart failure with cardiogenic shock cannot be resolved).
- Strictly futile treatments should not be provided (eg, dialysis in the absence of renal failure). Legally proscribed treatments should not be provided.
- Lead public engagement efforts and advocate policies and legislation about when life-prolonging technologies should not be used.

These recommendations frame the discussion of conflicts that can arise about care at the end of life in the ICU. The specific approach recommended for an individual situation in which intractable conflict occurs may include[27]:

- Enlisting expert consultation to continue negotiation during the dispute-resolution process
- Giving notice of the process to surrogate (family)
- Obtaining a second medical opinion
- Obtaining review by an interdisciplinary hospital committee
- Offering surrogates (family) the opportunity to transfer the patient to an alternate institution
- Informing surrogates (family) of the opportunity to pursue extramural appeal

- Implementing the decision of the resolution process

It is obvious that the process as described cannot be implemented by a single individual. It is important that the entire multidisciplinary health care team be involved in any discussion and work cohesively. Because of the complexity involved in deciding when an intervention is futile or potentially inappropriate, the Society of Critical Care Medicine's Ethics Committee developed a related policy statement with guidance[28]:

- Appropriate goals of ICU care include:
  - Treatment that provides a reasonable expectation for survival outside the acute care setting with sufficient cognitive ability to perceive the benefits of treatment.
  - Palliative care that provides comfort to patients through the dying process may be an appropriate goal of care in some ICUs.
- ICU interventions should generally be considered inappropriate when those goals cannot be met.
- At times, it may be appropriate to provide time-limited ICU interventions to a patient even when the above definition is met if doing so furthers the patient's reasonable goals of care.
- If the patient is experiencing pain or suffering, treatment to relieve pain and suffering is always appropriate.

Decisions about care at the end of life in the ICU are complex. Multiple factors related to the patient, the family, and the multidisciplinary team affect decisions. Because of this complexity, design of research studies to test interventions to improve end-of-life care can be difficult. Several studies have identified potential interventions with promise. Use of an evidence-based screening tool to trigger palliative care consultation can increase the number of referrals.[29] End-of-life and palliative care education training sessions are well received by interprofessional team members, improve symptom management and communication, and provide support to clinicians.[30] Training in end-of-life communication improves comfort and performance.[31] These intervention studies are small but can provide direction as clinicians work toward improving end-of-life care in the ICU.

RECOMMENDATIONS FOR END-OF-LIFE CARE IN CARDIOTHORACIC SURGERY PATIENTS

The expectation for almost all cardiothoracic surgery patients is that they will experience a short period in the ICU, recover, and return home. Preoperative symptoms are expected to be resolved, or at least significantly improved, following recovery from surgery. When these expectations are not met, the situation is stressful for the patient, family, surgeon, and the rest of the multidisciplinary health care team. Although all are aware of the potential complications and risk for mortality with a given operation, patients and families most often do not expect that they will be the ones to experience those complications. Ivarsson and colleagues[16] (2008) describe how families of deceased cardiac surgery patients transitioned from hope and expectation to despair, and eventually to ending and relief.

Clinicians have a moral obligation to provide optimal care for patients and their families. Following cardiothoracic surgery, this involves routine ICU care and aggressive treatment of any complications. Identifying the point in time at which treatment becomes futile or potentially inappropriate is difficult. Communication between all members of the interdisciplinary team, the patient's family, and the patient (if the patient is able) is essential. Acknowledgment that end-of-life care is appropriate may come first from the patient, the family, or any member of the health care team. It is crucial that members of the interdisciplinary health care team resolve any differences of opinion concerning prognosis and further treatments before discussion with patient and family. Conflicting opinions from various clinicians serves to increase confusion and stress for the patient and family.

End-of-life care in cardiothoracic surgery can be thought of in 3 overlapping stages. First, acknowledgment that end of life is near. This acknowledgment must eventually be a shared knowing by the surgeon, other multidisciplinary team members, the patient's family, and the patient if able. Next, comfort care. Comfort care consists of symptom management with specific treatments depending on the individual patient needs. This care should be managed by the attending surgical service. Palliative care consultation is helpful if that service is available. Comfort care/symptom

Table 1	
End-of-life care recommendations for cardiothoracic surgery patients	
Overlapping Stages of Care	**Specific Recommendations**
Acknowledgment that end of life is near	Regular communication between patient/family and multidisciplinary team
	Weekly family meetings in cases of prolonged ICU stay
	Clearly communicate realistic expectations
	Clearly communicate rationale for withholding or withdrawing potentially inappropriate treatments
	Consider cultural factors that influence conversation/decisions
	Proactive ethics or palliative care consultation in cases of disagreement
	Follow ATS/AACN/ACCP/ESICM/SCCM policy statement in cases of protracted disagreement[27]
Comfort care	Pain management: continuous narcotic infusion
	Agitation: intermittent or continuous benzodiazepine
	Dyspnea/respiratory distress: intermittent or continuous benzodiazepine
	Positioning for comfort
	Remove nonessential lines and tubes
	Allow family privacy with patient but provide mechanism to call for assistance
	Provide support to family: physical, emotional
Withdrawal of treatment	Discussion of options: withdraw treatments vs do not add new treatments
	Vasoactive infusions
	Ventilator support
	Dialysis/renal replacement therapy
	Oxygen
	Medications except for management of symptoms
	Anticipate need for management of symptoms that occur in response to withdrawal of treatment
Clinician support	Education on end-of-life and palliative care
	Opportunities to develop resilience skills (eg, mindfulness training)
	Training in communication skills
	Organizational culture that promotes multidisciplinary team
	Adequate staffing to meet patient needs

Abbreviations: AACN, American Association of Critical-Care Nurses; ACCP, American College of Chest Physicians; ATS, American Thoracic Society; ESICM, European Society of Intensive Care Medicine; SCCM, Society of Critical Care Medicine.

management should be provided even while the team moves through the initial acknowledgment phase. In addition, there is withdrawal of treatment. Note that clinicians never withdraw "care"; they withdraw treatments that are no longer effective to meet the patient goals of care. This withdrawal could include extubation/removal of ventilator, discontinuing vasoactive medications, or stopping mechanical circulatory support. In addition, consideration must be given to support for the clinicians involved in care of the patient and family. Specific recommendations are summarized in **Table 1.**

Nurses are often viewed as the "medical liaisons, facilitators, supporters, and patient/family advocates"[15] in end-of-life discussions. In cardiac surgery, nursing may be a bridge between surgical providers and patients and their families to initiate end-of-life discussion and complex decision making, in both the preoperative and postoperative settings. Providing transparency with regard to potential surgical complications, including death, may help in dismantling the misconception that surgery is without obstacles and can restore a patient's health. In addition, it could aid in reducing the frequency of patients and families experiencing unexpected shock and anguish in the event of a postoperative death.

REFERENCES

1. D'Agostino RS, Jacobs JP, Badhwar V, et al. The Society of Thoracic Surgeons adult cardiac surgery database: 2018 update on outcomes and quality. Ann Thorac Surg 2018;105:15–23.

2. Seder CW, Raymond D, Wright CD, et al. The Society of Thoracic Surgeons general thoracic surgery database 2018 update on outcomes and quality. Ann Thorac Surg 2018;105:1304–7.

3. Seder CW, Wright CD, Chang AC, et al. The Society of Thoracic Surgeons general thoracic surgery database update on outcomes and quality. Ann Thorac Surg 2016;101(5):1646–54.

4. Kouchoukos NT, Blackstone EH, Hanley FL, et al. Kirklin/Barratt-Boyes cardiac surgery. 4th edition. Philadelphia: Saunders; 2013.

5. Lonchyna VA, editor. Difficult decisions in cardiothoracic critical care surgery: an evidence based approach. Switzerland: Springer; 2019.

6. Bojar RM. Manual of perioperative care in adult cardiac surgery. 5th edition. Hoboken (NJ): Wiley-Blackwell; 2011.

7. Katz NM. The evolution of cardiothoracic critical care. J Thorac Cardiovasc Surg 2011;141(1):3–6.

8. Lobdell KW, Haden DW, Mistry KP. Cardiothoracic critical care. Surg Clin North Am 2017;97:811–34.

9. Michaelis P, Leone RJ. Cardiac arrest after cardiac surgery: an evidence-based resuscitation protocol. Crit Care Nurse 2019;39(1):15–25.

10. The Society of Thoracic Surgeons Task Force on Resuscitation After Cardiac Surgery. The Society of Thoracic Surgeons expert consensus for the resuscitation of patients who arrest after cardiac surgery. Ann Thorac Surg 2017;103:1005–20.

11. Mazzeffi M, Zivot J, Buchman T, et al. In-hospital mortality after cardiac surgery: patient characteristics, timing, and association with postoperative length of intensive care unit and hospital stay. Ann Thorac Surg 2014;97(4):1120–5.

12. Hua M, Scales DC, Cooper Z, et al. Impact of public reporting of 30-day mortality on timing of death after coronary artery bypass graft surgery. Anesthesiology 2017;127(6):953–60.

13. Rubino A, Costanzo D, Stanszus D, et al. Central veno-arterial extracorporeal membrane oxygenation (C-VA-ECMO) after cardiothoracic surgery: a single-center experience. J Cardiothorac Vasc Anesth 2018;32(3):1169–74.

14. Song MK, Kirchoff KT, Douglas J, et al. A randomized, controlled trial to improve advance care planning among patients undergoing cardiac surgery. Med Care 2005;43(10):1049–53.

15. White P, Cobb D, Vasilopoulos T, et al. End-of-life discussion: who's doing the talking? J Crit Care 2018;43:70–4.

16. Ivarsson B, Larsson S, Johnsson P, et al. From hope and expectation to unexpected death after cardiac surgery. Intensive Crit Care Nurs 2008;24(4):242–50.

17. Freeman RK, Arevalo G, Ascioti A, et al. An assessment of the frequency of palliative procedures in thoracic surgery. J Surg Educ 2017;74(5):878–82.

18. Nelems B. Palliative care principles for thoracic surgery. Thorac Surg Clin 2013; 23(3):443–6.

19. Klinedinst R, Kornfield ZN, Hadler RA. Palliative care for patients with advanced heart disease. J Cardiothorac Vasc Anesth 2019;33(3):833–43.

20. Warraich HJ, Hernandez AF, Allen LA. How medicine has changed the end of life for patients with cardiovascular disease. J Am Coll Cardiol 2017;70:1276–89.

21. Berlin A. Goals of care and end of life in the ICU. Surg Clin North Am 2017;97: 1275–90.

22. Campbell ML. Ensuring breathing comfort at the end of life: the integral role of the critical care nurse. Am J Crit Care 2018;27:264–9.

23. Davidson JE, Aslakson RA, Long AC, et al. Guidelines for family-centered care in the neonatal, pediatric, and adult ICU. Crit Care Med 2017;45(1):103–28.

24. Beckstrand RL, Mallory C, Macintosh JLB, et al. Critical care nurses' qualitative reports of experiences with family behaviors as obstacles in end-of-life care. Dimens Crit Care Nurs 2018;37(5):251–8.

25. Beckstrand RL, Hadley KH, Luthy KE, et al. Critical care nurses' suggestions to improve end-of-life care obstacles. Dimens Crit Care Nurs 2017;36(4):264–70.

26. Mehter HM, McCannon JB, Clark JA, et al. Physician approaches to conflict with families surrounding end-of-life decision-making in the intensive care unit: a qualitative study. Ann Am Thorac Soc 2018;15(2):241–9.

27. Bosslet GT, Pope TM, Rubenfeld GD, et al. An official ATS/AACN/ACCP/ESICM/ SCCM policy statement: responding to requests for potentially inappropriate treatments in intensive care units. Am J Respir Crit Care Med 2015;191(11): 1318–30.

28. Kon AA, Shepard EK, Sederstrom NO, et al. Defining futile and potentially inappropriate interventions: a policy statement from the society of critical care medicine ethics committee. Crit Care Med 2016;44:1769–74.

29. McCarroll CM. Increasing access to palliative care services in the intensive care unit. Dimens Crit Care Nurs 2018;37(3):180–92.

30. Graham R, Lepage C, Boitor M, et al. Acceptability and feasibility of an interprofessional end-of-life/palliative care educational intervention in the intensive care unit: a mixed-methods study. Intensive Crit Care Nurs 2018;48:75–84.

31. Zante B, Schefold JC. Teaching end-of-life communication in intensive care medicine: review of the existing literature and implications for future curricula. J Intensive Care Med 2019;34(4):301–10.

Moving?

Make sure your subscription moves with you!

To notify us of your new address, find your **Clinics Account Number** (located on your mailing label above your name), and contact customer service at:

Email: journalscustomerservice-usa@elsevier.com

800-654-2452 (subscribers in the U.S. & Canada)
314-447-8871 (subscribers outside of the U.S. & Canada)

Fax number: 314-447-8029

Elsevier Health Sciences Division
Subscription Customer Service
3251 Riverport Lane
Maryland Heights, MO 63043

*To ensure uninterrupted delivery of your subscription,
please notify us at least 4 weeks in advance of move.

Printed and bound by CPI Group (UK) Ltd, Croydon, CR0 4YY

03/10/2024

01040406-0004